Imagery for
Pain Relief

Imagery for Pain Relief

A Scientifically Grounded Guidebook for Clinicians

David Pincus and Anees A. Sheikh

Foreword by Ernest L. Rossi, PhD

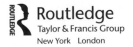

Routledge
Taylor & Francis Group
New York   London

Routledge
Taylor & Francis Group
270 Madison Avenue
New York, NY 10016

Routledge
Taylor & Francis Group
2 Park Square
Milton Park, Abingdon
Oxon OX14 4RN

© 2009 by Taylor & Francis Group, LLC
Routledge is an imprint of Taylor & Francis Group, an Informa business

Printed in the United States of America on acid-free paper
10 9 8 7 6 5 4 3 2 1

International Standard Book Number-13: 978-0-415-99702-7 (Hardcover)

Library of Congress Cataloging-in-Publication Data

Pincus, David, 1969-
    Imagery for pain relief : a scientifically grounded guidebook for clinicians / David Pincus, Anees A. Sheikh.
        p. ; cm.
    Includes bibliographical references and index.
    ISBN 978-0-415-99702-7 (hardback : alk. paper)
    1. Imagery (Psychology)--Therapeutic use. 2. Pain--Treatment. I. Sheikh, Anees A. II. Title.
    [DNLM: 1. Pain--therapy. 2. Imagery (Psychotherapy)--methods. WL 704 P647i 2009]

RC489.F35P56 2009
616'.0472--dc22
                                                                                        2008041603

Visit the Taylor & Francis Web site at
http://www.taylorandfrancis.com

and the Routledge Web site at
http://www.routledge.com

In loving memory of David Grove

He delighted and inspired us with his *joie de vivre*, his lively
curiosity, his sense of humor, and his genius as a therapist.
He left us much too soon, but his contributions will live on.

How could we forget those ancient myths that stand at the beginning of all races—the myths about dragons that at the last moment are transformed into princesses. Perhaps all the dragons in our lives are only princesses waiting for us to act, just once, with beauty and courage. Perhaps everything that frightens us is, in its deepest essence, something helpless that wants our love…. Why do you want to shut out of your life any uneasiness, any miseries, or any depressions? For after all, you do not know what work these conditions are doing inside you.

Rainer Maria Rilke

in Letters to a Young Poet (1984, pp. 92–93)

Contents

Foreword

The significance and timeliness of this excellent volume on *Imagery for Pain Relief* reveals an inconvenient truth about the helping professions. Secretly, many psychotherapists, emergency and rehabilitation personnel, social workers, nurses and doctors in all areas of medical specialization remain cowards in the face of pain even after many years of professional training. From their earliest childhood experiences with what appeared to be "unjust pain" to their confrontations with the prospect of encroaching "shameful debilitation and death," many clinicians would rather not deal with pain in themselves or others. Even after extensive clinical experience, many psychotherapists are still hesitant and reluctant to accept pain patients.

As an independent participant/observer and presenter of professional training workshops in therapeutic hypnosis and psychotherapy for over 40 years, I have noticed the numinous awe with which many students and professionals regard their training in the application of psychological and cognitive-behavioral approaches to the relief of pain. While confident in their training and clinical expertise in all other areas of clinical work, many professionals still stumble in the face of pain. We must wonder why. Is it because of their unresolved personal issues with their own difficult experiences with pain? Is it because they are not able to resolve the dilemmas and conundrums of the Cartesian gap between mind and body?

In the face of such difficulties, the plain and simple truth is that many students and professionals tend to avoid the scientific and clinical literature dealing with pain. Pain thus remains a shadowy and woebegone area of uncertainty in their training. This is a tragic mistake because advances in modern neuroscience currently are making great strides in understanding the psychophysiology of pain on all levels from mind to brain anatomy and even on the molecular-genomic level. This new look at pain research can bring profound relief and even joy to the hearts and minds of students and clinicians who know they really want to do the right thing for themselves and their patients.

Recent scientific research now can document how imagery, in particular, has hidden and unexpected efficacy in facilitating pain relief for many people. A research team led by Katja Wiech of the University of Oxford in England, for example, illustrates how imagery can reduce pain perception in the September 5, 2008 issue of the high-impact scientific journal, *Pain*. While their subjects viewed religious imagery, they perceived electric shocks to the back of their hand as less painful. This is an example of the efficacy of imagery as a powerful placebo that has real effects that can be scientifically measured with functional magnetic resonance (fMRI). Pain relief was associated with heightened activity in the right ventrolateral prefrontal cortex. This imagery research is consistent with previous studies that have found this area of the brain related to the capacity for emotional detachment and the cognitive-behavioral experience of control over pain.

How do we utilize such laboratory evidence to facilitate pain relief in everyday clinical situations in the hospital and consulting room? Can this book really give us any help when a lifetime of previous personal and professional experience may not have? This is where the practical clinical techniques presented by the authors, David Pincus and Anees Sheikh, prove their humanitarian worth. Their compendium presents a rich tapestry of verbal transcripts that bridge the mind-body gap with clear protocols for facilitating pain relief and human healing on many levels from mind to molecules that is entirely consistent with my own scientific work in this area.

Ernest Lawrence Rossi, PhD
Co-Editor with David Lloyd of the 2008 volume,
Ultradian Rhythms from Molecules to Mind:
A New Vision of Life

Preface

When the Buddha... was asked what his teaching was, he said that it was whatever led to true cessation of suffering.

Brazier
(1995, pp. 19–20)

Guided imagery has been used in pain management for centuries (Achterberg, 1985), and within modern scientific history, the practice has reemerged: Research from the past 30 to 40 years consistently has shown the benefits of imagery in pain reduction and in the promotion of health (Sheikh, Kunzendorf, & Sheikh, 2003). One would assume that such a long tradition in the healing arts, so much accumulated scientific evidence over such a short time, and so many possible interventions within the imagination would have inspired a guidebook for practitioners to help their clients to use their imaginations for pain relief. But this seems to be the first book of its kind.

Our first task is to prime you with a deeper understanding of pain, one that goes beyond its physical aspects to its emotional, cognitive (i.e., attention, perception, beliefs), and social character. Chapter 1 is designed to deepen your understanding of pain, how it impacts each of us, how it typically is treated, and how it may be caused and maintained over time.

Chapter 2 leads to a full and detailed understanding of mental imagery. You will gain a broad understanding of imagery, what it entails, and how it can be therapeutic. We also discuss the history of guided imagery, from the practice of the ancient shamans up to its use in modern medicine. One key area in this discussion is deconstructing the mistaken notion that body and mind are completely distinct and separate. This myth has a great impact on patients in pain, pain treatment, and attitudes toward the use of imagery that are held by patients and practitioners alike. Most people raised in the West are prone to wonder how on earth something as real and physical as pain can be treated within the imagination. Yet the research is consistent on this topic: Imagery can reduce pain and increase pain management. Chapter 2 seeks to reconcile this apparent conflict.

Chapter 3 aims to explore in greater depth the question of why imagery is well suited to pain management. The chapter begins with a scientifically rigorous yet practical analysis of the scientific literature on the effectiveness of imagery treatments for various types of pain. This review is aimed at enhancing your ability to think critically about clinical trials and other forms of evidence for treatments, at increasing your practical understanding of the methodologies and statistics used in these investigations, and at making clinically meaningful translations of research results to guide your day-to-day work.

The second half of Chapter 3 explores, through the lens of dynamic systems theory (also known as chaos and complexity theory), the question of how imagery works. Within this discussion, technical aspects from these cutting-edge systems concepts are presented to assist clinicians in developing general principles to guide the treatment process. The intent is to provide a unified theory to account for the effects of imagery on pain, namely that image therapies may change the flows of information, matter, or energy among injured regions of body–mind systems, allowing for renewed flexibility, healing, and relief. A deep understanding of these theoretical processes explaining how imagery works will allow clinicians to adapt techniques to fit each patient's unique set of clinical circumstances within the imagination.

Chapter 4 makes the transition from the more didactic information from Chapters 1, 2, and 3 on pain, imagery, and how they work together into the second half of the book, which is technique driven. Detailed information is provided for clinicians on how to obtain a pain-focused psychosocial assessment. The chapter outlines topic areas that should be covered with each client as well as methods for assessing each client's imaging abilities and methods that can be used to improve these abilities prior to the start of active treatment.

Chapter 4 also discusses initial therapeutic treatment planning from a relational perspective. In this chapter, you will become familiar with the process of treating pain with imagery, from the first session through the selection of techniques and on to termination. Not only will you learn the content of treatment (i.e., what to do, when, and with whom), but you will also gain a deeper sense of the process of treatment (i.e., a sense of how to be).

Chapters 5, 6, and 7 provide detailed descriptions of a large menu of useful imagery techniques. These techniques have been organized in three chapters according to different levels of intensity: simple, deeper, and deepest, because of the vast array of techniques that exists within the realm of therapeutic imagery (Sheikh, 2002). The simple techniques in Chapter 5 include the subtle use of imagery in everyday language, which health-care professionals may integrate into their standard care to maximize the positive impacts of intangible factors often ascribed to bedside manner. Simple techniques also include various relaxation techniques, simple sensory transformation techniques (i.e., numbness), healthy distraction techniques, and behavioral techniques focused on rehearsal and confidence building.

The deeper techniques in Chapter 6 focus on more symbolic-transformation techniques, including techniques that move pain within the body or to the outside of the body. Such symbolic transformations involve metaphors such as the rolling up of pain into a ball, the draining of pain from the body like sand from a sack, or the cleansing of the body with sources such as radiant light. Chapter 6 also includes a variety of ways a patient may be guided through travel within his or her body to interact with symbolic pain directly in the promotion of relief and healing.

The deepest techniques, presented in Chapter 7, generally require the greatest skill, the most time, and potentially the most emotional investment on the part of the client (e.g., working through traumatic memories in a symbolic fashion, spiritually oriented techniques aimed at deepening existential connections and enhancing life meaning). Each technique includes a contextual description that outlines how the technique was developed, for what types of pain it may be best suited, the basic theoretical mechanisms that may explain how it works, and vignettes to illustrate the language used by the guiding practitioner.

Chapter 8 presents information to allow the reader to adapt the information from prior chapters to the use of imagery treatment with children. The use of imagery in treating children's pain is an important applied area, since medications tend not to work as well with children as they do with adults and due to children's increased risks of harmful side effects. Furthermore, the available evidence suggests that imagery techniques may be particularly effective for children; they are naturally imaginative and playful.

Chapter 8 discusses children's cognitive development across the age spans and the ways imagery techniques may be modified (e.g., made more concrete) to allow children to effectively engage in the process. Next, special aspects of the process of treating children in pain are presented, such as ways to include the family in the treatment process and, similarly, ways that parents may inadvertently act to maintain pain problems in their attempts to be helpful. Finally, a number of different techniques appropriate for use with children are described.

The concluding chapter, Chapter 9, moves our discussion away from scientific and practical matters to broader philosophical and spiritual issues. It discusses in detail the possible opportunities the experience of pain and suffering provides for growth and how the clinician can be of significant help in this venture.

Throughout these chapters, you are asked to open your mind and simultaneously are provided with clear, evidence-driven rationales. You need not choose between traditional medicine and alternative medicine, between science and spirituality: On the contrary, each gains from the other. The eminent philosopher of science, Reichenbach (1938), has described two interacting contexts that underlie the scientific pursuit of knowledge: (1) the context of *discovery*; and (2) the context of *justification*. The context of discovery requires an open mind, allowing for the unlimited and creative development of theory in a universe filled with mystery and complexity. This is the context in which areas of scientific exploration are selected and in which theoretical framework are first generated. The context of scientific justification involves critically examining the evidence for these frameworks. It is this latter context that people usually equate with science. Nevertheless, open-mindedness is a key precursor to critical thinking. The two contexts of science complement one another, like yin and yang. The context of justification allows for procedures that complement the openness of free discovery, as different explanations are evaluated based on careful observation and logic, leading to new investigations, hopefully in the direction of truth and utility.

By embracing each context of investigation, we present you with a book that is firmly grounded in science in the truest and most balanced sense of the word (Kantorovich, 1993). The resulting expansion of your understanding of pain and imagery ideally will open you to new vantage points while at the same time allowing you to crystallize these views into useful forms: principles that may bring relief from pain. As you open up to new ways to experience, to relieve, and to manage pain, it is our hope that a parallel process of learning will find a way into your day-to-day endeavors.

Acknowledgments

Although only our names are on the cover, several others deserve to share the spotlight with us. We would like to express our deepest gratitude to our most loyal supporters, our wives, Kristin Kinsfogel and Kathy Sheikh. Kathy carefully read the entire manuscript and made significant stylistic changes to improve readability. Cei Davies Linn kindly agreed to review the section on the work of the late David Grove. She had worked with David for more than two decades, and no one understands his work better than she. We thank her for sharing her insights and valuable suggestions. We are indebted to Trish Johnson of the psychology department at Marquette University for her cheerful assistance with the numerous revisions of the manuscript. Without her invaluable help, the project would have taken much longer to complete. We also would like to recognize two students for their valuable assistance: Annette Metten saved us countless hours by her library research, and Jaimie Lex carefully checked the bibliography. We are also deeply grateful to our students and patients, who have illuminated various aspects and have led us to sharpen our focus over the years.

We are grateful to the staff of Routledge, especially to editor Dr. George Zimmar and editorial assistant Marta Moldvai for sound advice and guidance. Thanks are also due to Marquette University for granting Anees a sabbatical to work on this project.

The following publishers generously permitted us to incorporate our previously published work in this book:

Baywood Publishing Company for Pincus, D., Wachsmuth-Schlaefer, T., Sheikh, A. A., & Ezaz-Nikpay, S. (2003). Transforming the pain terrain: Theory and practice in the use of mental imagery for the treatment of pain. In A. A. Sheikh (Ed.), *Healing images: The role of imagination in health.* Amityville, NY: Baywood.

Brandon House, Inc., for Pincus, D. (2006). Dynamical systems theory and pain imagery: Bridging the gap between research and practice. *Journal of Mental Imagery, 30*(1–2), 93–112.

Last, we would like to express our pleasure in working together on this book. Undoubtedly each of us and the project were enriched by our collaboration.

CHAPTER 1

Pain

A Primer

> To lessen the suffering of pain, we need to make a crucial distinction between the pain of pain and the pain that we create by any thoughts about pain.
>
> **Dalai Lama and Cutler**
> *(1998, pp. 209–210)*

What is pain? This is a question we tend not to ask unless we are in pain, and then the answer is pretty simple. "Here?" the doctor asks, pressing with strong and knowing fingers. "Ouch! Yes that's it! And please don't do that again."

In a sense, this is what we will be doing in this chapter. We are going to take a deep and probing look at pain. This is something we don't ordinarily do. Although it is a universal human experience, we go to great lengths to avoid pain, to avoid talking or even thinking about pain. Let's take a few moments to do what we don't normally do.

Although we tend to point to affected areas that hurt and call that pain, pain is more than this. Pain is abstract. You can't see it or touch it directly. I know it hurts when you touch it, but there is much more happening. Pain is an experience, a universal experience of humans and other complex creatures (Kleinman, Brodwin, Good, & DelVecchio-Good, 1992). As such, pain is phenomenological at its core—which means that it is fundamentally a subjective and a private experience. There is no thermometer for pain. Just like colors, each of us experiences pain in our own way and must take it on faith that our perceptions are in line with those of others.

What is blue? How is it different from red? What is cold and what is hot? What is a dull ache or a sharp stab?

As a negative, repetitive, and inescapable part of our lives, each of us develops a relationship with pain. Like any other relationship, conflict and domination by pain may lead us to become isolated and worn down. Furthermore, to some degree each of us is in denial of our relationship with pain and of the inevitability of our upcoming pain experiences. This is especially true for those of us who enjoy long, pain-free intervals, allowing us to forget the inevitability of its return.

Yet pain marks the beginning and also the end of life (for most of us) and peppers our remaining existence with moments of suffering. When will you next feel pain? How long will it last? How many times will you feel it over the course of your life, and how much will *you* suffer? Will it hurt when you die? What about after death?

The experience of pain is like a visit from a ghost in some ways. Like a ghost, pain comes and goes in its own unpredictable manner, invisible and often undetectable by others—including the best modern medical technology. Like a ghost, pain reminds us of our frailty, connects us with our earliest sufferings, and is a specter pointing to our inevitable deaths. Like a visit from a ghost, pain is a private experience, somewhat indescribable and often scary. Talking about a pain experience with others will tend to turn them away from you, to be socially uncomfortable, and could lead them to question your honesty and your motives. While few of us will ever see a ghost, each of us will experience pain, and many of us will eventually experience a haunting.

Webster's dictionary defines pain primarily as punishment, and elaborates: "to impose a penalty on for a fault, offense, or violation (Merriam-Webster Inc., 2008). Further, *pain* and *punish* each share the same Latin root, *poena*, which means "penalty." Think about this connotation. Pain is equivalent to punishment? Penalty? One may reasonably ask, "So what's the crime?" If the pain sufferer is at fault, what was the violation or offense? It seems that blaming the victims of pain is nothing new, dating back at least 700 years to Old France (Douglas Harper, 2001), where the word *punishment* first emerged: it is entrenched even in the language we use to describe the experience we call pain.

Similarly, this one-word definition, "punishment," shines a light onto the social context of pain that most chronic pain survivors could describe readily. The experience of pain is usually accompanied by two related interpersonal processes: social stigma and self-doubt. People surrounding pain sufferers actively blame them, looking for reasons to justify the sufferer's suffering. If there has been a penalty, there must have been a foul. At the same time, friends and family tend to distance themselves psychologically and emotionally from the afflicted by finding differences of virtue between themselves and the sufferer, differences that will keep the ghost of pain from visiting them. It is human nature to try to make sense of senseless suffering.

As this process occurs on an interpersonal level, a converse process unfolds within the sufferer. Sufferers themselves tend to distort the context of pain in the opposite direction—desperately looking for external causes, ideally a physical cause, to explain away the pain. At the same time they tend to overlook any habits (cognitive, emotional, behavioral, or social) that might inadvertently be increasing their suffering. Pain sufferers are one of the few groups of people who are actually relieved to find out that something is physically wrong with them. This is a telling irony within modern culture and its difficulties in understanding pain.

At the same time, pain patients tend to ask themselves on a less conscious level, "Why me? What crime did I commit? When will my penalty be served? Maybe I am to blame?" What a load to carry around along with a raging set of aches and pains. No matter whether one is actively trying to make sense of pain by finding the crime for which the sufferer is being punished or one is a sufferer trying to escape judgment, pain automatically brings with it a social and personal wrestling match involving blame and stigma. Why is this necessarily so?

Social psychologists have identified two well-known processes that govern our social perceptions: the "fundamental attribution error" (Ross, 1977) and the "just-world bias" (Lerner, 1980). The fundamental attribution error is our tendency to blame victims, which research has repeatedly shown to be automatic, pervasive, and universal, barring some minor caveats in collectivist cultures (see Norenzayan & Nisbett, 2000). Our tendency to blame victims is not just a long-standing cultural tradition that has been folded into the etymology of our language for pain; it is a byproduct of our brains and really cannot be helped (Nispett & Ross, 1980; Tversky & Kahneman, 1974).

You see, brains are designed to make sense of the world and to reduce emotional discomfort. We blame victims not because we are unjust but because blame provides the simplest answer to explain a victim's suffering and in the process it makes the world seem safe and predictable for the rest of us. A safe and predictable world is generally a nice place to live. The downside of course is that the world is not really as safe or as predictable as we tend to imagine, particularly in regard to pain, which, again, you will experience.

Similarly, we have an inherent bias to believe in a just world, where bad people are punished (i.e., pain) and good people are rewarded (i.e., pleasure). Wouldn't this be great, if it were true? Alas, people who are in pain are, on the whole, just as worthwhile (or naughty) as everyone else—no more, no less. This imaginary world where pain equals punishment is, however, the most adaptive possibility for a meaning-dependent organ like our brains. In fact, we should thank our brains for reducing our fears of unpredictable and unjustified pain and suffering to the lowest level it is able to muster. This blame-the-victim, just-world fantasyland in which we all live to some degree allows us to move on to more pressing and complex problems.

Of course there is one time in which we make an exception to these neurologically based biases, when *we* are the ones who are suffering. When it happens to us, a third, well-known cognitive bias naturally kicks in: the *self-serving bias* (Bradley, 1978; Fletcher & Ward, 1988). The self-serving bias leads us to overestimate external causes and to underestimate internal ones, the opposite of the fundamental attribution error. This self-serving bias is adaptive inasmuch as it preserves our somewhat false sense of mastery over ourselves and our integrity while at the same time making things appear simpler than they really are. Again, the brain likes to keep things as simple as possible.

The downside of this simplicity, however, particularly with chronic pain, is a mind-set in the pain patient that the world is in fact unjust. Why else would someone be repeatedly punished for a nonexistent crime unless the world was cruel and mean? And if the world is unjust, doling out punishment in the absence of crimes, why would one foolishly hope for amnesty, for relief? Why would one try to free one's self from pain? Why would one listen to those who say, "You know there are some things you can do to relieve your suffering." Or even worse, "You know we're going to *imagine* your pain away; how does that sound?" More hollow words from a non-sufferer who doesn't understand the cruel nature of universal crime and punishment. After all, this is just another message calling for the admission of wrongdoing, personal blame, and a desire for repentance; it is just one more voice screaming not that it desires to help but instead that it is all your fault.

Ultimately, pain, particularly chronic pain, brings with it all of these negative connotations and multi-layered conflicts. Sufferers are in conflict with pain itself, with an unjust world, with others who appear to indict them for their wrongdoings, whether they are trying to help or not. Similarly, sufferers are in conflict with themselves on some level as they try not to focus on those things that would justify their punishments. After all, are any of us really that innocent that we couldn't search our personal histories and find some crime that is worthy of punishment?

Varieties of Pain

In Western culture we love to label things. This is especially true in science and medicine. Of course, labeling is not uniquely Western; all human cultures name things, and in so naming they shape and construct reality to some extent. Inasmuch as pain is a human experience firmly within the purview of Western science and medicine, there is no paucity of different ways to semantically slice and dice the experience of pain (for more detailed and technical classification systems for chronic pain, see Merskey & Bogduk, 1994; Turk & Okifuji, 2001).

One common strategy in typing pain is to use its location, as in lower-back pain, dental pain, joint pain, and pains in the neck. This allows us to come up with a plethora of types of pain from head to toe. Another common strategy is to type pain according to its cause, for example, inflammatory pains, neuropathic pains (i.e., related to nerve damage), even central pain (related to information processing in the central nervous system), which is the newer and less stigmatizing term for "all in your head." Cause-typing leads to problems as such, because pain is always multiply determined, with causes ranging across scales, from large-scale socioeconomics down to the level of molecules.

One broad and very important dimension we use in classifying pain is time, as in chronic pain, which lasts a long time, versus acute pain, which is shorter in duration. The length of time at which acute pain becomes chronic pain is a bit fuzzy, varying from expert to expert (Hardin, 1997). Merskey and Bogduk (1994) define chronic pain as "pain which persists past the normal time of healing…. In practice this may be less than one month, or more often, more than six months" (p. xi). The primary type of acute pain for which imagery has been shown to be effective is procedural pain, which arises from some medical treatment, for example, following knee surgery (i.e., Cupal & Brewer, 2001), cancer treatments (i.e., Syrjala & Roth-Roemer, 1996), or childbirth (Achterberg, Dossey, & Kolkmeier, 1994).

There are times when there is no initial physical cause for a pain condition, in which case the line between chronic and acute may be defined by duration, somewhere between 1 and 6 months. Of course some conditions, like arthritis, are chronic by nature, as is the pain that comes with them. Other specific examples of chronic pain include the pain that accompanies irritable bowel syndrome or headaches, which may then be further subdivided, for example, into tension-type, migraine, cluster headaches. Of course, most of these common examples are actually *recurring* rather than *chronic* per se. They come and go, with flare-ups, but never quite go away. Using the metaphor of the unwelcome houseguest, these types of pain will leave for a little while, leaving a mess behind them and then returning all too soon.

Because time is such an important factor in determining our experiences of and relationships with pain, a more useful distinction than simply chronic versus acute might involve the different manner in which chronic pains come and go. Pain that is always there is distinct from pain that comes and goes regularly and also from pain that comes and goes unpredictably. An unwelcome visitor who is always there must be managed differently from one that comes once per year or that pops in unexpectedly.

The key distinction between chronic and acute pain then is the relationship the sufferer forms with the pain. Again, pain is a familiar, emotionally charged, meaning-laden, unwelcome, yet inevitable visitor for all of us. The meaning of such a visit is completely different, if it is for an afternoon versus a weekend, if pain is going to stay only for tea, or if it is going to tag along with everything we do. On human experiential and relational levels then, the differences between chronic and acute pain run far deeper than an issue of duration.

Pain in Modern Medicine: Round Pegs and Square Holes

After the primary definition connecting pain to punishment, Webster's does in fact provide a more medical, less criminal, secondary definition of pain: "Usually localized physical suffering associated with bodily disorder (as a disease or an injury); *also*: a basic bodily sensation induced by a noxious stimulus, received by naked nerve endings, characterized by physical discomfort (as pricking, throbbing, or aching), and typically leading to evasive action; b : acute mental or emotional distress or suffering: GRIEF" (Merriam-Webster, Inc., 2008). Examining this sequence of definitions one finds that punishment comes first; next comes the physical manifestation of pain, related to injury and nerve endings, and the emotional and psychological elements are listed third. Generally speaking, this set of definitions is an accurate characterization of the way pain is interpreted by most of us. Our first reaction to pain is either, "Woe is me" (if it is our pain), or "Shame on you" (if it is someone else's); our second reaction is to look for physical damage, and finally we attend to the mental and emotional aspects of suffering. We usually ignore the social and relational aspects altogether.

Pain is viewed primarily as a physical phenomenon within Western culture. While pain is among the least likely reasons for seeking mental health treatment, pain is the most commonly reported symptom within physical health-care systems, and treatment costs are in the multibillions worldwide (Hardin, 1997). It would be accurate to say, then, that pain is one of the largest moneymakers for the world's health-care industry. In the United States it is estimated that between 24 and 80 million Americans (10%–30%) are suffering from significant pain of one sort or another at any given time. Take a moment to think about this in human terms. Imagine you are in a small movie theater, with 20 seats in each row. You would find two to five people in each row who are in significant pain. Of course, the people in the worst pain probably would prefer to stay home, but you get the point. So take a look around you the next time you are out, virtually anywhere, and you probably will be in the presence of several pain sufferers. If pain really is some sort of cosmic punishment, then naughtiness must be very widespread indeed.

The standard treatment for pain due to injury, medical procedures, and the like (e.g., relatively temporary pain that is to be expected) is to prescribe sufficient doses of pain medications to produce analgesia. However, when pain is the primary issue, such as with a chronic condition like back injury, headaches, or fibromyalgia, pain survivors often will obtain care at a clinic specializing in pain. Within such clinics, professionals including physicians, physical therapists, and mental health professionals will ideally work in multidisciplinary teams. Pain may be treated by mental health professionals in private practice as well. In either setting, integrating the care and interventions within a biopsychosocial framework is most important so that the left hand knows what the right hand is doing, so to speak. Ideally, patients' treatments should be individually tailored to fit the specific pains they are encountering and also to fit their own unique biopsychosocial makeup.

The physician might use assessments including scans, such as computed tomography (CT) or magnetic resonance imaging (MRI), blood tests, test of autonomic functioning, and electromyography. Physical therapists may assess for rigidities and flexibilities in the musculoskeletal systems using range of motion, vestibular perception, and other tests. Similarly, mental health professionals should obtain detailed accounts of patients' multiple psychosocial domains, including full developmental histories, personality assessments, and social assessments. Within and across each of these domains, you should listen carefully for information about your patients' relationships with their pains, what you might call their "pain narratives." Listening in this manner, you will gain all of the detailed information required for professional purposes, such as paperwork and reporting to the other members of the team. But in addition you will gain an experiential sense of the pain, a more human understanding. Your patients will also gain from having shared their experiences in a holistic manner such as this.

As you tune in and listen to this pain narrative, it will be important to observe your patient's *process* as well as the *content* of what is said. For example, understanding where and when the pain has been involved in the client's development of relationships with self and others would provide a deep level of narrative content. At the same time, understanding how the client reacts to and relates with the pain would provide a deep level of narrative process. Content in assessment represents the plot of the story, what happens, whereas process represents themes and symbolic meanings, how and why things are happening. You will want to determine the depth and breadth of the pain, how far it reaches across your patient's phenomenological existence in both time and space. How does pain come and go, and how extensive is its negative impact?

Clarity and objectivity in assessment are important as well. Analogue rating scales (e.g., 1–100) of pain intensity and interference across different times and life domains or visual analogue scales using colors to capture different pain intensities (e.g., red is intense and blue is less intense) and size to represent functional interference (from tiny to huge) are quite helpful in this regard.

No matter how medical and objective you may try to be, pain is so tied to perception and immediate social situation that pain assessment can never be completely objective. This often ignored fact is one reason why pain treatment has always been a thorn in the side of the prevailing biomedical paradigm in which it is frequently treated. Think about it. Pain is the most frequently reported symptom in medical practices across the world, yet physicians have no objective tools with which to measure it—no pain thermometer, no pain x-ray. Furthermore, it is unlikely that such a tool will ever be built, even in the era of high-powered brain and full-body scans. Given the focus the Western medical mind-set on material cause and reductionism, however impressive many outcomes may be, something as complex, idiosyncratic, and multiply caused as pain simply just doesn't fit very well. As a result, when dealing with its most ubiquitous complaint, traditional biomedical medicine has a very poor and at times destructive (i.e., iatrogenic) track record in pain management compared with many other areas (Osterweis, Kleinman, & Mechanic, 1987).

Because pain is complex, subjective, personal, and also invisible, the first and most important thing you must do in relating to someone with pain is to attend to his or her subjective experience with pain. Kleinman et al. (1992) describe this point elegantly:

> Personal and social responses to pain thus remake the everyday worlds of patients and their families.... Perception, experience, and coping run into each other and are lived as a unified experience. When reconstituted as a medical problem, however that experience is fragmented into a series of dichotomies that represent the deep cultural logic of biomedicine. Physiological, psychological; body, soul; mind, body; subjective, objective; real, unreal;, natural, artificial—these dichotomies ... are at the heart of the struggle between chronic pain patients and their care givers over the definition of the problem and the search for effective treatment. (p. 8)

They go on:

> Neither in the biomedical research literature nor in the pain clinic does the suffering of pain patients and their intimate social circles receive much attention as such, that is, as a moral burden or a defining existential experience. (p. 14)

Because pain is experiential and relational, the way you approach clients in pain creates a social context, which may impact subsequent experiences. As such, *you* as the treatment provider are entering the complex equation of pain cause and pain relief, so your process and mind-set may be as important as your client's. Why are you treating pain? How do you understand it? Define it? Assess it? When working with someone in pain, the way you *are* is likely to be at least as important as what you *do*, yet we typically apply much greater focus to what we do. We tend to focus on content over process.

Pain patients almost always come to a mental health provider as a last resort, carrying with them the demoralizing sense of pain as punishment and the shame of having a physical disorder that cannot be found by their physician. Deeper than the internalized mantra of demoralization, "It's all in your head," most of these clients will be left with very little explanation to go by other than shame, self-blame, and the twisted peephole through which they may still see traces of hope.

After negative or ambiguous lab and physical tests, as is often the case, they may be left with the only available alternative in our culture: They, their whole self, must be to blame. Unfortunately, the act of coming to you, a mental health professional, for help often will serve only to reinforce that notion. It is certainly rare that a pain sufferer jumps for joy at the chance to work with images, emotion, and habits as a way to decrease their long-held suffering that has outfoxed the best that medical science has to offer. They will rarely exclaim, "Yes! Hooray! I'm finally getting the mental health treatment that is at the root of my physical discomfort!" Instead, you will likely be seen as a place of last resort or limbo of sorts. As such, the importance of finding traces of hope, sparking remoralization (Frank & Frank, 1991; Orlinsky & Howard, 1986), will be even more important with your pain patients than with your nonpain clientele.

Similar to distortions created by the Western belief in a mind–body split, people seeking help for pain may also be hindered by an artificial Western dichotomy between science and spirituality. There is in fact no pervasive or fundamental conflict between the two, despite superficial appearances. The Western scientific revolution began more than 400 years ago, yet it appears that the human mind is still more drawn to appearances than to data, to imagination over critical examination. While this may be helpful within the realm of imagery treatment, this inherent human bias for imagination actually acts as a counterpromotion away from the selection of imagery approaches, and instead techniques with more "scientifical" (seemingly scientific on the surface) appearance toward, like biofeedback, transcutaneous electric nerve stimulation (TENS), and at times even medication.

Despite its stated values in empiricism and rational logic, science has filled the gap once held by spiritual and religious traditions in providing a culturally based and institutionalized authority to the healing arts (Frank & Frank, 1991). This is fantastic if empiricism and rational logic remain the measuring stick for sanctioning treatments. Unfortunately, as humans we tend to fall back to old habits and to apply our old spiritualistic biases to the new context of science. As such, most Western practitioners and clientele will value things that have the appearance of science and technology and will ignore the logic and data behind these appearances. A healer and patient from a spiritually based culture without knowledge of modern medical practices may be likely to shy away from a pill in favor of a ritual or to explain the effectiveness of a pill based on spirits and energies rather than pharmacokinetics. Conversely, individuals from Western modernist cultures are likely to shy away from anything that appears nonscientific and to explain the efficacy of approaches like imagery based on some potentially oversimplified neurochemical process.

At the same time, our minds are out of sync with our culture, still operating more like the spiritualist than the modernist. We rarely actually look at the evidence for a particular treatment. Instead, we defer to approaches that appear the most scientific, with science taking on the role that religion and spirit once occupied. It doesn't help matters that the pain treatment research is so complex and contradictory, making the process of examining evidence for clear conclusions more difficult. This ambiguity in the research may lead to even greater skepticism in regard to holistic and naturalistic approaches like imagery, which actually tend to consistently show strong positive results.

To be fair, the problem is not just with the mainstream, scientific approaches to pain treatment. Alternative practitioners and psychotherapists, including those who use imagery for pain, are not without oversimplifications of their own. For example, psychotherapists tend to exclude the body to a large degree, focusing too much on mental and emotional processes for pain that is indeed located primarily within the physiological systems of the patient. Apart from a hearty handshake at the end of a successful course of treatment, most psychotherapists want to duck for cover at the very idea of laying hands on a client: "Go ahead and tell me things you wouldn't tell your best friend, but please don't touch my hand or arm or I'll need you to sign a waiver." While psychologists across the United States are fighting with psychiatrists for prescription privileges, they certainly are not fighting physical or massage therapists for the right to perform a far less risky set of therapeutic procedures. At their best, therapists try to touch their clients' beliefs, values, even their spirits in as deep a manner as is necessary, while anything regarding their bodies is strictly off limits. We definitely are not suggesting that you touch your clients superfluously during psychotherapy, and professional boundaries are indeed important for the safety of our clients and for the therapeutic process. Nevertheless, it may be helpful to recognize the impact of the strict body–mind boundaries within modern medical practices.

We must not fall into an error of attribution ourselves in blaming a class of practitioners, saying the problem is with the "science types," the "spiritual types," the physicians, or the hypnotists. The actual problem is larger and lies in the worldview derived from the Western cultural soup in which we swim. This worldview distorts the clarity of our vision of pain as completely as the water distorts the reality of a fish living in a bowl. A body-versus-mind, slice-and-dice mentality is simply counterproductive to our patients in pain. Kleinman et al. (1992) describe a sort of nether-world that exists between body-medicine and mind-medicine that leads to a fragmented, disconnected, and at times obfuscated view of our patients' experiences of pain:

> The dichotomy between mind and body upheld by both medical and psychological research is invalid and unavailing. Yet it is the viewpoint of many practitioners, most researchers, and not a few patients. (p. 11)

They go on to describe pain as being:

> so densely interrelated and multileveled and of such astonishing complexity that the reader (social scientist or health scientist) must despair at ever grasping the processes that mediate a pounding headache or that transform a social stigma into the nauseating cramping of abdominal distress. With such a vast network of "variables," whose resonances and results are so poorly charted, it is not surprising that researchers have defined (or created) a subject matter they can actually study with available conceptual and methodological approaches. Thus arises the recent interest in chronic pain and the diverse disciplinary approaches to its study. (p. 13)

People in pain feel its impacts, spanning the continuum of day-to-day life experiences, from the most physical aspects to the most spiritual. Even an apparently tangential factor like socioeconomics, for example, can be critical to understanding chronic pain. Specifically, poor, unskilled workers are more likely to become disabled by equivalent levels of chronic pain than wealthier sufferers with white-collar jobs, even accounting for different work conditions. Further, rates of pain-related disability covary with rates of unemployment and other global financial indicators. Furthermore, these large-scale socioeconomic factors are not subtle. In fact, these relationships are so robust that social factors predict rehabilitation better than biomedical tests (Syrjala & Abrams, 2002). Getting "kicked while you're down" by hard times, layoffs, or poverty may at times be experienced in a somewhat literal manner.

Surrounding the individual pain experiences of each patient lives a dynamic web of causation (Pincus, 2006). Yet we struggle with accepting and working with this plain reality. Our patients describe pains in these terms, but we analyze their stories in terms of details that fit within discipline-specific frames. In the age of space travel and 100-year life spans, how did we end up becoming such strangers to our ancient, familiar, and universal companion, pain? The answer lies in the history of our relationship to pain, to healing, and to some unfortunately overblown assumptions of the scientific revolution such as mind–body dualism and reductionism (which is discussed in detail in Chapter 2).

But let's not be too extreme on this point about complex cause, assuming that everything causes everything else and simple causes don't matter. The scientific approach, which has focused on small and simple causes, has been quite fruitful, particularly given the fact that serious study of pain only dates back about 50 years. To understand the myriad ways that imagery impacts pain, for better and for worse, it is important that we deepen our understanding of the distinct psychosocial factors that impact the pain experience. By first looking at the simple causes of pain, we can work toward an understanding of how these factors build to form a unique pain system for each individual client (Pincus, Wachsmuth-Schlaefer, Sheikh, & Ezaz-Nikpay, 2003).

What Causes Pain?

Some caveats are in order before we dive into the discussion of the causes of pain. First, we are going to ignore more than 20,000 years of oral and written knowledge and focus instead on the past 50 years of scientific inquiry. As absurd as this may seem, at least we are pointing out this omission of roughly 19,950 years of acquired wisdom. In addition, we are going to begin our discussion with a one-by-one focus on single causal factors even though we already know that there is really no such thing as a *single* cause when dealing with pain—just as there is not any universal set of causes that applies equally to everyone. Finally, we are going to almost completely ignore bodily causes, like tissue damage, central and peripheral nervous processes, diet, and metabolism. We will do so, however, knowing full well that although this is a bit ridiculous, it is standard practice in alternative medicine. If that's not a good enough excuse, we can claim genuine ignorance of physical causes and provide a reference instead (see Merskey & Bogduk, 1994, for a more complete discussion of physical causes of pain). The identification of numerous psychosocial causes of pain does not diminish the importance of physical causes, nor do there need to be predominant psychosocial causes for imagery to be an effective pain reducer. Pain from surgery (e.g., procedural pain) is about as physical a cause as possible, yet imagery is effective for procedural pain. Causes and effective treatments do not necessarily coincide.

Gate Control

The gate-control theory (Melzack & Wall, 1965, 1996) was the first prominent theory linking psychosocial factors with physiological processes in pain perception. The *gate* in the theory, connecting mind and body, was believed to be the dorsal horn of the Substantia Gelatinosa of the spinal cord, thus the name *gate control*. Efferent (downward moving) psychological factors theoretically modified the sensitivity of the spinal chord to afferent (upward moving) nociceptive signals, thereby opening or closing the gate on the intensity of the pain experience.

On a broader, more psychological scale, the theory specified three somewhat distinct yet interacting dimensions of the pain experience: *sensory-discriminative, motivational-affective*, and *cognitive-evaluative*. The first dimension, sensory-discriminative, involves nerve activity at injury sites and resulting pain sensations. This is the tissue damage and resulting nerve activity that most Westerners first look for in understanding pain. Although it is the most body centered of the three dimensions of pain, imagery may target the sensory-discriminative dimension through simple transformational or dissociation imagery, such as by imagining that one's injured arm is made of wood or rubber or that the pain is spreading throughout the body and thus becoming more dull and diffuse. Thus, this dimension of the pain experience rests in the numerous cognitive processes involved in sensation and perception.

The second dimension of the pain experience is motivational-affective, referring to the feelings and desired actions resulting from the pain experience. Negative feelings, like sadness and fear, intensify and worsen the experience of pain (Ahles, Blanchard, & Leventhal, 1983; Stevens, Heise, & Pfost, 1989; Worthington & Shumate, 1981). Similarly, pain will intensify if the pain brings relative rewards, such as pain that blocks one's ability to return to a job that has been unsympathetic toward the sufferer of an on-the-job worker's compensation injury. Mental trips to exotic beaches or favorite places represent one common class of techniques aimed at blocking the motivational-affective dimension of pain by inducing relaxation and other positive emotional states.

The third dimension of pain is cognitive-evaluative, which refers to the meaning of the pain with respect to severity, negative implications, or expectations. This dimension may involve one's sense of being broken, damaged, or punished. Imagery aimed at shifting the cognitive-evaluative dimension of pain could include imagery focused on reframing pain as a sign of healing, images that focus on the temporary nature of pain such as rising and falling waves during labor pains, or images that place pain in a different relational context, like adventure images. On the deepest levels, transformational imagery involving existential self-world narratives can change one's experience of pain within this dimension as well.

According to gate-control theory, pain depends on these three separate but interacting dimensions that regulate the flow of sensory information between brain and body. Thus, if any one of these dimensions is shifted, the flow of pain information will shift, just as the flow of water through a river will shift along with the movement of banks or objects on the river bottom. For example, the experience of having one's arm slowly hacked off with a saw would strongly activate the sensory-discriminative dimension of pain. More subtly, a bruise to an athlete's leg that would end the chances of an Olympic gold medal, would strongly activate the cognitive-evaluative dimension, and anything that increases the negative affect involved would add fuel to the fire.

This model also suggests that each of us learns how to experience pain and that this learning is developmental. Most people have seen a child fall down and get a "boo-boo," and if you observe closely, you may notice a common yet remarkable thing. Children often pause and look around after they tumble or bump themselves. What are they looking for? They are trying to figure out whether it hurt. Of course if they fall really hard and the sensory-discriminative dimension is heavily represented, they will cry regardless of the adult reactions. Nevertheless, this model also helps to explain why kissing the boo-boo is such an effective treatment.

Children definitely do feel pain. We don't want to restart the antiquated myth from modern medicine that they don't. However, the sensory and other cognitive dimensions of pain are less developed in children, and thus pain may be more ambiguous to them, particularly for a mild- to medium-level boo-boo. Consequently, they look to adults to make up for their lack of experience, which would otherwise inform their interpretation of the pain. So how hard they cry depends on (1) how hard they fall (sensory-discriminative); (2) their moods and the attention they may get (motivational-affective); and (3) the reactions of the adults around them (cognitive-evaluative). A tired, needy toddler who takes a hard fall followed by strong adult reactions equals a strong pain experience. An active, happy toddler who takes a light fall with little or no parental reaction equals a minor pain experience. Adults are not so different, except that we also tend to also look within for the meaning of pain. What do we find within? Predominantly we find images—images that modify, shape, and regulate our pain, just as do the reactions of adults to an injured child.

Melzack and Wall's (1965) theory is still the preeminent model for understanding pain. However, it is worth mentioning that other models have been proposed that rightly try to put the dimensions of pain back together into a more systems-oriented framework. Perceiving, feeling, and thinking are not separate processes in fact and cannot occur in isolation.

Melzack (1999) has come up with a modern, systems model, updating his original gate-control theory and calling it the "neuromatrix" theory. This model focuses on the body's stress-arousal systems and the functional role of pain in maintaining homeostasis within key survival-related bodily systems. Melzack suggests that pain and stress act together and may be adaptive in the short term, acting as a kind of emergency brake preventing dangerous fluctuations in body temperature or blood sugar. However, as the old saying goes, you can't get something for nothing. The body's chronic overreliance on the pain–stress response to maintain homeostasis may lead to structural damage in skeletal, muscular, and neurological systems.

One way to interpret Melzack's (1999) model is that the brain and the body each form memories of pain through repeated experience. The neuromatrix is a neural network containing coordinated activation patterns of millions of neurons that, over repeated experience, come to represent pain. What one gets is a sort of kindling effect, whereby each experience of phenomenologically similar pain makes subsequent experiences more likely to occur. In terms of body–memory, the affected tissues become increasingly subject to degradation when this neural network activates the hypothalamic-pituitary-adrenal (HPA) axis in the midbrain—the body's stress system. Cortisol and other stress-related hormones actually can damage tissue with repeated and long-term exposure, just as professional athletes suffer in the long run from repeated injections of synthetic anti-inflammatory medications.

The pain and stress systems once linked to one another are designed to assist the body–mind in reacting to short-term environmental stressors. The problem lies in chronicity. When repeatedly and rigidly activated, the pain and stress—those pesky unwelcome guests—find a home in the body–mind.

Personality Factors

Before we go too far toward a comprehensive, systems-oriented understanding of pain and the uniqueness of each client (which we explore in more detail in Chapter 3), let's take a step back and continue to look at one of the first and most extensive areas in the study of psychosocial factors on clinical pain: personality (Gatchel & Epker, 1999; Weisenberg & Keefe, 2002). The interest in finding enduring characterological patterns that can be flagged as "pain-prone personalities" is likely fed as much by the basic human bias toward dispositional attributions as by a desire to be helpful. As discussed already herein, we all really need to watch out so as not to further stigmatize our pain patients by adopting oversimplified attitudes suggesting that their personalities are the primary cause of their pain. After all, this is really only a small step away from the concept that pain is punishment—not a good mind-set for a healer: "Well, it's not your pain, Tanya, that is actually the problem; you see it's your personality that is to blame." Furthermore, the problem with the nature of pain-prone personality is not just one of being nontherapeutic. Like most areas of pain research, the variability in specific manifestations of clinical pain has made general patterns difficult to identify. Realistically speaking, there is no single pain-prone personality.

We do realize, however, that there can be some merit to understanding personality factors that may be involved with pain. First, both Axis I (i.e., common psychiatric diagnoses such as depression and anxiety) and Axis II (i.e., broader personality styles that lead to dysfunction known as personality disorders such as dependent, avoidant, and borderline) disorders are about three times as frequent in pain patients compared with matched controls (Weisenberg & Keefe, 2002). However, the causal relationships have not been established, which means that it is not clear whether the pain causes the disturbance or the disturbance causes the pain or whether both are caused by some third factor. This is your all too common chicken-or-the-egg scenario that occurs with numerous clinical syndromes.

In the case of chronic pain, it is likely that research will be unable to ever really tell us if people with psychiatric and personality disturbances are more likely to suffer from chronic pain or if the cause works in the other direction. You see, our methodologies are not very good at dealing with things that evolve over time, such as chronic pain and psychiatric disturbance. The most likely situation is that the two cause each other and that this process happens in a somewhat unique way for each individual. Similarly, traditional research methodologies struggle with accounting for complex cause and individual uniqueness.

These are not the only difficulties. First, chronic pain symptoms are frequently woven together with the Axis II diagnostic criteria (Weisenberg & Keefe, 2002). This means that the symptoms used to make the diagnosis overlap with features that would be expected in anyone experiencing chronic pain. For example, borderline personality disorder includes "suicidal gestures or threats," "affective instability," and chronic "feelings of emptiness" (APA, 1994, pp. 654); each of these would be expected in higher frequency in people dealing with chronic pain. Similarly, dependent personality disorder includes feeling uncomfortable or helpless when alone due to exaggerated fears of being able to care for himself or herself; urgently seeking another relationship as a source of care and support when a close relationship ends; and being unrealistically preoccupied with fears of being left to care for himself or herself (APA, pp. 668–669). Avoidant personality disorder includes the following symptoms: showing restraint with intimate relationships due to fear of being shamed or ridiculed; being inhibited in new interpersonal situations because of feelings of inadequacy; and being unusually reluctant to take personal risks or to engage in any new activities because they may prove embarrassing (APA, pp. 665). To be fair, if the diagnosing clinician saw each of these symptoms as arising solely due to chronic pain, they are not supposed to make the personality disorder diagnosis. However, such a distinction is difficult to make in the case of chronic pain.

A second problem is that the personality measures most often used in pain-personality research are biased because they contain questions with somatic (physical symptom) content and because they have questionable links to *Diagnostic and Statistical Manual of Mental Disorders*, 4th ed. (*DSM-IV*; APA, 1994) diagnoses, for example, the Minnesota Multiphasic Personality Inventory-2 (MMPI-2) scales. So someone might come up in the dysfunctional range based on a personality trait, but in reality this dysfunctional trait might not be related to a personality disorder but rather to the pain.

A third problem is the dubious diagnostic reliabilities for *DSM-IV* (APA, 1994) personality disorders as a whole. In fact, there is so much overlap among the symptoms of the 11 personality disorders described in the *DSM-IV* that two people with different disorders may have more symptoms in common than two people with the same disorder.

With these caveats in mind, some interesting results have been found (for a thorough review of the existing literature connecting psychiatric problems, personality, and chronic pain, see Gatchel & Dersh, 2002). In studies that look at patients over time, there is in fact a great deal of evidence to suggest that psychiatric symptoms improve as pain decreases and that these psychiatric symptoms are far more prevalent in patients with chronic pain than in patients with acute pain.

On the other hand, there is a great deal of evidence showing high frequencies of Axis I and Axis II disorders among pain patients, far more than one would expect to emerge as a result of being in pain. Similarly, many pain patients show evidence of prepain psychiatric and personality morbidity. Taken together, these results suggest a chicken-and-the-egg conclusion. Dysfunction leads to pain and pain leads to dysfunction, and the specific dynamics of this interaction differ from individual to individual over time.

Gatchel and Dersh (2002) also have come up with a sophisticated model based on their results, which could set the stage for future researchers to bring pain research and clinical sense closer together. What they suggest specifically is that the most common path to chronic pain begins with pain that triggers idiosyncratic psychological reactions, depending on the psychiatric and personality dynamics of the individual, which they label as "Stage-1." At "Stage-2," these psychiatric and personality-style problems exacerbate both the pain and the original psychiatric dysfunction: The chicken–egg dance begins. This leads to "Stage-3," the final stage, where a stable, chronic time course for the pain emerges along with the adoption of a sick role, enabling pain to find a home in the person's day-to-day dealings with self and others. Finally, research has shown high levels of substance abuse are found in chronic pain patients, which may be considered to act as an accelerant on the entire process. As addiction and pain settle in together, the remedy for each becomes more difficult to find.

Despite all the caveats listed at the beginning of this section on the pain-prone personality, it is crystal clear that pain and other psychiatric difficulties often coincide. Therefore, therapists need to be alert to specific diagnostic categories and personality styles during assessment and treatment of pain. For example, Weisenberg and Keefe (2002) report a range of 31% to 59% in the prevalence of Axis I disorders in chronic pain patients. The disorders most often accompanying pain are mood and anxiety disorders, which makes clinical sense.

Due to the troublesome overlap between the diagnostic criteria for different personality disorders, it is more useful to describe personality clusters (groups of three or more specific personality diagnoses joined based on similarity) and styles that tend to go along with pain rather than specific personality disorders (APA, 1994; Widiger, Trull, Hurt, Clarkin, & Frances, 1987). The most prevalent cluster is Cluster C, "Anxious-avoidant-type." This cluster consists of the specific personality disorders of avoidant, dependent, and obsessive-compulsive personalities. Cluster B, "Dramatic-emotional-type," is the next most common cluster seen in chronic pain patients and consists of the specific diagnoses: borderline, narcissistic, and histrionic personalities.

Apart from diagnostic categories, four interrelated traits may best describe a common profile for the personality styles of people dealing with chronic pain: threat avoidance, dependence, helplessness, and emotional dysregulation (Weisenberg & Keefe, 2002). People with chronic pain tend to cope with stress by overusing avoidance, to adopt a one-down, dependent role in relating to others, and to experience the byproducts of these imbalanced coping styles: helplessness and emotional dysregulation.

These four traits may be a common thread among pain disorders, depression/anxiety syndromes, and the B and C personality clusters. Avoidance and nonassertion as coping styles are leading causes of anxiety (Levis & Brewer, 2001) and depression (Pettit & Joiner, 2006). Yes, there's serotonin too, and norepinepherine. But you hear about neurotransmitters all the time in television commercials. Imagine a television commercial for cognitive-imagery therapy:

Depression, anxiety, chronic pain, and other body–mind disturbances are believed to be caused by an overreliance on avoidance in
coping with life's problems. When there is an imbalance in avoidant
behaviors, one may be hindered in developing confidence and efficacy, leading to overdependence on others, to helplessness and ultimately to the physio-emotional dysregulation thought to underlie
depression, anxiety, and chronic pain. Cognitive therapies, like
guided imagery, are thought to correct these behavioral and personality imbalances, restoring one to a joyful state of health [cut to the
picture of an older couple smiling as they bend to take a generous
sniff of some roses growing in their backyard garden].

There would be no need for a long list of side effects at the end of this ad, yet
it is not something you will encounter on the television. Someday perhaps?

Pain research suggests that the primary culprits are indeed an overreliance on avoidance, misguided attempts to avoid pain, and other uncomfortable experiences. So pay attention to personality, along with anxiety,
depression, and the rest when you assess your pain patients. But don't
try to overexplain the pain based on these related syndromes or, even
worse, blame the patient's pain on his or her personality or coping styles.
Instead, blur your clinical vision a bit and see the general dysregulation
that stretches from the social to the neurochemical realms. See the suffering this dysregulation causes, your client's understandable tendency
to continue to try to avoid these varied types of pain, and the strains on
their psyches as they invariably try their best to put these problems out
of awareness. Once you can do this, your clients will no longer be alone,
painted into corners through the process of avoidance. From a shared vantage point of this corner, the two of you may begin to share a vision of the
way out, through letting go and falling gently and slowly back into the full
range of experience.

Behavioral Learning Factors

Think of personality as the garden in which pain grows, like a troubling
weed that chokes away the fruits of enjoyment, friendships, and competence. Within this metaphor, behavioral learning factors are like the soil,
fertilizer, sun, water, and perhaps even the gardener. Behavioral learning
provides an indispensable vantage point for understanding pain. Moving
beyond firm distinctions between operant and classical conditioning, one
may take a more down-to-earth (and probably more accurate; see Donahoe
& Vegas, 2004), ecological approach to behavioral learning by asking: What
function are these pain problems serving, and how is the pain maintained
over time within your clients' day-to-day lives?

Pain, although by definition punishing, may actually be reinforced if it provides some form of reward, which overrides its inherent discomfort (i.e., positive reinforcement), or if the pain provides escape from some aversive experience that is more threatening than the pain itself (e.g., negative reinforcement). If pain becomes reinforcing, it does *not* mean that your patients want to be sick. Instead, it means they are stuck between a rock and a hard place, a painful place both literally and figuratively. Once pain finds a source of relative reinforcement, it may use that source to feed a self-sustaining process. The pain then becomes a relatively functional part of the client's life, because its removal would lead to some greater general loss. The pain then is much like a parasite, sucking away at the lifeblood of reinforcement in the patient's life and making a comfortable home for itself within the life space of the body–mind.

Some concrete examples of gains (i.e., positive reinforcers) that may feed parasitic pains include disability wages, a means of relating to others, a means to obtaining sympathy, and worst of all, a coherent sense of self- and life-narrative. There also are a plethora of noxious factors that pain may assist one in avoiding (i.e., negative reinforcement), including avoidance of work, avoidance of feared people or feared interpersonal situations, avoidance of unpleasant activities such as exercise, avoidance of rejection, avoidance of painful emotions, avoidance of responsibility for life's invariable downturns, and, most generally, avoidance of the existential pain of many human experiences. Pain may shield a person from any or all of these experiences, making itself increasingly indispensable over time. (Incidentally, this process is fed through overreliance on avoidance as a coping style as was described in the previous section on personality factors).

You may have heard of people who are self-injurious, for example, people who cut themselves in response to their own painful experiences and strong negative emotional states. The available evidence suggests that most "cutters" do not hurt themselves for sympathy or to manipulate, as many assume. On the contrary, most people who cut go to great lengths to avoid this embarrassing habit. What cutting actually seems to do is to bring relief to these individuals within the various systems of the body–mind, from physical relievers like endogenous opiates that are released just prior to and during the act of cutting to existential relievers such as a concrete shift away from "metaphysical" bleeding to "actual" bleeding (Haines, Williams, Brain, & Wilson, 1995). Chronic pain may come to serve such a role in the lives of patients as well, except that the act of cutting is not necessary for them, because they are already hurt. The physical pain comes automatically whenever it is needed to cover up a larger, nonphysical, existential pain.

More simply, this process may be cued or triggered in an automatic sense, also known as classical conditioning. Like all negative, emotionally charged experiences, pain has the potential to form strong and enduring paired associations with other experiences. On a neurobiological level, this occurs because experiences containing strong negative emotions lodge themselves deep within the brain's neural circuitry (Perry, 2002), which is generally adaptive because it is important to remember negatively charged experiences so that you can learn from them. If you are mugged in a dark alley, it is good to remember the incident so that you will avoid that alley in the future.

When it comes to memory, your brain processes pain in a similar manner as a mugging. The more intense and emotionally charged the pain experience is, the deeper the pain will dig itself down into the lower areas of the brain that process emotion (i.e., limbic) and govern attention (i.e., brain stem). These deeper brain areas are less changeable, having lower *plasticity*, or recoverability, from physical changes. As such, painful experiences, like other traumatic memories, are stored across deeper layers of the brain and are less able to be washed away with subsequent experiences. Pain is a very "sticky" experience in this respect, easily linking itself to a variety of triggers.

Thus, pain may be maintained over time through repeated paired associations between pain sensations and some internal or external cue. The more intense or upsetting the pain, the stronger these paired associations will become. Furthermore, the law of contiguity states that the more frequent and specific the pairing, and the more intense the pain, the stronger, or "stickier," these linkages will be. Anyone who has been a smoker can attest that the experience of nicotine craving is particularly sticky, as cravings for a cigarette become paired to the most benign array of day-to-day experiences such as drinking coffee, riding in a car, listening to music, having 10 free minutes of time, or, cruelest association of all, thoughts about cutting down. Just reading about cigarettes may cause cravings in those of you who smoke or used to smoke. Similarly, the experience of pain may latch on to any number of other daily experiences.

Because the various states of mind and body are linked through experience, both conscious and less conscious, classical conditioning represents one of the most common and obvious connecting points between the body and mind. For example, seeing or imagining someone getting sick can make a person feel queasy; seeing or imagining someone eating a piece of lemon can make a person's mouth water and pucker; and talking about waterfalls and rivers can be torturous to someone who needs to urinate during a long car ride. In each case one is giving a nudge to consciousness (or, if you prefer, to the brain's parallel distributed patterns of neural activation) toward some well-rehearsed state, whether it be queasiness, hunger, or urination. Triggers in the environment simply can nudge one's body–mind into a state of pain.

These examples of classical conditioning can be useful in helping clients understand the routine connections between body and mind. In addition, these examples may be used to demonstrate how common it is for bodily response to be triggered by perceptual experiences. The saliva produced by imagining a tart slice of lemon is not all in your head (actually it is in your mouth—which is in your head, but you get the point). If clients have some obvious classical conditioning mechanisms involved in their pain conditions, these may be illuminated to further remoralize them, to reduce their self-blame, and to set the stage for imagery treatment.

Some common classically conditioned triggers for chronic pain include negative emotions, traumatic memories, various other thought processes, specific behaviors, temporal cycles (e.g., daily, monthly), or even pain medications themselves. Indeed, through the power of classical conditioning, mind–body experience associations can and often do override analgesic pharmacokinetics. According to Salkovskis (1996, p. 256), "a reduction in pain may occur in as many as 40 % of pain patients when (prescribed and non-prescribed) medication is withdrawn." Moreover, this effect may be particularly pronounced if pain medications are taken below therapeutic thresholds and on an as-needed basis.

How does this work? When taken on an as-needed basis, patients use their analgesics when they experience pain, then the pain goes away, comes back, more meds are taken, and so on over time. This often leads to a conditioned association between the time interval for the next dosing of medication and increasing pain. This association can then act as an accelerant, leading to what are commonly referred to as rebound effects. In addition, medication-taking behavior is strongly negatively reinforced (removing the aversive condition of pain) through operant principles, leading to increasing reliance on and need for the medication over time.

These days, most physicians who are well informed will prescribe continual doses of medication at a sufficient strength to relieve pain as completely as possible (Hill et al., 1990; Portenoy, 1994) and will help patients wean themselves off medication as quickly as possible when an injury is healed (Salkovskis, 1996). This dosing strategy aims to keep the medication's effects ahead of or on top of the pain and then gradually allows the patient's natural body–mind pain-killing mechanisms to take charge again as quickly as possible.

Again, the law of contiguity states that the strength of a classically conditioned pain response will depend on the strength and specificity of the original pairing between the trigger and the pain, as well as on their continued and repeated pairing over time. For example, if pain emerges during an emotionally laden experience, it may strengthen itself over time as the pain and negative emotional states are reexperienced together in subsequent episodes. Moreover, if the pain is experienced while the patient is in a wide variety of negative mood states, the conditioned link may become generalized, spreading to a more diverse array of triggers over time.

However, through understanding how this pesky parasite of pain makes its home within the body–mind's consciousness, interesting ways to attack the pain become apparent. In the case of classical conditioning, one simply needs to reverse this associative process, known as counterconditioning or desensitization. In the case of mood–pain pairings, if the associated mood is experienced without pain, counterconditioning may occur, breaking the associated links and leading to decreasing pain over time in response to that emotion. Not coincidentally, this process involves a reversal of the tendency toward *experiential avoidance* that frequently accompanies pain, as was described in our discussion of the trait of avoidance (see Hayes, Strosahl, & Wilson, 1999, for a complete discussion of the putative role of experiential avoidance in mental health and psychotherapy).

Throughout each of these conditioning processes, both operant and classical, you may have noticed that time is of critical importance. All associations, reinforcements, and broader habit formations occur within the context of time. As repetition over time is essential in developing chronic pain, it similarly will be essential in treatment. A focus on time and repetition also allows us to consider the myriad ways classical and operant conditioning are actually inseparable and work in tandem over time, both to trigger and to maintain pain experiences. For example, imagine that a person develops leg pain due to stiffness on frequent, long drives to visit family. Originally, the pain might be due, more or less, to a physiological weakness such as bursitis. Over time, however, any long drive may come to trigger the pain through classical conditioning. At the same time, imagine that the pain becomes a serendipitous means of avoidance, allowing the person to skip unwanted family visits, or, more subtly, provides a pain-related role for the individual as well as emotional distance from troublesome family dynamics: "You know what, I'm going to have to hit the road a little early to head home; my knee is really starting to bother me. I'll see you next Thanksgiving."

Over time, the combined effects of association and reward result in greater specificity in the pairing between the pain responses and long drives in the car: "It hurts, so I won't drive, so it hurts, so I won't drive," and so on. Thus, classical and operant conditioning may reinforce one another in a reciprocal manner as reinforcements for the pain may lead to avoidance, which strengthens the specificity of paired associations between pain and a variety of experiences (e.g., driving, being with family). The specific dynamics will vary with each pain patient. But already it becomes clear how even a few simple factors, such as an avoidant personality style together with operant and classical conditioning, can interact cooperatively over time to intensify and maintain pain that would otherwise have dissipated naturally.

In a meta-analysis, Holroyd and Penzien (1986) found that behavior therapy, aimed at strategically shifting reinforcements and reversing patterns of avoidance, is generally effective in the treatment of pain, with an average improvement of approximately 50% in the reduction of pain symptoms and a statistically significant benefit over placebo-control conditions. Although the analysis did not separate out imagery techniques per se, most behavioral treatments use imagery as a medium in which to carry out a number of these behavioral procedures (e.g., paired-relaxation, covert desensitization, covert rehearsal of coping behaviors).

Coping Behavior

Maladaptive attempts at coping were identified briefly in the previous discussion of operant conditioning (i.e., avoidance), but they are so important that they warrant their own section. In addition, they represent additional down-to-earth examples for your clients of ways psychosocial factors connect to bodily pain.

Maladaptive coping occurs when a client attempts to respond to pain in a positive manner but, without intending to, paradoxically makes the problem worse. As we already have discussed, the most frequent maladaptive coping behaviors are avoidant behaviors (Salkovskis, 1996). As a reminder, anytime we look at specific avoidant behaviors of our patients, we should also be mindful of the likelihood that these behaviors exist within a broader context of personality styles involving low efficacy, helplessness, dependency, and affective dysregulation.

A clear and prevalent example of coping gone wrong is prolonged avoidance of physical activity in response to pain. Taking it easy may in fact be functional in the short run, particularly if a person has pain related to some physical injury. However, prolonged inactivity can result in continued pain through direct impacts on physiological systems, such as the atrophy of muscles and the tightening of connective tissues.

For example, imagine a patient who goes to bed every time she feels the pain of her fibromyalgia flaring up. As she lies there, she becomes increasingly frustrated as her attempts to get out of bed are met with increasing soreness and stiffness, which reinforces her continued avoidance. The patient gets caught in a spiral of circular cause, like a snake swallowing its own tail. Over time, this patient goes on multiday stints in bed, getting up only briefly to use the bathroom, to get food, and so on. Physical activity becomes increasingly difficult and painful for her over the long term, as her muscles and joints tighten and weaken in their own maladaptive coping spirals.

In addition to avoiding physical activity, other maladaptive coping behaviors may include overmedicating, seeking pathological levels of support, physical overcompensation (e.g., overreliance on a cane), quitting work, or alienating significant others who refuse to accommodate to the patient's sick role.

Nevertheless, the answer is not as simple as just getting out of bed, going back to work, or pretending that one is not actually in severe pain. There is a delicate balance between gradually expanding life domains and recklessly reinjuring one's body–mind through overexertion. It also will not be helpful to replace behavioral avoidance (e.g., lying in bed) with experiential avoidance (e.g., telling oneself that it doesn't hurt as much as it actually does). This is where detailed assessment, clear treatment strategies, and a collaborative healing relationship can really pay off. Invariably, you will be assisting your patients in expanding their ranges of free movement. Just as the physical therapist works with range of motion in affected limbs, you will be assisting your clients to gradually expand their physical, social, and vocational activities, along with their emotional experiences, both positive and negative, and ultimately their sense of themselves and their worlds.

Expansion and change can be difficult and risky propositions, even when one is not injured. Your patients will carry the added burden of repeated experiences of punishment and failure in past attempts at expansion. Just try to prescribe daily exercise to your patient lying in bed all day with fibromyalgia, and she will tell you all about the various ways she has tried such things in the past and how miserably each attempt has gone.

Attentional–Perceptual Dynamics

One connecting point between people's mind-sets and pain perceptions lies in selective attention mechanisms that result in perceptual biases. Among the cognitive processes, we would suggest that the dynamics of attention and perception form the most basic and rudimentary level of consciousness building. For example, perceptual biases can lead people to experience their worlds in an excessively *top-down* (belief-driven) manner, such as through the filter of pain-related mind-sets. In this way, pain may be experienced even in the absence of *bottom-up* perceptual factors like nociception (the stimulation of pain receptors). Research in the area of signal-detection theory (Green & Swets, 1966; McNicol, 2005) has demonstrated clearly that perception is anything but an all-or-nothing phenomenon but is in fact probabilistic. As a result, false perceptions are a common everyday occurrence, not some bizarre process involving hallucination and the like.

Due to the constant bombardment of our sense modalities with information, the ability to selectively attend to some bits of information while ignoring others is necessary for day-to-day functioning. Research based on signal-detection theory has demonstrated that people's attention levels will shift depending on such top-down factors as expectations, beliefs, images, affective states, needs, and other motivations. For example, a child who goes to bed on Christmas Eve may hear bells or hoof steps on her ceiling at some point during the evening. This child is not crazy. Instead, her mind-set has created an attentional and perceptual bias, allowing her to perceive Santa-related noises in the absence of any physical sound. The same thing might happen to you as you hear noises in your house after a scary movie or as you notice the annoying habits of your spouse more intensely during an argument.

These same processes can increase or decrease one's experience of pain. Take a moment right now and scan your body for any pain that may be present. You probably will be able to locate some uncomfortable area even if you have no injury. Start with your head and move down through your face, neck, shoulders, arms, hands, down through your back, buttocks, legs, and feet. Actually, I've got a bit of pain right now in my right upper jaw, the back of my throat (just a bit), my right arm, and definitely my knees. I shouldn't type on the floor with my legs crossed—but enough about me. What did you find? Focus on your strongest pain site. Now, focus on this pain-filled area, and think about your inability to manage this pain. Feel the negative affect that results, and imagine the impact of some maladaptive coping response, like staying at home all weekend. Imagine that this perceptual process, cemented by negative affect and beliefs, is repeated day after day. With sufficient repetitions, one will acquire a dysfunctional schematic mind-set for a pain disorder triggered by little direct tissue damage (Salkovskis, 1996).

Of course, it is important to note once again that this attention-driven induction of pain happens automatically and is, thus, no more purposeful or conscious than clinical pain resulting primarily from a physical injury. Despite this fact, it remains relatively easy for people to grasp the idea that pain may change one's focus of attention, yet it is quite hard for them to grasp the opposite.

Researchers have not yet examined pain-related attention biases through signal-detection theory per se. However, there is ample indirect evidence supporting signal-detection processes in modulating pain. For instance, as simple distraction techniques can work as pain reducers, particularly distraction from the affective-motivational dimensions of pain (e.g., Ahles et al., 1983; Spanos & O'Hara, 1990: Stevens et al., 1989). Furthermore, strong support for the role of attention lies in the fact that clinical-pain patients frequently demonstrate somatic attentional biases (Barsky, Goodson, & Lane, 1998; Geisser, Gaskin, Robinson, & Greene, 1993; Okifuji & Turk, 1999). On the other hand, hypochondriacal individuals tend to respond to experimental pain stimuli with more physiological arousal, stronger subjective pain reactions, and even lower temperatures (during a cold-water immersion paradigm) compared with control participants (Gramling, Clawson, & McDonald, 1996). It seems that the spotlight of attention not only can influence pain perception but also can actually heat or cool our living flesh—so much for all in your head.

However, the specific healing mechanisms of distraction continue to elude pain experimenters (e.g., Farthing, Venturino, Brown, & Lazar, 1997), as do the specific situations, clients, and desired outcomes for which distraction is most helpful (Boothby, Thorn, Stroud, & Jensen, 1999). We would suggest that the elusive nature of these research questions lies in the isolated examination of attention and perception, which again are small-scale phenomena within the larger cognitive systems of individuals. As such, the impacts of attention and perception would be expected to be swayed depending on the larger contexts in which they are nested, such as mind-sets, affects, environmental situations, and also the intensity of the pain itself. One can more easily ignore a fly on one's arm than an elephant. Finally, as a small-scale process, attention-perception dynamics would be expected to be more ephemeral, working and then not working over time. For example, while engrossed in writing text for a book on pain, one may become so engrossed as to miss leg cramping from a poor sitting position, until the topic is mentioned directly, prompting a nice long stretch … Oh, yes. That's much better.

Beliefs

On a larger scale than cognitive processes involving attention and perception lie discrete information structures, better known as belief systems. There has been extensive research isolating and examining the roles of various beliefs in amplifying and maintaining pain over time (for a comprehensive review see Boothby et al., 1999). As with other more or less solitary factors, a muddy picture emerges from the research: It supports general conclusions, but it contains numerous null findings, in part due to the real-world backdrop of individual variability among patients. Similarly, experimenters have had a difficult time manipulating people's mind-sets to a sufficient degree to carry out experimental tests, which would be used to support causal inferences between beliefs and pain. Again, the issue of cause and effect is difficult to examine scientifically, especially when body–mind processes are involved.

However, general and theoretically logical patterns of results do emerge and center on two well-known belief systems in psychology: *self-control* (Rotter, 1954, 1990) and *self-efficacy* (Bandura, 1977, 1986). The problems of control are much broader than pain and are arguably at the center of the human condition (Burger, 1991). Beliefs about control underlie nearly every psychiatric disorder in the book (i.e., *DSM-IV*), from alcohol and other drug abuse to anxiety and mood disorders and even to neurologi-cally driven thought disorders like schizophrenia. On a universal basis, each of us has a limited ability to control the events in our lives, both exter-nal (e.g., obtaining food, human interactions, activities) and internal (e.g., thoughts, feelings, behavior, and bodily states). As the common motto from Alcoholics Anonymous suggests, the resulting challenge is to discern the things that can be controlled, the things that cannot, and to manage most everything that falls somewhere in between (Alcoholics Anonymous World Services, 1953).

Pain as a human experience is no exception. A person's sense of con-trol over pain or lack of control can contribute to the continuing problem through the mediating influence of coping behavior and negative emotions. For example, if clients' beliefs support overdeveloped needs for control, they may set themselves up for failure through misguided direct attempts to force their pains to subside. When these attempts invariably fail, one's sense of the pain gets a little bit bigger, as one's sense of self gets a little bit smaller in comparison. Conversely, patients may believe that they have no control over pain at all and thus will give up and stop trying altogether. Interestingly, opposite beliefs about control lead to the same end: big pain, small self, and an assortment of negative feelings and ineffective coping behaviors that result. In addition, people may flip-flop between over- and undercontrol. Or they eventually may settle into the latter, perhaps to the point where an undercontrolled, avoidant, passive, and dysregulated per-sonality style begins to infiltrate an otherwise healthy self-system.

A related set of beliefs is efficacy expectations (Bandura, 1977, 1986), which is a fancy name for self-confidence. If people lack confidence in themselves or the ability of their treatments to help them cope with pain, then treatments generally will be less effective (Marino, Gwynn, & Spanos, 1989; Philips & Hunter, 1981; Raft, Smith, & Warren, 1986; Spanos & O'Hara, 1990; and see Benson & Stark, 1996, for a more general discussion of the way hope and expectation impact health and wellness).

For example, Manyande et al. (1995) helped surgical patients prepare for postoperative pain through guided imagery as a means of enhancing their sense of control over the pain and their confidence in using pain management techniques. Compared with a control group, the coping-imagery patients had higher perceived coping ability, increased nora-drenaline and decreased cortisol levels (both positive physiological signs indicating decreased physiological stress), less postoperative pain, and less distress from the pain they did have. All of these effects were observed in the absence of group differences in self-reported anxiety and physiological arousal indexes. This means that the benefits of this imagery treatment did not appear to arise simply due to relaxation. Rather, their body–minds appeared to tune in to alternate states of consciousness that held less pain, both physically and perceptually. The tuning mechanism in this study appeared to be coping beliefs.

Like most experimental results, this outcome makes common sense when you consider it after the fact. Imagine the pain of a cut when you can put pressure on it and when you can't. The tissue damage doesn't change when you put that bandage on, yet the pain decreases right away. Similarly a mother's kiss on a boo-boo doesn't contain any analgesic ingredients, but it's one of the best painkillers a banged-up youngster can hope for. Does a marathon runner's pain hurt more when she is 10 miles from the finish line or 10 feet? In each of these examples, it is clear that confidence and control are miracle cures for pain. Like so many psychosocial factors in pain, they are so obvious in fact that we seldom even notice them.

Schema

In the broadest cognitive brushstrokes, many studies have looked at the ways that *pain schemata* can influence the experience and maintenance of pain disorders. A schema is a fancy name for belief system or mind-set, and the study of schemata helps us to understand the circular ways perception builds experience and experience builds perceptions, all of course as consciousness evolves over time. In a more technical sense, schemata are defined as networks of information or knowledge that guide each person's construction of subjective reality (Smith, 1998), from broad reconstructive processes in memory (beginning with the seminal work of Bartlett, 1932) to more elemental constructive processes in perception and recognition (McClelland & Rumelhart, 1985).

Schemata are the mental outpourings of complex temporal neural firing patterns distributed hierarchically and in parallel throughout the brain. Just as lifeblood flows through the pumping heart, consciousness-building information flows through the neuronal firings of the brain. Our schemata have been shown to frame perceptual process and generate belief structures, regulating the entry and flow of information through consciousness. Since a stream of images flows constantly through consciousness, the study of schemata provides a nice avenue for understanding the ways pain, consciousness, and imagery are connected.

Specifically, a schema may either allow or disallow the experience of pain to varying degrees. Furthermore, a different schema may be invoked through some associated internal cue, such as emotional states (e.g., anger), thoughts (e.g., self-denigration), memories (e.g., episodic trauma), sensations (e.g., pain), or more generally through the paralleled activation of a number of these cognitive factors in concert within an associative network (Berkowitz, 1989, 1993; Berkowitz, Cochran, & Embree, 1981; Berkowitz & Heimer, 1989). As such, schemata, and the images that flow therein, represent an arena of sorts in which pain exacts its influence over one's consciousness. In human terms, this means that different mind-sets may be either triggering *of* or triggered *by* pain or, more commonly, triggering of each other over time. Broader than the older notions of classical conditioning, consciousness is "sticky" business as well, forming new associations and new meanings over time.

On the smallest scale, perceptions clump together to build thoughts, which clump together to form beliefs, which further clump, branch, and network into schemata, the broadest and most enduring aspects of consciousness. Two interesting overlapping metafeatures of this system are the *will*, through which one exercises intentional behaviors, and *attention*, as described previously. Both will and attention are interactive with one another. Generally, one must pay attention to some degree to carry out intentional behavior. Each level of cognition is involved in the creation of experience, from perception up to schema. Across these levels individuals may utilize will and attention to examine and at times to modify our perceptions, beliefs, and so on. For example, one may intentionally focus attention onto beliefs and associated emotions, potentially changing relational experiences with each, opening up to novel flows of information during the process. Similarly, we may intentionally shift our attention to the boundary between sensation and perception, which we experience as a shift from internal information flows to flows in the external world. As such, redirected attention in and of itself can modify sensations, beliefs, and other substructures within a schema. Similarly, intentionality may change the context of any behavior, for better, as in the case of mindfulness exercises, or for worse, as in the attempt to perform a complex automatic task, like hitting a golf ball. These changing flows of information that result from shifts in attention and will have the potential to change consciousness at any scale, from the phenomenological level all the way down to the level of basic perception (for a detailed discussion of the neurological processes involved in intentionality see Freeman, 1995).

As one moves up the cognitive ladder of consciousness, from small-scale perceptions up to a schema, emotional and behavioral activation patterns of increasing strength mirror the increasing strength of cognitive structures, adding even greater structural resilience to the system of consciousness as a whole. Once formed, these schemata tend to be self-perpetuating over time, as they entrain the lower-level cognitive processes and serve as a hub for the branches of the body–mind's various interconnected systems, from the physiology of individual joint and muscle systems to one's sense of spiritual connection, values, and meaning. When one activates pain schemata, which interact in parallel with other relevant schemata.

Numerous studies, including both treatment outcome studies (e.g., Narduzzi et al., 1998; Raft et al., 1986) and experiments using functional brain imaging (e.g., Howland, Wakai, Mjaanes, Balog, & Cleeland, 1995) have supported the role of schemata in people's experiences of pain as well as the potential of imagery techniques to modify the pain-related schemata.

Affect

Negative affect serves to intensify pain not only indirectly by enacting and strengthening pain-related schemata but also directly as one of the central components in pain perception itself (Melzack & Casey, 1968). However, negative affect can't simply be put in the "bad" column, as a pain intensifier. An apparent paradox lies in the outcomes of some experimental studies that have shown the efficacy of negative affect (e.g., fear and anger) in "ameliorating" pain. This beneficial result from induced negative affect is thought to occur somewhat indirectly, due to distraction (e.g., McNeil & Brunetti, 1992) and perhaps due to the short-term release of endogenous opioids and cortisoids, which act as analgesics, within a sympathetic nervous system response. Indeed, when one analyzes the various studies of affect on pain together, it appears that the benefits of negative emotion seem limited to the rather brief arousal-response period: approximately 10 minutes. More frequently, when negative affect associated with pain sensations is enhanced through focused attention, the negative affect tends to intensify the pain experience (Ahles et al., 1983). Conversely, blocking the affective dimension of pain through pleasant imagery tends to bring relief (Stevens et al., 1989; Worthington & Shumate, 1981).

Outside of the lab, in studies of actual patients, it appears that any affect that serves to intensify the affective-motivational aspects of pain will intensify the experience of that pain (for a review see Robinson & Riley, 1999). As such, longer-term feelings of sadness, anxiety, or hostility and anger will tend to make pain worse, particularly when these feelings are associated with the pain experience itself. Thus, helping clients to face, to lean into, and become integrated with their negative pain-related emotions represents another broad area where imagery may be beneficial.

The Sick Role

The sick role was discussed already within the context of other single causal factors. However, it requires its own discussion. For just as schemata represent the arena in which consciousness is built, role and identity systems form the arena for the construction of larger-scale self and social systems. Further, as body–mind hubs (highly interactive information crossroads), these arenas are places where pain can be especially destructive in trying to carve out a home for itself.

People learn about themselves just as they learn about others, through self-observations and the communicated observations of people around them (Baumeister, 1998). These self-referent experiences are mediated through self-schemata (Markus, 1977), whereas experiences with others are mediated by relationship schemata (Baldwin, 1995). Again, both sets of schemata are fed by the experience-filtering processes of mental sets previously described as well as by behavioral sets, which limit a person's range of possible behaviors. Thus, a cycle emerges in which schemata limit experiences, and then subsequent experiences build subsequent schema. This symbiotic constriction process between experiences and worldviews occurs both within and across the individual and social domains. For example, experience builds the self-concept, which influences role taking in social situations. Within these various processes, the self must have a sufficient degree of flexibility (Marks-Tarlow, 1999; Rafaeli-Mor & Steinberg, 2002) to be adaptive and functional across social contexts (Turner, 1989; Turner, Oakes, Haslam, & McGarty, 1994) as well as across time periods (Markus & Nurius, 1986).

Theoretically, one of the most insidious processes that can impinge on a person's social and personal flexibility is the tight coupling of the self and relationship schemata to a dysfunctional pain schema. In other words, for some individuals, pain becomes a dangerously large part of their personal and social identities and thus is sustained over time by feeding off of the same social-cognition processes, which normally feed a person's sense of self. Again, pain acts like a parasite, except within this context it feeds off of one's sense of identity, growing bigger and stronger as it devours the nutrients of increasingly frail, rigid, and limited self and other experiences.

We suggest that these unfortunate pain patients are precisely those individuals who tend to get labeled with *DSM-IV* personality disorders (i.e., Axis II syndromes previously described), exhibiting rigid cognitive and relational styles involving avoidance, helplessness, dependency, and emotional dysregulation. These four characteristics do not emerge through serendipity but are each natural by-products of a battle-weary sense of personal identity.

In a meta-analysis of the effects of behavior therapy on clinical pain, Holroyd and Penzien (1986) were surprised to find that the strongest client variable in predicting response to treatment was age, which accounted for 30% of the variance in treatment outcome, with younger patients responding better than older ones, controlling for differences in age-related physiology and general health. One reasonable explanation for this result is that pain patients experience themselves as becoming increasingly incapacitated with the passage of time, rendering effective treatment more and more difficult. The longer one has pain, the more the pain colonizes the individual's sense of identity.

Just as a cancer may grow and spread over time, eventually the pain schema may take over so much of these formerly healthy self and relational schemata that its removal would cause victims to lose their identities, vital organs within the psychological realm. Beyond metaphor, chronic pain clients increasingly may focus their social lives, from minute interactions all the way up to social roles, on their pain as the years pass. They also might develop difficulties in imagining themselves without the pain, since it has become the focal point for movements throughout each of their life domains.

One particularly influential life domain within Western, capitalist cultures is the financial and occupational realm. In fact, potential financial incentives for pain, like unsettled worker's compensation claims, represent some of the strongest negative predictors in effectiveness studies for various pain treatments (Gatchel & Epker, 1999). Although malingering undoubtedly occurs, it is important to point out once again that financial and social incentives may contribute to *actual* pain experiences without the conscious intent of a victim. Again, affect-motivation is an intrinsic dimension of pain, just as is direct pain sensation.

Overall, the pain experience has a significant influence on the development of the sick role and vice versa. Therapeutically, a sufficient change in either one or both is necessary to promote health. The more difficult question is how one can most effectively and efficiently promote such changes through imagery. Read on.

CHAPTER 2

Imagery

More Than Make-Believe

It is in imagination that we begin to make ourselves into who and what we will become.

Harris
(2007, pp. 86–87)

Imagery is traditionally defined in psychology as "quasi-sensory or quasi-perceptual experiences of which we are self-consciously aware and which exist for us in the absence of those stimulus conditions that are known to produce their genuine sensory or perceptual counterparts" (Richardson, 1969, p. 2). The prefix *quasi-* indicates that imagery is similar to sensation and perception but a bit different. It involves conscious awareness, and it occurs despite an absence of outside sensory information from the world. If we are to become practitioners of imagery, we must probe further than mere definition and consider some deeper questions. If imagery is different from other sensations and perceptions, how is it different? Are these differences qualitative, quantitative, or both? Are there things that can be done within imagery that cannot be done within other perceptual experiences and vice versa? Are we sure that imagery is always conscious, or could imagery be occurring on an unconscious or preconscious level as well? Does imagery occur in the space between sensory stimulations? Or may imagery in fact occur all the time, outside of sensory stimulation, and also together with sensory stimulation, providing shape, nuance, and meaning to our experiences within our world?

Pink Space Bears and Other Contents of the Imagination

Before moving to the ideas of others, let's do a thought experiment together. Imagine a family member or close friend. Now imagine the animal that best fits with that person, based on physical resemblance or personality traits. Perhaps someone in your family is a monkey and someone else is a frog. Do you have a friend who is like a giraffe in some way, or maybe a lemur? Take your time and just allow your image of that person to merge with that animal, whichever one comes to mind. Were you able to do it? How hard was it? It is likely that you were able to do this imagination exercise rather easily. Or if you had difficulty, it is likely that you could switch to a different friend, family member, or coworker who had more of an animal resemblance to facilitate the task.

Let us try it the other way. Imagine three animals: a bear, monkey, and lion. Think about the one friend, family member, or coworker who most closely resembles each. Next time you see any of these people, do you think you would be able to imagine them as those animals while they are physically present? For almost everyone, the answer to this question is yes. It is clear that images may happen without any sensory input and that they may also mix with sensory input.

Which animal are you: a monkey, bear, lion, or lemur? You may visualize your "inner animal" in your mind, or you may do it while looking in the mirror. Certain aspects of your visual self-perception may guide your answer. The shape of your shoulders, the look in your eyes, the length of your arms may steer you toward being more of a bear than a monkey. Invisible aspects of your self-perception may be influential as well—aspects of your personality that make you bearish, monkey-like, or lionesque.

So it appears that imagery may combine with external information but is not confined to it or by it. Sensation is finite, but imagery is infinite. Moreover, to the degree that imagery mixes with sensation, sensations may also be stretched toward infinity. Furthermore, imagery is not fused to time as are present-bound external experiences. Imagery is timeless. Therefore, it may be imposed upon the past, the present, or the future.

At the same time, imagery is somehow weaker than external sensations. When you imagine yourself in the mirror, you see more of you than you do of monkey (or bear or lion and so on). The world is not a blank canvas. Nor are our lives cartoons created purely out of will; there is a stimulus pull from our physical senses that typically supersedes our imaginations. As such, imagery is quantitatively different from sensory stimulation in at least two ways: Imagery (1) is larger than stimulation in its range but (2) is smaller in its intensity. Furthermore, when imagery and external sensation mix, each impacts the other in a quantitatively consistent manner: The lower the intensity of sensory stimulation, the higher the intensity of imagery and vice versa. For example, imagine that your skin is bright green. If you can look at your arm, your mental image of it being green is less strong. If you cannot see your bright green pallor, or if you close your eyes, your skin will become brighter and more vivid.

The final question is in what level of conscious awareness does imagery exist? This is more difficult to examine directly; however, it appears that imagery may range across different levels of conscious awareness, from unconscious to conscious. Were those earlier animal images already somewhere in your mind before we did our experiment, or did we create the animal–person associations right then, from scratch? It is likely that it felt as if the image was already there for the monkey-mom or the bear-dad. Identifying images typically involves a process of letting go rather than engaging the will in an active manner; therefore, your experience was likely one of tuning in rather than conjuring up. Indeed, the available evidence from experimental cognitive psychology confirms that we can form images unconsciously and without effort and that these unconscious images may significantly impact judgments formed within the brain as well as bodily responses (for related reviews see Kahneman & Tversky, 1996; Richardson, 1983; Richardson-Klavehn & Bork, 1988; Schacter, 1987).

Zahourek (1988, p. 54) provides a broader, more modern description of imagery as "a private, non-observable inner process involving a neural activity within the brain associated with memory, perception, and thinking ... aris[ing] from both internal and external stimuli." Based on this description, imagery appears to be a connecting point for all mental processes, whether internally or externally generated. Imagery appears to be the arena in which past memories, present experiences, and future expectations join together in the construction of perception, thought, and ultimately meaning.

Let us suppose all of this is true. Imagery is always active. We experience it at a lower level when external stimulation is high and at higher levels when external information is low. Our bodies react to imagery in a manner equivalent to, though typically at a lower level than, actual experience. The contents of imagery are infinite and free from the bounds of time. Inasmuch as imagery may mix together with external experience, external experiences may be stretched toward infinity as well (Zahourek, 1988). Finally, imagery may be unconscious, occurring right now, for example, in the back of your mind as you read, or conscious, as you shift right now to become mindful of your current spontaneous imagery.

How can imagery do all of this within the bounds of physical neural processes? In other words, the brain is a roughly 3-pound organ. It is made of physical stuff: fats, proteins, and chemicals. How can something like the brain generate something that is as mystical as imagery? Though we are only beginning to gain an in-depth understanding of the brain, there are some pretty clear clues located within the architecture of the brain, which is in fact infinite.

The brain is made up of between 100 and 500 million neurons and each individual neuron is connected to approximately 1,000 other neurons (Kosko, 1993). As such, your neural architecture, which generates imagery, is composed of an information-processing web of more than 100 billion connections. Consciousness appears to be generated from distinctive firing relationships of groups of neurons called neural networks (Deadwyler & Hampson, 1995; Ferster & Spruston, 1995; Freeman, 1995; Kosko, 1993). To grossly oversimplify, imagine neuron A fires (sends an electro-chemical signal to a neighboring neuron) at a frequency of 4 pulses per second, which triggers neuron B to fire at 10 pulses per second, which triggers neurons C though G to fire at varying rates, together in a coherent manner. That is basically how a neural network works to generate imagery. Let us say that this group of neurons, when they fire in this specific manner, generates the conscious image of a bear.

Now for the infinite part: In reality, neurons may fire up to 100 times per second, and neural networks are composed of various groups of tens of thousands of neurons at different areas of the brain with feedback mechanisms (neurons that trigger other neurons that feed back to regulate the original neurons and so on) across brain layers. When one considers patterned firing over time among groups of neurons, the complexity of neural networks does not end with 100 billion connections. One must also consider varying rates of firing and the number of possible combinations of neurons involved, from a few (say only 10,000) up to a million. To consider mathematically the possible neural networks of the brain, the number of possible states of consciousness, in terms of combinations, is computed roughly as $100,000,000,000 \times 99,999,999 \times 99,999,998$ and on down to 1.

Each neuron is one little physical cell in the brain having two possible states, firing or resting—very simple. Yet as part of a system more complex than anything else on our planet, this finite little cell assists in the generation of an infinite number of patterns, an infinite number of states of consciousness, and an infinite variety of images. Add a few thousand neurons to your bear image, and you put a nice hat on him. Add some others, and you can see him fishing in a stream, with his hat on. Add a few more from your auditory cortex, and you can hear the splashing and growling as he grabs a fish. While we are at it, let us make it a pink space bear that flies back to his den using a jet pack. Now you have just experienced your own infinite cognition, an image you have never had before. You have also created a memory for your pink space bear (though likely a weak one), and within your brain you have linked a group of neurons that have never fired together in quite that manner ever before.

If pink space bears are not your thing, indulge one additional metaphor to assist in putting the brain's power into perspective. The earth contains approximately 6 billion people. Imagine instead a planet with 100 billion beings, about 20 times the number on Earth. Next, imagine that these beings are extremely social, communicating simultaneously with up to 1,000 other people at a time and at a rate of up to 100 times per second. (Ideally, they will get a very good rate from their telephone carriers.) Furthermore, these beings live in an advanced democratic social system: They form a multitude of political parties that vote together in blocks on highly specialized issues. For instance, those in the temporal lobes are particularly concerned with the nature of sounds, whereas those in the lower limbic regions make up the committees on emotion. Try to imagine the sociopolitical climate of such a planet: how much they may accomplish together, how many bills will become laws, how many laws will be repealed or improved, how many new committees and subcommittees and allegiances will be forged and how many conflicts will be resolved. Such a society of neurons exists within your skull, and such a sophisticated political process begins to approach the tremendous capacity for your brain to create images.

One needs to look no further than the workings of neural networks within the brain to observe the connection between the finite and physical realms of the body and the metaphysical and infinite realms of mind. When viewed in this manner, the brain and its imagery each may inspire awe and curiosity, perhaps even a sense of spirituality grounded in science. This spiritual sense may be even stronger when one considers that the infinite experiences of the imagination feed back to shape and reshape physical neural architecture in a circular manner. Experience shapes the brain, and the brain shapes experience.

Science is beginning to gain a more satisfying understanding of the physical processes of the brain to create images and of how these images may feed back to shape the brain. However, our understanding of the mind–body relationship is not new, and it is not limited to recent scientific discoveries. Our understanding of the role of imagery in health did not begin with the scientific revolution in the 1600s or with the invention of psychology in the 1900s. On the contrary, the understanding of imagery within psychology and science in general is better characterized as a struggle rather than as a smooth road to discovery, similar to the struggles that modern medicine has had in understanding pain. Therefore, to truly understand the modern role of imagery in science and medicine, one must understand the historical context of the struggle between science and the imagination.

Ancient Spiritualism

The practice of imagery is as old as human culture, and its role in healing, growth, and spirituality reaches back at least 20,000 years (Achterberg, 1985; Zahourek, 1988). Modern Western culture has created firm conceptual boundaries separating body and mind, individual and group, real and imaginary, scientific and spiritual; these boundaries did not exist for most of humankind's cultural evolution. Consider that in the shamanic tradition of ancient times, which was very consistent across cultures, healing practices provided what we might consider today a means of bio-psycho-social-spiritual transcendence. Access to the infinite experience bound up within the imaginary realms provided opportunities for connecting to a larger source of information beyond everyday individual experience that could engender healing of body, mind, social, and spiritual processes.

The term, *shaman* comes from the Russian word *saman*, which means "ascetic," describing "someone who practices strict self denial as a means of personal and especially spiritual discipline" (Merriam-Webster, Inc., 2008). Essentially, the shaman was the all-around go-to person within a tribal or kinship-based community, who would handle political, social, medical, psychological, spiritual, or business (e.g., agricultural) imbalances. Within the holistic and integrated folk-communities that defined most of human history, these purposes were manifestations of a single underlying process, and inasmuch as there was no division among these various life domains in traditional human life, it made perfect sense that the shaman would serve these varied purposes. It was the shaman's role to restore integrity to these various aspects of human life, and imagery represented a primary tool in this respect, drawing its power by providing a transcendental path to unity (Sheikh et al., 2003). In a sense, the shamans bridged the gaps to living with unity and harmony, moving through imagery as if it were a portal with the ability to transport humans to sources of wisdom that lie beyond the limits of our individual perspectives.

The shamanist perspective viewed imagery not as make-believe, like the connotations of our current understanding of imagination; rather, shamans were skilled at dialing in to a deeper level of reality, an infinite and unmoving shadow of the subjective personal consciousness. Thus, shamanic traditions relied heavily on ritual, shifts in consciousness and trance states (Achterberg, 1985; Sheikh et al., 2003). From the more recent Judeo-Christian perspective, the spiritual destination of imagery may be seen as moving the individual closer to Eden, a time when humans were closer to God and to the natural world. From the perspective of science, shamanic imagery practices were similar to modern scientific practice, except that the imaginary journey was focused inward and in the direction of holism rather than outward and in the direction of reductionism. In other words, like the scientist of today, the shaman sought truth, or at least information that would be useful and beyond subjective impressions.

Each of the modern (past 5,000 years or so) religious traditions retains a more mystical and spiritual set of rites and beliefs, which are somewhat distinct from mainstream practice and include the essence of shamanist practices, imagery in particular (Epstein, 1986; and for a full review see Sheikh et al., 2003). Specifically, the Jews have Kabalistic traditions (Scholem, 1961), the Christians have Gnostic traditions (Samuels & Samuels, 1975), and Muslims have Sufi traditions (Corbin, 1970). Even within the more mainstream veins of these traditions, one can find references to visions being used in ways consistent with the more ancient shamanistic practices from which these religions emerged. For example, in the Old Testament, one may find reference to the vivid dreams of the Egyptian Pharaoh involving 7 gaunt cows devouring 7 fat cows, which Joseph interpreted to be prophetic of 7 years of plenty followed by 7 years of famine across the land. The deciphering of this image brought widespread economic balance to Egypt by prompting the people to store grain in preparation for famine.

The communion ritual of Christians is another example of imagery used for restoring balance within the individual worshiper (Sheikh et al., 2003). At the moment of communion, images of Christ and the last supper allow the recipient to "commune" across space and time, to the infinite and unchanging spiritual realm to which Christ is believed to have ascended after the resurrection. This imaginary communion is by no means meant to represent some sort of once-upon-a-time type of fantasy activity. Neither do most Christians believe that the bread and wine literally turn into flesh and blood in their mouths. It is through faith that the imaginary connection in this symbolic act gains its power, leading to a transcendental communion experience with the larger spiritual realm, cleansing the individual and restoring balance to the eternal soul. One would be hard-pressed to identify a clear distinction between the modern practice of taking communion and the shamanist imagery of our past. It is occurring right there in our churches each Sunday morning.

Shamanist imagery practices are even more pronounced within the Hindu and Buddhist traditions, particularly within Indian Yogic and Tibetan Buddhist traditions; each of these has evolved a highly refined and specific set of imagery-based practices over the past several thousand years. For example, in the Samadhi tradition an individual focuses on an object with the aim of union with that object. From this process, the individual may lose the limiting sense of fusion with the self as an object and release through outer union a new transcendent sense of experiential reality.

The use of radiant light, within the Tantric medicine practices of ancient Tibet, as a source of healing energy that could penetrate the body is a classic technique that still finds use in mainstream medical practice today.

Sheikh et al. (2003, p. 11) describe one common light-oriented imagery technique derived from this tradition:

> At the center of the mandala, a radiant Buddha sits in lotus position on a 1,000-petaled lotus, which in turn is perched on a jeweled throne. In his right hand he is holding the myrobalan plant, and in his left hand a begging bowl filled with healing nectar. In this exercise, one imagines that one is sitting in a beautiful landscape and offering to the Buddha all that is precious. Now one asks him to bless one's being and to sit on the top of one's head. Then one senses the Buddha's rays of brilliant light stream into the body, dissolving illness and suffering.... One imagines brilliant light, generally white or blue, radiating from the deity and flowing through one's being, purifying it both mentally and physically. If the meditation is used for a personal ailment, the light is directed to the diseased area; if the exercise is used for the healing of others, the light is sent out into the universes.

Examples of imagery practices exist in ancient Western traditions as well. They are aimed at bringing unity and health through the transcendent connection of the individual to health-related deities, such as the Greek Asclepius, his wife, Epione (the soother of pain), and his daughters Hygeia and Panacea, who were goddesses of health and medical treatment, respectively. One may find countless other examples from around the globe. Yet despite the variations across different cultures, all of these practices have a number of factors in common. Mainly, they all involve visualization, an emphasis on clarity and immersion with the imagery, transcendence, union, balance, and a release from various ego structures toward spiritual health, which is believed to impact physical health.

Apart from the use of deities, which are generally not called on today, the ancient Greeks seem to have used imagery in a manner similar to how it is used in modern Western culture. Typically after the failure of physically directed interventions, an afflicted individual would be guided into a trance-like state to explore healing visions related to a specific ailment. These practices are supported by the ancient Greek philosopher Aristotle, who believed that images were central to the body's emotional processing systems, and Hippocrates, whose teachings focused on the physician's role in activating the body–mind toward intrinsic healing involving natural strengths and mechanisms of resiliency.

The Hippocratic viewpoint, which ostensibly has formed the foundation for modern medicine, was actually in line with modern complexity theory (West, 2006) and biopsychosocial models (e.g., Engel, 1977) that have been used as a foundation for modern alternative medicine practices. Specifically, Hippocrates viewed biological, psychological, and social systems as highly interactive, with a mixture of complexity and integrity. This flexible yet integrated structure of the body–mind was thought to allow for robustness against the various challenges to integrity that come from experience within the world. Disease was considered to be a movement away from integrity and toward fragmentation and rigidity. The healing potential of imagery was believed to lie in its ability to activate the unique biopsychosocial systems of the diseased individual toward self-healing, renewed integrity, and potential growth (Achterberg, 1985).

Following from this tradition, Galen was the first to create a systematic record of how imagery was believed to work. His conceptualization of imagery involved the existence of diagnostic information that would emerge spontaneously from guided imagery in symbolic form. An imbalance involving stomach pain, for example, might emerge in the form of hot stones burning their way through a sheepskin bag. Galen suggested that the process of imbalance and rigidity flowed in a cyclical manner, with mental images impacting the body and the body impacting subsequent images within the mind. Interventions, whether they were physical, mental, or combined, called for increased stretching of these cycles outside of their ever-tightening spirals toward increasing disease (Achterberg, 1985).

Throughout the Anglo-Saxon Middle Ages in Western history, the Catholic Church carried on the Greek healing beliefs and traditions, disallowing the ancient folk practices of nonchurch officials. Folk healers, predominantly women, who continued to use imagery techniques became increasingly subject to persecution, as the church considered these alternative techniques to be witchcraft. By the 1500s, the widespread torture and murder of these women signaled the beginning of a major shift in Western culture, which for the first time in human history moved imagery out of its prominent role in healing.

This shift away from traditional folk medicine was driven by numerous factors including politics, religion, economics, gender relations, and the birth of modern science. These factors drove the movement toward a more segmented and diversified set of roles and role relations that exists in Western culture today. Relatively recent examples include the demarcation of professional and private roles, movement toward the nuclear family and away from communal living, the separation of mind from body, and the split between religious and scientific sources of knowledge. Each of these divisions impacted the practice of imagery in healing; however, the split between religious and scientific domains may have been the most influential. Indeed, the current difficulty many of us may experience in conceiving of the mind and body as one could be considered to be the epistemological legacy of an agreement that was reached between the church and the scientists that founded modern medical practice. The power split that was brokered during the 17th century was so powerful that we may barely recognize its pervasive impact on our individual worldviews 400 years after the fact.

The Dualist Revolution of René Descartes

Early Western medicine was based on the philosophy of the Greeks. Aristotle postulated the existence of a biologically based soul from which psychophysiologic events emerged (McMahon & Sheikh, 1986, 1996). If one substitutes the word *brain* for *soul*, it appears that Aristotle was spot-on with respect to the best modern neuropsychological research. This biological soul was believed to guide both physiological and psychological events, with imagination, sensation, digestion, and reason each falling under its purview. Continuing through the Middle Ages, Western medicine viewed body and mind as interactive components of a body–mind complex, with various interactive mechanisms that served to maintain and restore balance within the human. Images were believed to play a role similar to emotions, to be integrated within the larger biopsychosocial system toward the goal of general balance and health in human life. Of course, the specific mechanisms of colored bile and evil spirits are not supported by mainstream science or even modern religion. However, on a metaphorical level the early Western notions of mind–body interaction fit quite well with modern physiology. Just as the brain may be thought of as equivalent to the biological soul described by Aristotle, the positive feedback of electrochemical messages leading to hyperarousal and stress between the hypothalamic-pituitary-adrenal (HPA) axis of the brain and the vagus nerve may be considered, metaphorically, to serve the same destructive role as the "evil spirits" of the Middle Ages.

McMahon & Sheikh (1986) describe the circular interactions among image, emotion, and physiology that were part of everyday health philosophy prior to the 17th century:

> What we interpret today as the expressions of emotions, such as tears, sighs, respiratory changes, and redirection of blood flow, were understood during this period as functional processes. They operated as homeostatic mechanisms to restore balance or equilibrium (p. 9)

They continued:

> Because imagination sets the circular arousal sequence into operation, the image had greater powers of control than sensation or perception. Anticipation of a feared occurrence was presumed to be more damaging than the occurrence itself.... During this era of holism, prior to the modern definition of mind, all illness was regarded to be psychosomatic (p. 11).

At this time, there was no stigma due to a lack of a clear physiological cause for illness: There was no "all in your head" mentality, there was no sigh of relief at the discovery of physical tissue damage to excuse your experience of pain, and there was no issue with the inclusion of imagery in the clinical assessment of illness, disease, and pain.

In 1673 Descartes (1637/1958) changed all of this when he argued that the mind and body are separate, saying that the mind "consists entirely in thinking, and ... for its existence, has no need of place, and is not dependent on any material thing.... This soul is entirely distinct from the body ... and would not itself cease to be all that it is, even should the body cease to exist" (p. 119). This was to become arguably one of the most revolutionary and influential ideas in the history of human healing practices. Indeed, Descartes's idea reversed more than 19,500 years of traditional belief, with a somewhat disastrous result.

Within this dualist philosophy, body and mind were now separate. Like any great thinker, Descartes's influence stemmed not only from his ideas but also from the relevance of those ideas within the broad social and political context of the time. Specifically, religion and science needed some clear-cut separation. Descartes's dualist philosophy was just what was needed to demarcate the necessary boundaries: The soul was to belong to the church (off-limits to the scientists), whereas science would have free and unfettered access to understanding the mechanics of the body.

Furthermore, at the time of Descartes scientific knowledge was limited. Physiologists had only just discovered that the heart functioned essentially as a pump rather than as the seat of the soul. It is possible that the physiologists of the early 1600s expected to find some radiant supernatural-looking substance within the heart that they could call the soul. Instead, they found valves, pumps, and wire-like nerves. Even the most holy of organs appeared quite mechanistic, devoid of anything resembling the unlimited realms of imagination. It is within this context that Descartes (1641/1958, p. 237) concluded:

> I am a thinking thing. And although possibly I have a body with which I am very closely conjoined...in so far as I am only a thinking unextended thing, and ... in so far as it (my body) is only an extended unthinking thing, it is certain that I am truly distinct from my body and can exist without it.

Metaphorically, one may view the entire matter as a large-scale divorce between science and the church, which may prove beneficial to the parents as they move on to greater success through independence. Indeed, the early medical practitioners and researchers experienced great success in viewing the body in a purely mechanistic manner. This viewpoint has culminated in modern medicines, advanced scanning devices, fantastic surgeries, the promise of gene therapies and nanotechnologies, and artificial limbs and organs. The modern church flourished as well, enjoying unfettered access to the spiritual lives of individuals, to the soul and the infinite, to the holistic experiences beyond the body, particularly the body-free afterlife.

However, as in most divorces, the children suffer. Because of its central role in connecting the mind and body, the imagination was one of the major casualties of the Cartesian split. Technically, the church retained primary custody over imagery, inasmuch as imagery was deemed a nonphysical process associated with the soul. Yet within these constraints, imagery was no longer acknowledged as having influence over bodily systems and general biopsychosocial health. Imagery as an aspect of spiritual transcendence was deemphasized, and its healing potential was largely discounted, as the church moved people away from traditional folk practices, particularly those with roots in shamanism. Neither did the emerging field of modern medicine want much to do with imagery, treating it as a bad absentee father, angrily pushing imagery out of its new life as an independent discipline, free to focus on bodily systems, physical medicines, and advanced surgical procedures.

Since the teachings of Aristotle in ancient Greece, imagery had been considered to be a central component within physical health; with the split of Cartesian dualism, this central position was now lost deep within a wide schism. Once the centerpiece of ancient healing, imagery had been removed from modern medicine (Zahourek, 1988).

Yet an undercurrent of dissatisfaction has remained, despite great medical advances. This dissatisfaction derives from the sense that something is amiss on a philosophical level. Cartesian dualism suggests that the activities of the mind and body are correlated but that the activities of one do not in fact cause the other. This correlation exists through divine intervention, with God maintaining the illusion of connection, where actually the two are separate and distinct. This idea of a correlation maintained through divine intervention is difficult to swallow. From either a scientific or religious viewpoint, it stands out as a gap in the logical integrity of the human being. Why would God create and maintain such an inefficient arrangement between mind and body? Why would scientific laws and principles apply to everything except the mind? As a result, a lingering interest in folk medicine continued on the fringes of Western culture. Even the mainstream church continued to recognize and work with the power of prayer and faith in healing both the body and the spirit, and science eventually began to take a look at the mind in the emerging discipline of psychology in the late 19th and early 20th centuries.

Revival: Imagery in Psychology and Modern Medicine

Imagery enjoyed approximately 20,000 years of prominence in shamanistic healing, was banned from medical science for approximately 250 years, and was then rediscovered a little more than 100 years ago, in the late 1800s when science began to encroach upon the territory of philosophy and religion in the emerging disciplines of psychology and psychiatry. Unfortunately, the Cartesian error has remained within the cultures of mental and behavioral health, despite overwhelming research supporting the notion that the mind emerges from the brain and that the brain is shaped by experience (for complete accounts of this emergent interaction view of the mind–body relationship see Schwartz & Begley, 2002; Sperry, 1993).

Indeed, the all in your head way of thinking remains pervasive, serving to stigmatize diagnosis and treatment of physical illness within psychiatric practice. Imagination is still considered to be something more useful to a creative writer than to a health practitioner and still connotes fantasy or make-believe. Mirroring the split between body and mental practitioners, physical and psychosomatic ailments have been defined categorically, as one or the other, losing the range and reciprocal influences that actually exist. Imagination always impacts the body, and the body always impacts imagination. One cannot occur without the other. The hope of regaining and perhaps even improving on our shamanistic heritage may rest within the behavioral sciences.

Bain (1872) was the first of the behavioral scientists to suggest that the brain responds in a similar manner to imagery as it does to actual experience. However, the idea did not really catch on until Jacobson's (1931) studies of muscular tension and relaxation in response to specific images. To understand the suppression of early imagery research such as Bain's and the limitations that have been placed on subsequent work such as Jacobson's, one must understand the political climate that has dominated the field of psychology for the past 100 years.

The early history of American psychology involves the dominance of radical behaviorism, which espoused the unbending belief that internal mental processes did not really exist or were at best epiphenomena to behavior, serving no functional purpose (Watson, 1919). Indeed, one could argue that radical behaviorism was a defensive attempt to embrace a most intense form of Cartesian dualism to allow the emerging field of psychology to stave off threats from the more established scientific disciplines. Jacobson's (1931) research was careful and well controlled, involving sensitive physiological instruments, and the results were clear-cut: Relaxing images resulted in decreased muscle tension, whereas the imagination of specific physical activities resulted in specific muscle contractions (e.g., arm muscles contracting in response to throwing an imaginary baseball).

Although the initial reaction from American behavioral psychologists to this research was hostile, its irrefutable nature prompted the behaviorists to take the general position that thoughts (including images) were actually behaviors, carried out at extremely low levels. In this sense, the behaviorists suggested that imagining throwing a baseball was equivalent to actually throwing the ball, except that the observable movement was so minor it could only be detected by physiological recording instruments. Similarly, the behaviorists suggested that relaxation involved the subobservable stretching of muscles and that thought was actually subvocal speech (Watson, 1920). Psychology took a first step toward ending the 200-year-old prohibition on the imagination. Yet to appear scientific, early behaviorism placed a strict ban on the study of the imagination within psychology.

This ban, however, applied primarily to the United States. The European psychological communities were more open to considering the role of the imagination in health, although Cartesian dualism did limit this examination somewhat to the role of the imagination in mental health only rather than in body–mind health. Prior to 1900, Sigmund Freud was still considering the role that the imagination would play in his emerging theories of personality and psychotherapy. However, he eventually gave up on using the imagination in any central fashion in his theory or techniques because he was finding that imagery contained too much raw, unconscious, primary process material (Zahourek, 1988). Freud, a physiologist by training, was building a theory that made the biological process primary within the psyche, retaining to some degree the split between mental and physical causes, despite his central interest in psychosomatic medicine.

Freud's protégé, Carl Jung, on the other hand, was trained in a more philosophic tradition and in fact did his dissertation on the occult healing practices of traditional cultures. As such, Jung carried on with the exploration of the imagination, particularly after his relationship ending conflict with Freud and a subsequent psychotic break during the period from 1912 to 1917. It was during this period that Jung explored the depths of his own internal imagery, developing his most abstract concepts, such as the collective unconscious, the archetypes, and the use of active imagination. In describing the mind–body relationship, Jung (1960, pp. 325–326) writes:

> The psyche consists essentially of images. It is a series of images in the truest sense, not an accidental juxtaposition or sequence but a structure that is throughout full of meaning and purpose; it is a picturing of vital activities and just as the material of the body that is ready for life has a need of the psyche in order to be capable of life,

so the psyche presupposes the living body in order that its images may live.

Within these words, it is apparent that Jung believed that the mind is actively engaged in layers of imagery in an unending, flowing manner. These images are not epiphenomena but are vital, meaningful, and deterministic. The body and its actions in the physical world were believed by Jung to be the end results of imagery. The imagination is considered the wellspring of creativity for the mind and the body.

Jung's Active Imagination

Jung's process of active imagination was the first modern approach to reclaim the central role of imagination in the creation of identity. Therefore, it is worthwhile to examine this process in greater detail, as we attempt to understand the true role of the imagination in health and healing. Active imagination was developed by Jung in the years following his conflict and separation from his closest colleague and mentor, Sigmund Freud. During this period, Jung's work became less precise and scientific, likely due to his bouts with psychotic depression (Stevens, 1999). As a result, Jung used many different terms in describing active imagination and was far from linear or clear-cut in his writings on the subject. In its current usage, the term *active imagination* most often refers to the act of tapping into the deep and spontaneous images emerging from the psyche rather than to the broad theoretical conceptualizations of the imagination that were developed by Jung (Chodorow, 2006). The practice of active imagination involves directing clients to focus attention inward, usually on some affect or bodily state, and then focusing awareness on the symbolic form this experience takes within the imagination. The process continues with the expression of meaningful reactions to these symbols in relation to the self (Schaverien, 2005).

It is important to examine in detail the distinction Jung made between ordinary imagination and active imagination. According to Jung, ordinary imagination typically uses imaginary fantasies that do not have real substance and depth but rather are an unconscious strategy aimed at separating from reality or avoiding particular experiences (Colman, 2006). By contrast, active imagination is focused on increased presence, a process of falling into and joining with one's internal experience. Ordinary imagination or fantasy is more or less driven by the will of the superficial self or ego, whereas active imagination is not invented by the individual but emerges from the portion of the self that transcends individual boundaries through connection to the infinite unconscious reservoir of the collective. As emergent structures arising from the collective unconscious, beyond the bounds of the ego, active images are thought to have a life of their own; this is why they are referred to as *active*.

More recent imagery approaches and Jung's original active imagination practices share some common features. First, the narratives that emerge through active imagination are believed to contain important information relating to a client's motivational system. Second, the conscious processing of symbolic imagery can bring about new and deep insights. Finally, these insights are considered to be more easily obtained than with verbally oriented therapy methods, due to their relatively unfiltered or undefended nature. The sensory and symbolic contents of the active imagination are considered to be more primary than information that has gone through the process of linguistic symbolization. Each of these factors provides a number of practical advantages for particular clients, such as those who tend to avoid affect, those who tend to stall within their treatment process due to interpersonal rumination about their relationship with the therapist, and those who are not cognitively sophisticated enough to hold on to abstract verbal-linguistic therapy material.

The process of active imagination is inherently dialectical, as was Jung's broader theory of balance through the union of opposites (Stevens, 1999). During active imagination, the will is applied to letting go, as one becomes mindful of potentially painful internal experiences without becoming fused with these experiences (Colman, 2006). In each of these respects, active imagination is identical to modern imagery approaches as well as to the ancient shamanistic practices.

Most contemporary writers focus on the use of active imagination in dream interpretation; however, it may also be applied to the analysis of bodily sensations, including pain (Chodorow, 2006). Both negative and positive images are useful within the procedure, as negative images are allowed to flow toward positive transformation with conscious analysis, whereas spontaneous positive images are brought to bear directly to promote healing (Eisendrath, 1977). Such healing is considered to happen immediately or over extended periods of time involving multiple sessions. The therapist's role is to assist clients in remaining within the confines of their own deep imaginary processes, so the therapist gives minimal direct instruction (Schaverian, 2005).

Just as in contemporary image therapies, Jung recognized that various art forms could be used toward the expression of therapeutic imagery, including drawing, painting, dancing, writing, modeling, and composing music (Chodorow, 2006). Likewise, Jung recognized that imagery involved not just visual content but the full range of human experience, including emotion and physical movement. In these respects, along with the process of active imagination as already described, each of the image theories and techniques described within this text should be considered to be follow-ups to Jung's work in this area.

The Cognitive Revolution

In the United States, the behavioral paradigm began to loosen its hold on psychological research and practice in the late 1960s and early 1970s. It is typically called the "cognitive revolution" in psychology and represents the first widespread study of internal processes such as attention, memory, verbal thoughts, and imagery. After more than 30 years of selective focus only on directly observable phenomena within the behavioral paradigm, psychology had finally discovered thinking.

The buildup to the cognitive revolution actually began several decades earlier, with the development of cognitive therapies (e.g., Ellis, 1958) and research investigating cognitive learning in animals (i.e., Tolman, 1940). Indeed, even the staunchest behaviorists were using the imagination in their earliest desensitization treatments and were assisting people in imagining feared events to reduce fear and increase confidence (Locke, 1971). The rigid behavioral theory of the research labs was simply unworkable once therapists were faced with actual clients in need of practical assistance. Imagery was indispensable in even the simplest behavioral treatments, for example, if an individual was afraid of something that could not easily be brought into the treatment room (e.g., animals, planes, war).

Nevertheless, acknowledgment of cognition and its study did not rapidly increase until the 1970s, along with the mainstream use of cognitive approaches to therapy, which focused on opening up people's belief systems to new information to improve emotional and behavioral functioning. Yet despite the changes that have come with the cognitive revolution, imagery to this day generally has been treated as more of a superficial tool than as a deep and central approach. As a result, most modern forms of therapy use imagery without incorporating it into their explanations of change, and the full potential of imagery in healing has rarely been explored. For example, cognitive therapists used imagery as a medium for mental rehearsal (Bandura, 1986) and the restructuring of rigid beliefs (Ellis, 1977); the psychodynamic therapists used imagery to examine sources of unconscious developmental memories and beliefs to identify and resolve internal conflicts. Finally, somatic (e.g., Ahsen, 1984), experiential (e.g., Gendlin, 1981), and transpersonal (e.g., Assagioli, 1973) approaches began to reemerge, each including varying degrees of ancient mystical tradition that were repackaged to allow for modern secular understanding. These latter approaches have provided a deeper perspective on the imagination. Yet the more central the treatment of the imagination, the less mainstream the approach tends to be and the less research it stimulates.

Each tradition suggested its own explanation concerning the manner in which the imagination impacts functioning. The behaviorists suggested that imagery impacted beliefs about control, that it allowed for classical conditioning, and that it allowed for the covert rehearsal of specific coping skills. The psychodynamic therapists suggested that imagery was better able to bypass defenses compared with verbal cognition, allowing for greater opportunities to approach emotionally charged material. The somatic, experiential, and transpersonal approaches were based on the multidimensional nature of imagery compared with relatively narrow and sequential verbal reasoning. Of course, none of these explanations is mutually exclusive, nor are they comprehensive.

Along with the expansion of the use of imagery in therapy, behavioral scientists in the 1960s and 1970s were beginning the first scientific examinations of imagery. They were finding that imagery acted as a mediator for classical conditioning, both consciously and unconsciously. In other words, the strength of associations between bodily responses, such as stress, and stimuli from the environment is determined by ones image of the stimuli, not by its actual physical characteristics. As William Shakespeare suggested, a rose by any other name would smell so sweet. However, it appears that a rose on a casket may smell far different from a rose on a lover's bed.

Similarly, evidence was accumulating to suggest that differential responses to biofeedback and hypnosis for relaxation were due to the spontaneous imagery that people generated and that imagery could be used to enhance the effects of biofeedback (McMahon & Sheikh, 1986). Furthermore, it was becoming clear that neither biofeedback nor hypnotic suggestion was necessary to impact bodily responses, such as relaxation, changes in blood flow and pressure, electromyographic (EMG) responses or muscle tension, immune response, contact dermatitis, and even breast enhancements (see McMahon & Sheikh, 1986, for a review of this research). Currently, the most intriguing research is examining neuroplasticity and the ways distributed societies of neurons shift their firing patterns and locations within the brain along with shifts in the imagination. With advanced brain scan technology, such as functional magnetic resonance imaging, the coming decades should bring far greater understanding of the ways the mind and brain interact through the imagination (Turner, Lee, & Schandler, 2003).

Full Circle

From the earliest moments of our primordial history, humans have had a deep and profound relationship with the imagination. Living within the bounds of a finite world of physical experience and moving ever forward with the unstoppable momentum of time, human beings turned their attention inward to discover the boundless and timeless realms of the imagination. From the early polytheistic religions to the tradition of Abraham to even the most modern constructions of theology, the spiritual realm has been defined by the infinite, the timeless, and the indefinable. Aristotle defines God as the "unmoved mover," the ethereal force that reaches into the physical world to spark creation and destruction, union and separation, and growth. Deep within the universal spiritual bedrock of all the world's traditions lies the ancient knowledge that the imagination represents a bit of the spiritual realm within our physical beings. Even through the lens of critical thought, of scientific empiricism and rationalism, it is clear that the imagination has at least two irrefutable qualities: it is unlimited, and it impacts the body–mind.

Indeed, history is repetitive, but in the best of circumstances history is also evolutionary, improving slightly with each cyclical pass. As scientists, we are just beginning to rediscover the imaginary processes at the core of phenomenal human experience. Our tools are great: We have categories of reasoning and hierarchies of evidence with which to construct a truer (or at least more useful) understanding of nature. Yet we are still neophytes, having just stuck a toe into this ocean in which our ancestors would dive and swim, and in which we exclaim simply, "It appears to be wet!"

What might we find as we delve deeper into the realm of imagination, with our tools, both mental and physical, ready at hand? Perhaps Descartes was correct and there is essentially nothing to discover—the connection between imagination and the physical world is only the clever handiwork of God creating an illusory correlation for no apparent purpose? Or perhaps we will rediscover a deep sense of unity that was shared among our ancestors? Perhaps within the depths of our consciousnesses we will find a single consciousness, something that lies even beneath the archetypes described by Jung. Perhaps we will find a unity between the living and nonliving, life and death, ashes to ashes, and learn that the nature of consciousness is both a neural and spiritual product? Perhaps the imagination is the road back to the Eden, except this time we will have handy our recording equipment and our "mythical snake repellent."

Why is imagery so ubiquitous? Why has imagery emerged within nearly every modern psychotherapeutic tradition of the last 100 years and yet has not been the central focus of theory and practice in clinical psychology? One explanation is that imagery is simply too large and vast; imagery is beyond theory. Imagery is as ever present and central as behavior itself, as broad as thought, emotion, or physiology. Physiology itself is not a "theory" of medicine; it is the subject on which medicine directs its practice. Similarly, imagery is the stuff on which psychotherapy acts. It is the arena in which psychotherapy takes place. Just as air is not a manner of breathing, imagery is not a manner of therapeutic technique.

Yet if we are to come full circle, the trajectory in which history will likely take us is on a scientific exploration of consciousness within psychology. Sheikh, Kunzendorf, and Sheikh (2003) outline major challenges for a society poised on the brink of a spiritual and scientific reunion, which aims to inject some of the holistic wisdom of the shamanic era into modern medicine.

The first challenge will be to do away with the dualist notion of disease and the prohibition on the use of imagery without doing away with all of the powerful knowledge, technology, and medicine that modern science has produced. Clearly the shamans did not possess the technical medical knowledge to which we have access today. Yet it seems that, in the process of gaining physical knowledge, we may have turned our backs on other sources of healing:

> The shamans not only knew of no reason to isolate the spirit from the body, but they even recognized the danger of doing so. In their view, the primary problem was not the pathological change in the body but the decrease in personal power that led to the intrusion of disease. In other words, disease was a concrete manifestation of a spiritual crisis. (Sheikh et al., 2003, p. 4)

Individuals in pain will clearly understand the message this quote conveys. Pain hurts, yes; however, pain hurts far worse when it steals your life, your identity, and your connection to others and derails your life journey in general. Moreover, when a pain patient encounters the medical system, a narrow focus on the body may potentially lead to a further insult to the spirit of that person, making the pain experience worse. We must remember the wisdom of the shamans without throwing away our science and technology; we should use machines to heal the body yet not mistake the body for a machine itself. For the spirit, once damaged, does not heal easily.

The second task on the road back to shamanic wisdom is to reclaim the gift of imagery: "Basically they [shamanic practices] consist of healing by imagination or, more specifically, by using visualization to bridge the gulf between the individual and the universe" (Sheikh et al., 2003, p. 4). Our best science to date suggests that pain can be caused by very small physical processes, such as chemical signals within the receptor cites of nerve cells. Medicines should be used to treat such identified causes. At the same time, our best science suggests that pain can also be caused by much larger-scale processes, such as the imagination acting within the broader consciousness. Just as chemicals are used to treat small chemical causes, imagination should be used to treat broad and potentially spiritual causes.

Finally, to achieve full integration of shamanistic wisdom with modern science we must reexamine and possibly alter our entire notion of health, including the meanings of words like *disease, treat,* and *heal.* The shamans' definitions of *healthy* and *unhealthy,* of *well* and *unwell* were much broader than the biomedical focus on physical viability today, which we owe to Cartesian dualism and its mechanistic view of the body. For the shamans, "health consisted simply of being in harmony with creation" (Sheikh et al., 2003, p. 4). Clearly, this is a radically different concept, and we will need to reshape our expectations accordingly. Imagery is not made of the same stuff as chemical medicines, it does not work in the same manner, and, most broadly, it does not fit well within the narrower restriction of health only of the body. Imagery does not fit well within the mechanistic tendency to find what is broken and fix it through direct means of repair.

The key distinction between the ancient traditions and the newly emerging holistic approach to medicine is that the body and mind were considered as a single unit within the ancient world. At a minimum, they were considered to be densely interconnected systems (Sheikh et al., 2003). Inasmuch as the body–mind may develop a particular path to illness in response to external triggers (e.g., viruses), the body–mind may also provide its own momentum to the healing trajectories of an external healing agent (e.g., medicine). At a deeper level, the health-promoting trajectories of the body–mind are enhanced through a balanced flow of information within the body and mind. This balance comes from an adaptive mix of integrity and flexibility, promoting unity and connection among the body–mind systems and the systems of the surrounding worlds, both internal and external. The ancient practitioners focused on spiritual health and strength, often using communal rituals to evoke group imagery experiences to enhance integration at the level of community.

The key distinction within these practices lies in their focus on the quality of life rather than its length:

> The shamans' primary focus was not on bodily well-being but spiritual health. They were not primarily concerned with prolonging life, but rather with improving its quality by restoring harmony. Their interest in disease sprang from their belief that illness pointed to a spiritual crisis. If it was handled incompetently, it could be destructive; however, it also could become the springboard for personal growth and vision. (Sheikh et al., 2003, p. 5)

From a Western perspective, the lack of focus on bodily health and longevity may sound like a cop-out or may even seem reckless. In clarification, bodily health and longevity were indeed a focus of the shamanic practitioners. They simply were not the primary focus. Rather, the focus was either on healing or on being sick in a healthier way. The choice was not up to the shaman, the sick individual, or the tribe that shared their illness in a communal manner. If the disease then was due to a spiritual crisis, it would likely dissipate through the imagery practices. If the disease was primarily physical, the imagery rituals would allow the disease to enhance the individual's growth, connection, meaning, and transcendence through the illness on the pathway through life. Injury to the physical body and death are natural and inevitable occurrences; therefore, they are not tragedies in the same respect as injury or death to the soul.

Indeed, one may find within the various religious traditions a great emphasis on the practice of acceptance and its relation to soul healing. For example, the Judeo-Christian traditions contain numerous allegorical lessons in acceptance of our role as humans who are finite and mortal. We are taught not to question the ways of God, which are often mysterious. We are taught to have faith and to live in harmony and peace despite our limited efficacy, limited perspective, and, ultimately, our unpredictable path into injury or disease and then death.

Cartesian philosophy relegated acceptance to the church, and within the mechanistic world of modern medicine, there is an emphasis on controlling, changing, and dominating natural processes. As a relatively new branch of this scientific endeavor, psychology has been undergoing a general revolution in the opposite direction, toward the recognition that both acceptance and change are each powerful strategies and that they are even more powerful when they are united and synthesized toward the goal of healing and integrity (Walsh & Shapiro, 2006). This is not a new idea but rather a reawakening to the most basic approach to shamanic practice. Perhaps psychology is rediscovering this wisdom as it becomes acquainted with the decidedly nonmechanistic realms that were once the territory of the shamans and more recently the territory that was at the outskirts of the science–religion divide.

Whatever the case, this broader philosophy will need to accompany the use of imagery techniques in modern medicine if they are to reach their full potential. Imagery practitioners must be able to balance acceptance and change, as they delve into the imaginary realms. A surgeon would not open a wound only to light an incense stick and begin to chant or pray. Similarly, one should not enter the realm of imagination with the restrictive goal of physical repair. Rather than stitching up this or that or changing the chemical makeup from this level to that, the practice of imagery should be directed at broader healing. The shaman's role in the health process was in "making an imaginary journey in a quest of the sick person's soul, finding it and returning it to its owner" (Sheikh et al., 2003, p. 5). The result was broad acceptance and a restoration of integrity within the person and between the person and his or her world. The result will likely also be a decrease in pain. However, the impacts on the body must be of secondary concern. Achterberg (1985, pp. 19–20) describes this acceptance versus change distinction within the broader context of the shamanic traditions:

In shamanic society health is not the absence of feeling; no more so is it the absence of pain. Health is seeking out all the experiences of Creation and turning them over and over, feeling their texture and multiple meanings. Health is expanding beyond one's singular state of consciousness to experience the ripples and waves of the universe.

It is apparent from this passage that the healing use of imagery is so expansive that it places limitations on the attempted direct and mechanistic control that is the rule within modern medical practice.

In fact, when Cartesian philosophy meets Western notions of direct control, the result can be quite destructive when practicing within the imaginary realm. Specifically, the mechanistic view of illness can become combined with a bias toward change through direct control, leading to the viewpoint that an individual in pain has not only a broken body but also a broken spirit. This in turn may lead to the idea that they are weak or at fault not only in the physical realm but within their metaphysical realms as well. Approaching imagery practices with an "It's broken, and I'm going to fix it" attitude is most likely going to make "it" even more broken.

"If you can't have it, you've get it," is a commonly used phrase within the newer acceptance-based behavior therapies (e.g., Hayes, Strosahl, & Wilson, 1999), which suggests that attempts to avoid internal experiences will tend to backfire. What this means is that you can not unimagine something; trying not to think about something *is* thinking about it. Therefore, a journey into the imagination that sets out under the pretext of broken mechanisms and direct physical healing in isolation is likely to be doomed from the outset, because the images this journey conjures up will be negative and misguided. In image therapy we are seeking to open the mind, to explore the realms of consciousness that may bring deeper meaning and connection within an individual and between that individual and the transcendental. The direct search for physical healing and pain relief is by definition a closed activity that is grounded within a physical reality. This type of search is the opposite of transcendent. Therefore, the use of an acceptance-based secondary control strategy when using imagery is necessary even if, ultimately, one is solely concerned with practicalities.

Consider the language we use when we are sick. You feel *under the weather, down and out, off kilter, out of sync, dis-eased, dis-ordered, out of sorts, out of it,* and, ultimately, *not yourself.* The role of the shaman is to take you on a journey through your imagination, into the broader realms of consciousness to find *you* and then to bring *you* back to *you.* If your body is damaged beyond repair then that is you, but within the imaginary realm, knowledge as to the extent of damage or likelihood of healing is not readily available. Direct control, precision equipment, and "common procedures" are not the norm. Consequently, the agenda is more often informed by acceptance than it is by direct change. The source of healing is broad, infinite, and outside of time rather than sharp, pointed, and precise. To really come full circle, science will need to come to grips with this inherent paradox of working with the imagination.

Types of Imagery

Richardson (1983) and others (e.g., Sheikh, 1978) have worked toward developing procedures for classifying various types of mental images, particularly in regard to the various phenomenological qualities of images and the contexts in which they emerge. Identifying the various aspects and types of mental imagery has obvious practical significance for clinicians and cognitive researches alike. Furthermore, these lines of research explore the continuum of human experience as it emerges from the combination of sensory experience from the environment and stored information within memory. Richardson describes four broad and admittedly overlapping classes of imagery that may be distinguished with respect to qualities including clarity, vividness, stability, and relation to sensory perception. These four types of imagery are referred to as (1) after-images, (2) eidetic images, (3) thought images, and (4) imagination images. After-images occur immediately and spontaneously after sufficiently intense or prolonged exposure to sensory stimulation. Common examples include the image of a flash of light that persists after closing one's eyes, the rocking sensation one continues to feel after having been on a boat, or the sense that one is continuing to wear a hat even after it has been removed. After-images closely resemble the sensory information that triggers them, though with decreased intensity, clarity, and stability (e.g., they move along with movement of the eyes).

Eidetic images are similar to after-images, except that they generally have a longer duration and originate from some combination of memory or creative imagination rather than simply from prolonged sensory stimulation. Eidetic images are very intense and clear, similar to actual sensory stimulation, and are more stable than after images. This category of imagery is a bit confusing as the term has been used differently in different contexts. For example, Ahsen (1973) refers to these images within his original approach to treatment as intensely vivid developmental images with psychological and somatic significance, whereas experimental psychologists such as Haber (1979) operationally define eidetic images as single modality (e.g., touch, hearing) images that are experienced in full sensory detail without direct sensory stimulation. Most research in this area has focused on children, while it has generally been concluded that these types of images are exceedingly rare to nonexistent in adults (Sheikh, 1978). Nevertheless, Ahsen's variety of eidetics will be encountered quite commonly in the practice of image therapy, and the experimentally defined variety, although rare, could potentially occur in clinical situations as well.

Thought imagery (formerly referred to as *memory imagery*) is the imagery most people think of when they use the term *imagination*. Thought imagery may be produced in response to memory or during our ongoing interpretations of experiences. Thought images tend to be hazy and less intense than sensory stimulation, although clarity and immersion may be greatly enhanced through training (Richardson, 1983).

Thought images become clearer and more engaging of body and mind when one engages in relaxation and turns the attention inward toward the thought images and away from external sensory stimulation. This purposeful inward focus distinguishes *imagination imagery* from thought imagery, along with the resulting increases in intensity, clarity, and immersion that result. Imagination imagery is the predominant type used in image therapies.

The True Nature of Imagination

By this point, your understanding of imagery should be greatly expanded. You should have moved beyond the idea that the imagination is make-believe, child's play, and outside the realms of serious medical practice or scientific inquiry. At this point, you should be able to see beyond the dualist biases of the past. You should be able to keep your logic and scientific skepticism nearby and at the same be open to the exploration of the true nature of imagery and its potential role in the modern healing arts.

Along with many others (e.g., Zahourek, 1988), it is our position that imagery is at the center of consciousness. Furthermore, imagery is active, not passive. Imagery is occurring whenever one is conscious, regardless of the state of consciousness. It may occur automatically and spontaneously or under the influence of the will to serve the purpose of conscious goals. Imagery may be relatively nonverbal, or it may be well integrated with verbal thought processes. For example, when you think to yourself, "I'd love a glass of lemonade," images relating to lemonade are evoked automatically that impact your physiology (e.g., thirst), emotions, and broader motivations. Lemonade images may also occur without the verbal thought ("I'd love a glass"), which lead you to look in your refrigerator. In addition, the lemonade images that have just been made clear within your awareness may continue to flow on to other related images within the unconscious associative stream of your mind as you continue to read. Finally, you may influence your images and associated physiological responses in a willful manner. For example, if your imagined glass of lemonade is tall, cool, wet, and waiting for you next to a lounge chair overlooking the ocean you will have a different response from if it is half-empty, warm, and sitting in a kitchen sink. The choice is yours.

Beyond the ancient beliefs, the common sense, and the thought experiments discussed earlier in this chapter suggesting that imagery is a continuously unfolding process at the center of consciousness, there is some experimental evidence to this effect as well (Kahneman & Tversky, 1996; Richardson, 1983). Specifically, researchers have found evidence for the existence of unconscious images that may inform knowledge and guide behavior, the common experience of a "felt sense" or intuition about phenomena. These studies typically involve the examination of the reaction times of individuals instructed to use or not use imagination in responding to challenges that draw on the imagination. For example, one may be asked to judge whether a hand is left or right when it is presented visually at various angles, which presumably involves imagining one's own hand superimposed on the drawing. The general conclusion has been that the conscious use of imagery to solve such imaginal tasks does not lead to faster reaction times. Furthermore, in studies that have included measures of imagination and special ability, no differences have been found (Richardson, 1983). Richardson (p. 11) summarizes this line of research:

> The evidence, such as it is … suggests that human adults have a continual, night-and-day stream of imaginal events going on within them. Given the appropriate conditions, each of us can tune in and watch…. Just as an art teacher may bring the usually unnoticed effect of light and shade on the trunk of a tree to the students' attention, so the imagery trainer may help the weak imager to relax and pay attention to the sensory details of similar internally represented events.

As a centerpiece of consciousness, imagery is also intricately involved in ones experience of one's self. Zahourek (1988, p. 56) writes, "Imagination provides a bridge between the different levels of the self.… It mediates between past experience and future projections." In other words, imagery is at the crossroads of self-consciousness, the process by which we figure out who we are and who we want to be. Sensory memory lasts for about 1 to 2 seconds, and short-term memory (i.e., working memory) lasts less than 30 seconds. It is imagery that allows us to reach into memory and explore who we were in the past. Conversely, it is also imagery that allows us to imagine who we will become in the future. If it were not for our self-imagined projections into the past and future, we would be continually rediscovering ourselves every few moments throughout our lives. Therefore, the imagination may be considered to be the key process at the center of the development of personal identity, our health, and our wellness in the broadest sense of these words.

CHAPTER 3

Imagery for Pain Relief

How Does It Work?

I sometimes *feel* I am right, but do not *know* it. When two expeditions of scientists went to test my theory I was convinced they would confirm my theory. I wasn't surprised when the results confirmed my intuition, but I would have been surprised had I been wrong. I'm enough of an artist to draw freely on my imagination, which I think is more important than knowledge. Knowledge is limited. Imagination encircles the world.

Albert Einstein
(from an interview by George Sylvester Viereck, *published in the Philadelphia Saturday Evening Post, October 26, 1929*)

As the resident expert in the positive impacts of hope and the therapeutic alliance on treatment outcomes, the mental health professional is usually the leader within the treatment team in helping the patient to develop positive expectations about the benefits of treatment as well as in providing attention, empathy, and reeducation on the true nature of pain and on the role of mental health in physical health. Furthermore, patience on the part of pain practitioners is critical, as the movement toward rehabilitation at times will be slow and demoralization on the part of the patient may be great. This may be especially true in the more action-oriented and efficiency-driven health-care settings. In these situations, the therapist will need to be prepared to make imagery fit within a multidisciplinary treatment environment and to be able to help reframe the understanding of the patient and also other professionals in regard to imagery. Imagery is not a superficial or palliative treatment. It is not purely psychological, and it is not an alternative to more scientifically grounded treatment options. Our task in this chapter is to help to clarify that imagery is a scientifically based treatment and that it is particularly well suited for the treatment of all types of pain. Deep understanding of these issues will place the therapist in a position to educate patients and colleagues alike on the potential benefits of imagery in pain management.

Once each of the various health professionals involved in a case has completed the initial assessments, integration of the results is critical. Unfortunately, accounting for the whole person in treatment planning is rare, even in the best clinics. Specialization in science and practice leads to a refinement of knowledge, but it may also lead to a fragmented view of the patient. For example, an individual's developmental history, personality, and social context typically fall within the purview of mental health rather than medicine. As such, the goal of integration across disciplines using a model that is genuinely biopsychosocial should still be considered aspirational. Science is quite adept at taking things apart but far less equipped at putting things back together, particularly a phenomenon as complex as the biopsychosocial functioning of a human being.

In addition to the problem of integrating imagery within the broader treatment plan is the problem that imagery typically takes a secondary role in treatment planning. Although it has been used successfully for thousands of years and for at least 100 years within the context of modern medicine, imagery remains one of the most underused treatments available for pain (Baer, Hoffman, & Sheikh, 2003). This underuse has continued despite consistent scientific results supporting the effectiveness of imagery over the past 20 to 30 years (Syrjala & Abrams, 2002).

Science, Scientism, and Modern Pain Practice

One explanation for the aforementioned disparity is that people from Western cultures tend to be more easily swayed by things that appear scientific rather than by actual scientific evidence. Such a noncritical, quasi-religious belief in scientific appearances may be referred to as *scientism*. Ironically, scientism holds sway over practitioners as much as it does over patients. For example, two alternative treatment mainstays in specialty pain clinics are biofeedback and transcutaneous electrical nerve stimulation (TENS). Yet biofeedback (e.g., listening to a changing tone that responds to lowered heart rate) has not been found to add anything beyond other nontechnologically based relaxation techniques, such as deep breathing, progressive muscle relaxation, and relaxation imagery (Turner & Chapman, 1982).

Admittedly, it is nice to have some objective means, such as a tone, to determine if the patient is relaxed. However, widespread use of biofeedback equipment appears to suggest that its use is motivated by more than the perceived convenience of knowing in a more objective manner when a patient has achieved a state of relaxation. So why do clinics bother with the cost of the apparatus and the training in its use if biofeedback does not add benefits beyond those of deep breathing alone? Would clinics be likely to invest the same money in more comfortable furniture or in intensive training in guided imagery, each of which may actually enhance the relaxation abilities of patients beyond biofeedback?

An even more dramatic example is the widespread use of TENS in specialty pain clinics despite the fact that the best research evidence suggests that it does not work. TENS involves the stimulation of nerve endings with low-level electrical current. The current is not painful but can be felt so that the patient can experience that the electrodes are doing something. An entire industry is built around the production, sale, and marketing of TENS devices, which are used primarily for pain—although they are also marketed for other ailments including depression, fatigue, and digestion. TENS is the perfect example of the impact of scientism in modern pain treatment. It involves a sophisticated technological device, the rationale involves "sciency" factors like electricity and the stimulation of nerves, and it is body focused rather than mind focused. Yet despite the fact that TENS is a standard of care in pain clinics, the evidence for its effectiveness for pain is at best inconclusive (Johnson, 2001). Indeed, people are prone to have faith in appearances and to ignore evidence, even in the realm of modern science and medicine.

Does Imagery Work?

The primary question to answer before therapists ask patients to invest their hopes and expectations in imagery treatments for pain is whether it is likely to work. The answer is yes, imagery does work. Although imagery is underused in modern medicine due to the impact of scientism, the evidence supporting its use has been strong enough to push further into the mainstream over the past couple of decades (Syrjala & Abrams, 2002). For example, in the year 2000, just 2 years after the National Institutes of Health (NIH) established its National Center for Complimentary and Alternative Medicine (NCCAM), imagery had attained the highest status in terms of effectiveness among the most accepted approaches in behavioral medicine literature (Baer et al., 2003). Although imagery techniques do not require wires or electricity, they stand strong on firm scientific evidence.

We would not have written this book if imagery did not work. Yet the question, "Does it work?" is only the first and simplest question we need to ask. And the answer, "Yes it works; trust us," is an incomplete answer. Therapists who deal with issues like pain know from experience that nothing works for everyone all the time and that pain can be difficult to treat effectively. Pain patients know this even better and often have been misled into holding false hopes that result in demoralization, shame, and anger when treatments do not live up to expectations. Indeed, chronic pain patients will arrive at a therapist's office dragging a long history of failed treatments behind them.

It is important for the therapist to understand the nuances of treatment outcome research on guided imagery so that realistic and measured expectations may be conveyed to each patient. Deep and scientifically grounded knowledge about how imagery works for pain is crucial for the treatment process and enables the therapist to merge logic with clinical intuition to shape techniques that are most likely to benefit each particular patient. Some healthy skepticism about image therapy will shape more realistic expectations, will reduce the chance of letdowns, and will maximize the chance for pleasant surprises.

And who would not be surprised about these techniques? Despite our history lessons from Chapter 2, it may still seem difficult to accept the fact that the imagination can bring healing and relief for something as physical and real as pain. In our day-to-day experiences, we typically do not notice things in the imaginary world reaching into the physical world and making changes. Nevertheless, it is clear that the imagination can in many instances relieve pain. But the story is a bit more complex than that. Within that complexity lie the shades of gray that will bring about deeper understanding of how imagery works and what therapists and patients can expect from treatment.

Shades of Gray: Understanding Clinical Research

Research is simply a set of tools designed to find truth. For some problems, however, truth is harder to find, even with the best tools. When truth is hard to find, research may at least help us to discover what is *not* true, ideas that are misleading and thus potentially harmful. When used in this manner, research can be pretty useful, particularly in evaluating healing practices such as imagery. Psychology has a long list of therapies that research has shown to be essentially useless, leaving a trail of consumers with dashed hopes for relief. These bogus therapies exist today as well; you can find them on the Internet claiming to be effective for everything from pain, to ADHD, to depression, and more.

One of the reasons for the draw toward bogus healers is that truth is hard to ascertain in mental health research. Mental processes are hidden, individual, subjective, and inherently fuzzy. By *fuzzy*, we mean complex:

Research questions are difficult to formulate, observations are difficult to make, objectivity may not truly exist, and answers are often both yes and no rather than cut and dried. As a result, it is best to approach therapy research with an open mind. This point deserves clarification. An open mind does not mean that one should believe in everything, nor does it imply that more holistic explanations always are better than scientifically based explanations. Believing in everything equally does not make an open mind; on the contrary, it represents being closed-minded to the possibility that some things are not true. On the other hand, a truly open mind means that you examine evidence in an impartial manner, that you examine evidence in context, and that you realize that some things are truer than other things. It is in this spirit that we will attempt to understand if and why imagery is well suited for the treatment of pain.

Like any toolset, different research tools are good for different tasks. That said, there are two main types of tasks involved in examining treatment outcomes: experimental tasks and clinical tasks. Each tells us something different about how imagery works for pain. Experimental pain studies are usually done in laboratory or university settings, often using psychology undergraduates with what is called *analogue pain*, pain that is meant to be analogous to clinical pain. Analogue pain is usually induced by having the participants dunk their hands in ice water, known as cold-pressor pain, or by having participants' fingers squeezed with clips. The reason researchers use analogue pain is that in experiments, one must be very careful to control all of the conditions, including the pain stimulus. By controlling all of the factors, or *variables*, within the study, researchers can obtain the best possible evidence to inform the truth about whether the imagery tested within the study actually caused pain relief. The imagery in these studies is usually kept very uniform and simple; relaxing on a beach is the most common imaginary scenario. These experimental studies can be excellent for telling us that it was the imagery that brought about reductions in pain and not some other factor. This type of knowledge is referred to as *efficacy*, which addresses the simplest question: "Can imagery work?" Experimental studies addressing clinical efficacy are typically the first studies to consult when examining an alternative treatment approach, and evidence for efficacy based on well-controlled experiments is the most trustworthy evidence that exists within science.

There are, however, a number of downsides to experimental studies pertaining to treatment efficacy. First, there is the question of applicability of these controlled experiments to real treatment, referred to as *external* or *ecological* validity. *Internal validity*, the ability to establish as simple causal relationship by controlling other factors, often comes at the expense of ecological validity. For example, undergraduate psychology students imagining relaxing on a beach for 10 minutes while they stick their hands in ice water may not actually be comparable to the intense and multifaceted real-world pain encountered in patients. The risk in this situation is that you may be comparing apples and oranges. The results of the lab experiment may not apply to actual clinical practice. The internal validity is solid because of the use of a homogenous group of participants and simple procedures. Yet this homogeneity and simplicity limits the real world applicability of a study, or its external validity.

Consequently, *clinical* research that is carried out on real patients, often using more comprehensive imagery techniques, is vital. However, inasmuch as these studies try to control for other factors that could be reducing pain to identify imagery as the main cause, they too tend to oversimplify treatments and to homogenize patients to varying degrees and at the same time are less well controlled than true experiments. This issue of control and a focus on simple causes is a liability of the research process in general, as it makes the study of the unique individual and complex causes more difficult to examine. Nevertheless, clinical studies are useful along with lab-based experimental studies because they answer the *effectiveness* question, "Does imagery relieve pain in the real world of actual clinicians and real pain patients?"

In addition to issues of experimental control and validity, outcomes are important to consider as well. Research on imagery in pain management often involves measuring improvement in pain tolerance (amount of time the students can hold their hands in the water or remain in a finger clamp), pain thresholds (amount of time until they say it is starting to hurt) and discomfort (paper–pencil ratings of how bad the pain was after the fact). Skeptics might be asking, "What does 'improved' mean? What if the pain simply goes from 'very bad' to 'just bad'?" To tease this out, researchers rely on statistics, another tool in the research toolkit, which are quite helpful if used with skill and clarity of purpose. One important way that statistics can be misleading is that *significant* results, as in *significant reductions* in pain ratings, may actually have little to do with the actual degree of the improvement. This is because statistical significance depends upon three distinct factors: (1) the size of the effect; (2) the overall numbers of people studied; and (3) the degree of background variation or unique response among people in the study.

Size of the effect and number of people studied are two fairly straightforward factors. However, the background variation is a more nuanced issue that can have a major impact in deciding on the clinical relevance of a study. To reduce background variation, researchers attempt to ensure that participants in a study are as similar as possible; for example, investigators may look only at women within a certain age range, with no other conditions other than a particular type of pain. Similarity among participants is desirable because statistics are based on differences in numerical context or across a backdrop of variability. This background variation acts as a measuring stick to assess whether a reliable change has occurred as a result of a treatment. If everyone in the study is as similar as possible, then differences between treatment A and treatment B will show up more clearly, like a painting on a white versus a speckled canvas. It is easier to see the picture without all the distraction in the background. Unfortunately, this statistical strategy removes research from the real world of clinical practice, where each pain patient is unique and has problems that are typically quite complex. For all of these reasons, it is important to look at the population included in a study, the depth or simplicity of the intervention, and the actual size of the improvement—in other words, the *clinical significance*. Furthermore, background variance itself is interesting to examine for a couple of additional reasons. First, significant results that emerge despite high levels of background variation generally should be given greater weight in making clinical interpretations because they are harder to come by in research. Second, high levels of background variation point to the likelihood that individuals are having unique and idiosyncratic responses to treatment, a point explored in detail subsequently.

Before we proceed, let us review:

1. Research can be a helpful toolkit for finding truth, or, when truth is hard to determine, for steering us away from falsehoods.
2. Experimental research is good at figuring out if imagery can cause decreases in pain, whereas clinical research is good at figuring out if it actually works in a clinical setting.
3. Statistics work best in studies with many people who are similar to one another and worse in studies examining a range of individuals receiving individually tailored treatments.
4. Statistically significant results do not necessarily mean that the results are clinically significant, so actual outcomes in studies should be examined in detail.

And the Winner Is ...?

With these lessons in mind let us examine the nature of imagery and its role in pain management. First, imagery has consistently been found to be efficacious, bringing about statistically significant levels of improvement in experimental studies (for recent examples of such experimental studies see Borckardt, Younger, Winkel, Nash, & Shaw, 2004). Recall the undergraduate psychology students immersing their arms into ice water. Typically, researchers have found increases of approximately 100% (from about 100 seconds to 200 seconds) in the length of time the students can keep their arms submerged after training in a simple imagery technique. In addition to reaching statistical significance, these numbers appear rather impressive with respect to potential clinical significance, especially considering the superficial nature of the imagery that is used in these studies (e.g., imagining your arm changing color and feeling warmer and more comfortable) with only a few minutes devoted to receiving the imagery instructions and to practicing.

As tolerance goes up, reports of pain intensity go down as well, although not as dramatically. Reductions in pain ratings tend to be closer to 30%–40%, or, for example, from 12 to 8 on a scale of 0 to 20. So the cold water does not hurt as much, but it definitely does still hurt. The differential response between tolerance and intensity suggests that the physical properties of the pain, the pain sensations, are not modified to the same extent as people's ability to carry on with what they are doing in spite of the pain. This differential response probably is what one would expect from a purely psychological intervention.

However, before you conclude that imagery does not work as well on pain intensity as it does on tolerance, keep in mind that there is a problem (i.e., technically a *confound*) with the way these studies are carried out. The longer you hold your arm in ice water, the more intense the pain becomes. Increased tolerance brings more intense pain, as the students hold their hands in the water longer. Failure to account for this confound in numerous studies has left their results subject to question, whereas studies that have accounted for this confound tend to find even greater benefits on pain intensity than on pain tolerance (Borckardt et al., 2004). Consider the general finding that pain intensity after simple imagery is on average around 40% lower after 200 seconds of immersion in ice water than after 100 seconds for a no-imagery control group. This result is quite impressive, particularly when you consider the fact that ice water is a clear-cut physiological cause of pain. One would be hard-pressed to explain these results simply in terms of changes in levels of relaxation or confidence.

In clinical studies of pain, one finds similar magnitudes of effectiveness, suggesting that imagery does reduce pain, increase tolerance, and improve the lives of patients (e.g., Achterberg, Kenner, & Lawlis, 1988; Albright & Fischer, 1990; Gauron & Bowers, 1986; Mannix, Chandurkar, Rybicki, Tusek, & Solomon, 1999; Manyande et al., 1995; Philips & Hunter, 1981; Powers, 1999; Raft, Smith, & Warren, 1986; ter Kuile et al., 1994). Again, however, the truth is in the details. For example, in 1981, Philips and Hunter treated a group of patients with chronic and severe headaches using relaxation training over an 8-week period: Half of the patients used visual imagery along with the standard relaxation procedures (i.e., deep breathing and muscle contraction exercises). The study was aimed at determining if imagery worked better than relaxation alone. The only statistical difference they found between the groups was that the imagery group had more improvement in depression and sense of control over the pain. So in these two respects, imagery won over relaxation alone, albeit by a nose. However, the researchers had only eight people in each group, the imagery was superficial, and the groups were heterogeneous (i.e., real headache pain patients with diverse circumstances and treatment responses). Each of these factors makes it difficult to find statistically significant differences.

Other studies have compared, for example, imagery with distraction, self-talk methods, relaxation, and biofeedback. The results are usually the same, with imagery coming out as the most consistent performer (e.g., Achterberg et al., 1988; Albright & Fischer, 1990; Fors, Sexton, & Gotestam, 2002; Gauron & Bowers, 1986; Mannix et al., 1999; Manyande et al., 1995; Philips & Hunter, 1981; Powers, 1999; Raft et al., 1986; ter Kuile et al., 1994). For people in therapy, clinical significance is a more important issue. For example, in Philips and Hunter's (1981) pioneering study, the imagery + relaxation group's headache intensity dropped by 300%, the number of headaches per week dropped by 100%, duration dropped by 25%, emotional distress dropped by 100%, avoiding activities and complaining about pain decreased by 75%, depression about pain dropped by 90%, and sense of control in reducing pain increased by 300%. Subsequent studies have shown similar magnitudes of positive change. Most clinicians would be pleased to observe results of this magnitude on average across their patients, particularly after only 8 weeks of relaxation training combined with simple relaxing imagery.

To summarize, for most people, imagery does decrease pain intensity, increase pain tolerance, and improve the associated psychosocial factors (e.g., relationships, depression, confidence) in their lives. In the experimental studies, where the physiological cause of the pain is crystal clear (e.g., ice water), the biggest improvements tend to be in both pain tolerance and pain intensity. However, the pain does not disappear as it often does with medications. So it is not helpful to oversell the results of these studies. The pain will not be suddenly and completely imagined away for good, especially when dealing with a clear-cut physical injury. But it is probable that the pain will become far less intense, less distressing, and less of an obstacle in day-to-day functioning.

Imagery versus Hypnosis

Hypnosis is a common treatment for pain, yet many practitioners and patients are unaware of its true nature or its relationship to guided imagery. Before beginning to practice imagery for pain, it is important that the therapist understands the relationship between imagery and hypnosis so that this information may be conveyed effectively to patients either who may specifically request hypnotherapy or who, conversely, will specifically request that they not be hypnotized.

Simply stated, imagery and hypnosis are equivalent. If you were to read a hypnosis script and an imagery script, you would be hard-pressed to identify which was which. The reason that people typically assume that hypnosis is distinct is because of misconceptions about the nature of hypnotic states. A hypnotic state is a state of relaxation and high suggestibility. Hypnosis is not a trance, and you cannot be hypnotized unless you want to be hypnotized. Not everyone is susceptible to hypnosis, even if they want to be hypnotized, and you cannot make people do things under hypnosis that they would not otherwise do. Finally, you cannot leave someone permanently hypnotized through posthypnotic suggestion, nor are the effects of hypnosis necessarily any longer lasting than any other psychological intervention. Each of these myths is due to people's misconceptions about hypnosis, which are propagated by the fact that hypnosis is used in stage shows, films, and television programs as a vehicle for entertainment. Clinically, imagery and hypnosis are equivalent in effectiveness: Each produces the strongest and most consistent effects across studies with various types of pain compared with all other psychological treatments (Fernandez & Turk, 1989; Syrjala & Abrams, 2002).

Again, hypnosis is a state of relaxation and high suggestibility. For example, a common hypnotic induction is to tell the subjects to stare at the tip of a flame or at the hypnotist's finger and then to instruct them that their eyes will become heavier and heavier. What the hypnotist is doing is working with the body's own natural reactions. Staring at a solitary object fatigues the eyes. It is only natural to feel like closing our eyes during prolonged staring. Continuing the induction, the hypnotist uses increasing levels of suggestion to continue the body in the direction of relaxation, suggesting to subjects that they should close their eyes as their lids become heavier, take deep breaths, and experience increasing levels of relaxation with each breath. At this point, hypnotherapists working with pain typically begin to use imagery techniques, like draining the pain out of an area, spreading the pain out so that it becomes more diffuse, suggesting the imaginary experience of numbness in an area, and so on. The only difference between hypnotic imagery and nonhypnotic imagery then is that hypnosis involves more suggestive statements during the induction phase, whereas imagery approaches may use less suggestion. Each begins with relaxation, moves the patient to an internal focus, and then guides the imagery of the patient toward healing and relief. If one feels the need to distinguish the two, hypnosis may be considered to be a special case of imagery involving greater degrees of suggestion in the induction phase, or imagery may be considered to involve a more collaborative process of treatment. There is, however, no clear line that distinguishes one from the other.

As a result, most researchers now consider relaxation and imagery to be synonymous (see Nolan, Spanos, Hayward, & Scott, 1995; Spanos et al., 1993 for recent examples of well-controlled empirical test demonstrating the equivalence in procedures). Furthermore, studies generally have suggested that imagery is the factor that accounts for reductions in pain during hypnosis, even when other procedures such as relaxation are being used as well. For example, Gay, Philippot, and Luminet (2001) examined the pain reduction in an older adult population, 64 years old on average, with moderate to severe osteoarthritis pain. These patients were given either a set of eight 30 minute hypnotic imagery treatments or a series of eight 30 minute relaxation sessions. The researchers examined the relationship between levels of improvement and the hypnotizibility (proneness to entering a suggestive state) and imagery abilities of patients. The relaxation treatment was simple progressive muscle relaxation (having patients tense and release distinct muscle groups to decrease tension), whereas the hypnotic-imagery treatment involved going on a relaxing vacation for 5 minutes and then spending 25 minutes within a memory from childhood in which the patient had full joint comfort and mobility (e.g., running in a field at age 10).

Both treatments decreased pain significantly over time compared with a wait-list control group (i.e., no treatment). The hypnotic-imagery treatment brought quicker improvements (4 weeks vs. 8 weeks). Individual differences among the patients in imagery ability moderated the maintenance of improvements at a 6 month follow-up assessment, as did hypnotizibility to a lesser degree. Specifically, the average decrease in ratings of pain intensity went from 4.16 to 1.97 on a scale from 1 to 10 after 4 weeks of the hypnotic imagery treatments. The results held at a 3 month follow-up, but average levels of pain crept back up at the 6 month follow-up. On close examination of the details of the results, however, it seems that imagination ability was the key factor among those who maintained improvements and who relapsed. Specifically, the standard deviation in pain ratings (i.e., the average variability in people's ratings around the average) went from 1.49 to 2.47 between the 3 and 6 month follow-ups. This suggests that some peoples' pain reduced even further at the 6 month follow-up whereas some of the patients deteriorated, perhaps in some cases due to progression of their osteoarthritis condition.

Imagery ability was a strong predictor of who the long-term improvers were, with a correlation between imagery ability and pain levels at the 6 month follow-up equal to −0.71. Correlations range from −1 to +1, so this result suggests that there was a large long-term beneficial effect of the treatment for those patients who came into the study with strong imagination abilities. Moreover, imagery ability had an equivalent degree of relationship to improvement at 4 weeks in the relaxation only group. This suggests that those who improved from relaxation alone likely were experiencing spontaneous healing imagery during their relaxation sessions and that it is imagery that accounts for improvement in this treatment within the same time frame as the improvers in the hypnotic imagery treatment.

Another interesting outcome from this study was the finding that confidence in treatment did not predict outcomes. In fact, confidence in the treatment in this study on average was quite low. On a scale from 1 to 3, the average rating among these patients was 1, corresponding to the description, "I do not believe in the treatment you propose." Apparently belief in treatment was not important. Patient buy-in may not always be as important as we assume.

Altogether, these results suggest that imagery is the active ingredient in hypnotherapy and relaxation therapies, that skepticism with treatment should not be seen as a deterrent at the outset of treatment, and that imagery ability is an important factor to assess at the outset of treatment and to use in treatment planning (e.g., prescribing imagery training exercises prior to therapy, using booster sessions to maintain improvements for low imaginers).

"You Are All Special, Just the Way You Are"

Pain comes in all shapes and sizes: back pain, stomach pain, muscle and joint pain, fibromyalgia, even pain in limbs that no longer physically exist (i.e., phantom limb pain). People come in all shapes and sizes too: older and younger, male and female, anxious and calm, big and small. Treatment settings, therapists, and techniques all vary. In view of all of these factors to consider, the questions of what works for whom, when, and to what degree are difficult to address. Many researchers have attempted to tackle these questions in research (e.g., Beers & Karoly, 1979; Fanurik, Zelter, Roberts, & Blount, 1993; Fernandez & Turk, 1989; Holroyd & Penzien, 1986; Marino, Gwynn, & Spanos, 1989; Spanos & O'Hara, 1990; Stevens, Pfost, & Rapp, 1987; Tan, 1982; ter Kuile et al., 1994; Turner & Chapman, 1982). Yet we have not learned much. It appears that factors that make treatment more effective include being younger, being less distressed, having less pain, being more engaged with treatment, and not dropping out of treatment. You might have guessed each of these without the bother of carrying out a formal investigation. However, the lack of exciting conclusions from these studies is not the fault of the researchers. These types of questions are very difficult to address with research.

Yet one potentially interesting result that is typically overlooked is that different people appear to have very different reactions to imagery, even to the simple types of imagery techniques that are typically used in these studies, such as lying on a beach. This result tends to be overlooked because it is not the result that researchers are seeking; typically researchers aim to find universal laws that will hold up across individuals. Yet, from a clinical perspective, the uniqueness of individuals may be quite interesting, suggesting that the words of Mr. Rogers from the old PBS program apply to pain management: "You are all special, just the way you are."

The specific result that researchers tend to ignore in experimental studies of imagery for pain is differences across people, known technically as *error variance* or *scatter*, because they are looking for average differences, which are harder to find when everyone is doing his own thing in response to a treatment. Usually when researchers mention "scatter," they do so at the end of an article to suggest that it is a methodological problem that must eventually be overcome. Variance across people is assumed to be caused by random factors, which is why it is called "error" variance. However, an alternate interpretation is that the variation among people is interesting in and of itself and that it is our research methodology that is the problem in these types of studies, not the variance. The typical result that has been observed consistently across studies is that variance increases from two-fold to fourfold among individuals following treatment (Hackett & Horan, 1980; Stevens, 1985; Stevens et al., 1987; Worthington & Shumate, 1981). This is a very large increase. To illustrate, if a hypothetical group of 50 people come in for 8 weeks of lie-on-the-beach imagery training, we might expect their average ratings on a scale from 1 to 100 to drop from 50 to 20. However, if we examined the variance in pain ratings, we may observe a change in range from 55 to 45 before treatment to 40 to 0 following treatment; some individuals experience dramatic improvements whereas others see very little. These results may fit with the experience of clinicians treating pain, but they are unacceptable for researchers whose research methods mislead them into thinking that these differential responses are caused by random factors. On the contrary, the fact that these variance increases occur consistently following treatment suggests that they are not random at all. A more reasonable explanation is that the treatment is producing a unique effect within each individual. For traditional research methods, this creates a barrier to answering the questions of who benefits when and why.

Answers to these questions will probably stay hidden until researchers begin to examine more realistic treatments, treatments that are more patient specific, as they are in actual clinical practice. Researchers also need to recognize that they must embrace the unique reactions of individuals. Paradoxically, unique responsiveness actually may be the general law they are seeking (see Allport, 1968, for a complete discussion of this topic in the field of personality). Nature can be greedy with her secrets and is not easily manipulated, which keeps modern health care well within the realm of art as well as science. Yet nature might have a message in her responses to these studies. In addition to suggesting that some patients are highly prone to the benefits of imagery whereas others are not, it also seems logical to assume that if such simple imagery can have such large effects, then deeper imagery ought to have the potential of working even better. If 10 minutes on the real beach helped your headaches, you might be inclined to try a 5-day trip to the Caribbean. Why would we not expect the same from the imagination?

An additional nonobvious conclusion from these studies is that beach imagery does not fit everyone. If you went to a travel agent looking for a ski trip to Aspen, and she told you that she was going to send you to the beach instead because people who go to the beach report an average 100% increase in satisfaction, what would you do? You might reconsider, but you also might say, "No thank you; I'm really sure I want to go skiing in Aspen." The same logic may be applied to imagery therapy for pain. The differential responses to treatment that are so typically observed suggest that patients should be actively engaged in the treatment process and that imagery procedures should be made as unique as possible. Everyone's pain is unique, even if it has the same apparent cause (e.g., cold water immersion); and everyone's imagery is unique as well.

Stevens (1985; Stevens et al., 1987) found direct evidence to this effect. Specifically, 68% of participants who were trained and instructed to use specific imagery strategies came up with their own unique set of strategies, ignoring the strategies in which they were trained and spoiling the primary questions of the investigation to determine which type of imagery works best. It appears that the type of imagery that may work best is imagery generated to some extent by the patient rather than being selected by the practitioner (for similar empirical examples see Avia & Kanfer, 1980; Hargadon, Bowers, & Woody, 1995; Worthington, 1978). Not only is it a natural tendency for people to dislike being told what to do, but they also know inherently that burning fire pain will respond best to water, that a wooden arm image will best protect them from cold that feels like needles, and that deeper psychological wounds require a transformation in imagery from victim to survivor. The beach is a lovely image, but it is not a panacea.

Furthermore, it appears that research participants have a hard time not using imagery automatically as a way of coping with pain. For example, in experimental studies comparing the effectiveness of imagery versus other treatment (e.g., rational self-talk) and control conditions (e.g., backward counting), one typically finds a strong tendency for individuals to use imagery regardless of specific instructions to the contrary. Such tendencies typically shows up in *manipulation checks*, procedures designed to investigate whether the results of the study may be considered valid. The consistent outcome of these manipulation checks across studies is that people do not do as instructed, which calls into question the results of treatment comparisons. Rather than sticking to their assigned strategies, it is typical for most individuals to use multiple strategies, such as relaxation, self-talk, distraction, and imagery, looking for the combination that is most beneficial to them.

This phenomenon was first examined explicitly by Hackett and Horan (1980), who found that people were naturally inclined to use calming imagery, doing so in a pretest before any imagery training or assignment to a treatment condition in 100% of the cases. Furthermore, they found that everyone in their study continued to use imagery during a pain induction despite specific instructions not to do so. Conversely, they found that rational self-talk skills (e.g., telling yourself that you will be okay or that it is just a sensation) were the least popular. Only 55% of individuals assigned to this group used their self-talk training as their primary strategy despite specific instructions to do so. Furthermore, it seems that people are intrinsically pulled to use multiple strategies, with 93% of participants admitting to the use of all three strategies employed within the investigation (i.e., imagery, breathing, and coping self-talk) to some extent. Imagery most often takes the role of primary strategy, despite training or experimental instructions to the contrary. Worthington and Shumate (1981) found similar results: Only 25% of individuals used self-talk skills following specific training. On the contrary, 80% of individuals in their study used imagery skills following training. These results and those that follow are particularly important to consider in clinical practice settings, where rational self-talk training is among the most common procedures described within cognitive-behavioral approaches to pain management.

Indeed, there is some evidence that imagery is more effective than self-talk even for people who are strongly verbal in their thinking styles, who one would expect would prefer verbal treatment. Stevens et al. (1987) matched people to self-talk or imagery treatments according to cognitive style (preference for verbal versus visual thinking) and found that self-talk did not work for the visualizers or the verbalizers whereas imagery worked for both groups. It is particularly interesting to note that matching the highly visual people to the imagery treatment did not result in the usual scatter in improvement that was discussed earlier. As a group, the visualizers not only improved on average but also did so far more consistently. The verbalizers improved in response to imagery too, but the scatter became four times larger after the treatment, as is typical in these types of studies. These results suggest that there may be a small subgroup of strong verbalizers that will require some additional training to benefit from imagery or for whom imagery may not be the first option in treatment.

In an attempt to account for the general preference for imagery over self-talk of individuals in pain, Worthington and Shumate (1981) suggest that people might be prone to use self-talk spontaneously and then figure that they have "tried that already" and conclude that it will not work. A simple alternative explanation is that people intuitively realize that self-talk does not work and imagery does and that the motivation of relieving actual discomfort supersedes experimental instructions. Indeed, self-talk may even interfere with the positive effects of imagery for some individuals. For example, Hackett and Horan (1980) found that although imagery increased pain thresholds, the same imagery did not work in an experimental group instructed to use it along with self-talk. The results seem to suggest that self-talk detracted from an otherwise effective imagery intervention.

Although we would not want to formulate overly firm conclusions from a small set of studies, the idea that imagery would be the most effective cognitive treatment strategy for pain, preferred by patients over self-talk methods, makes logical sense. The multisensory nature of imagery (e.g., sight, sound) should be far more potent and engaging than a strictly auditory verbal monologue, no matter how reassuring that monologue is. As the saying goes, a picture is worth a thousand words. You would not expect a person leaving a film to say, "I didn't really get drawn in by those action scenes, but the narrator's voice was truly amazing." Furthermore, as the arms of research participants are submerged in buckets of ice, it may begin to seem ridiculous to them as they try to keep saying words to themselves such as, "I'm okay; just relax" while images of freezing glaciers and sleeves of needles spontaneously come into their minds.

Most studies have not examined people's lack of compliance with experimental instructions and have continued in vain to try to urge people to do just one thing for pain. Even worse, most studies do not even use manipulation checks, which might help to explain why it rarely pays for a researcher to make a bet on any of the studies comparing different techniques. It is logical to suggest that different approaches such as these are actually inseparable and that this is why researchers struggle so hard to unyoke them. Breathing and other signs of relaxation change automatically along with verbal thought patterns and images. The participants in these studies are probably not stubborn or difficult people. Images might just be the easiest thing for people to focus on as they try to cope with pain in a multifaceted manner. Rather than fighting the wisdom of the inner doctor (Cousins, 1980), researchers should acknowledge her existence and examine her methods scientifically.

One final point should be made concerning the often overlooked results of clinical research on imagery and pain. What would be your reaction to the assertion that researchers have proven conclusively that effective treatments do not have to address the causes of pain? Indeed, this result is so obvious that researchers neglect to point this out. The cause of pain in experimental studies is purely physical, such as cold water or some similar device like finger-pinchers. Taking one's hand out of the water is the most effective cure for cold water pain. However, imagery and other interventions work too and have nothing to do with removing the arm from the tank. Research has looked at different sources of pain, including burns, operations, and headaches, and indeed imagery tends to work, regardless of the cause of the pain. This inherent potential for imagery to relieve pain together with people's natural drive to use imagery may be one place where people are more alike than they are unique.

In the helping professions, we generally realize the uniqueness of the individual when we are doing our best work. However, the desire to have clear answers sometimes causes us to forget this fact. When working with people's unique worldviews, we do not have the answers for them. We can't. Instead, we have the questions that need to be asked. This situation makes psychotherapy, including imagery, such a strange job at times, particularly in knowledge-oriented health-care settings. The more you learn over time with each clinical experience, the less you find that you know at the outset with each new patient. It may be difficult for nontherapists to understand this or to understand why we find it difficult to explain what we do. If we are honest with ourselves we can admit that neither the patient nor the therapist often really knows exactly what is going on at many points during treatment. The answer to questions such as, "What approach do you use?" and "What would you do with this patient?" should be "I'm going to do as little as possible." The most beneficial stance an imagery therapist probably can take is to work along with the inner physician and assist the natural healing tendencies of the imagination. This outlook may assist in taking the pressure off the healer, but in a professional setting it may run counter to our expectations of the healer to be the direct conduit for healing change.

Indeed, it is ironic that the latter half of this book is focused on techniques—what to do. As you read these chapters, and more so as you apply them with patients, remember to collaborate. Therapy is most effective when it is tailored to patients and their unique situations, when patients help to generate the rationales and procedures, and when patients are maximally confident in their ability to do their part as well as in your ability to do yours. This mutual confidence is like that between ground control and an astronaut. The astronaut can see what is going on out there in space, while the ground control has the technical knowledge and is able to see the bigger picture more clearly from Earth.

How Does Imagery Work?

The dorsal horn of the Substantia Gelatinosa is proposed by Melzack (Melzack & Wall, 1965, 1996) to be the physiological gate between body and mind for pain. Images might be considered to exist just across this divide on the mental side of the gate. Why images? Images are experiential thoughts, and therefore they would be considered to be the mental equivalent of physical experience. Just as the Substantia Gelatinosa is a gateway through which physiological pain signals pass on their way from the body to consciousness, images are the gateway through which conscious experiences travel back into the physical body. In summary, imaginary experiences activate image-relevant behavioral, cognitive, neurological, and other physiological processes.

The evidence for this proposition is extensive and unequivocal (for a review see Baer et al., 2003). For example, Hugdahl et al. (2001) used functional magnetic resonance imaging (fMRI) to observe activation of both motor and sensory cortex, as an amputee performed painful imaginary movements with his missing fingers. The neural activity of these individuals was responding as if the painful movements were actually occurring. While your imagination cannot reach out into the physical world and grow back a missing hand, your imagination can reach out and affect the neurophysiology underlying the experience of a hand, including the experience of movement and pain.

To review, it is well established that imagery is effective in reducing pain and in increasing coping. It is also well established that the imagination impacts the brain and associated physiological processes in a manner that mirrors sensory-driven experience. However, the practical question of exactly *how* imagery works in reducing pain remains. Although it is a difficult question to address, much less to answer, it is important to try. Beyond science, on a practical level, clinicians need to be able to improvise, to go off the trail and coinvent new techniques with their patients, depending on the practical demands of a treatment situation. Again, uniqueness is the rule in people's pain, their pain-related images, and their responses to image therapy. Therefore, to use the techniques within this book most effectively and most flexibly, it will be important to acquire a deep understanding of how imagery works.

The general answer we will suggest is that imagery works in a systemic manner, utilizing the body–mind's own momentum toward integration, flexibility, and adaptive growth. Indeed, we are in good company in making this suggestion. Cousins (1980, pp. 68–69) describes a conversation with Nobel Prize-winning physician Albert Schweitzer in which Dr. Schweitzer expressed a similar opinion:

> When I asked Dr. Schweitzer how he accounted for the fact that anyone could possibly expect to become well after having been treated by a witch doctor, he said that I was asking him to divulge a secret that doctors have carried around inside them ever since

Hippocrates. "But I'll tell you anyway," he said, his face still illuminated by that half smile. "The witch doctor succeeds for the same reason that all of us succeed. Each patient carries his own doctor inside of him. They come to us not knowing that truth. We are at our best when we give the doctor who resides within each patient a chance to go to work."

Benson and Friedman (1996) describe this internal doctor as well, along with the research that supports its power within the framework of *remembered wellness*. Remembered wellness is suggested as a replacement for the term *placebo*, which has come to carry negative connotations through the familiar Cartesian distortions of mind versus matter. Specifically, remembered wellness refers to a process wherein positive beliefs and expectations induce healing and recovery. In reviewing the scientific literature on the remembered wellness response, Benson and Friedman find that positive benefits have been observed in between 60% and 90% of medical illnesses, apart from any physically oriented medical intervention. They interpret these results as suggesting that "remembered wellness has been one of medicine's most potent assets and it should not be belittled or ridiculed. Unlike most other treatments, it is safe and inexpensive and has withstood the test of time" (p. 193).

Baer et al. (2003) describe this process as well, providing still more detail as to how the inner doctor operates within positive expectations and the doctor–patient relationship:

A key tenet of mind–body medicine is that health is not the mere absence of disease; it is the dynamic integration of our environment, body, mind, and spirit. Therefore, an essential difference between medical models that uphold dualism versus those that uphold a mind-body-spirit unity (nondualistic models) is the emphasis in treatment on curing versus healing the diseased state. One may be healed without being cured of the pathogenic state; one may suffer physically from chronic or terminal illness but nevertheless maintain a sense of dignity and inner peace throughout. Similarly, a person may be cured of a disease without being healed, and elimination of a pathogen does not necessarily eliminate feelings of fragmentation or imbalance. (p. 144)

None of these researcher-practitioners are suggesting that Western medicine is bad or that mind–body–spirit integration should replace surgery for torn ligaments or painkillers following surgery. What they are suggesting is that the simple-cause, simple-cure, materialist-reductionist paradigm of modern medicine leaves out some essential elements. Specifically, what modern medicine has neglected is the fact that simple and material causes are surrounded by larger systems involving multiple causes from both the physical and the metaphysical aspects of the body mind. When practitioners are able to recognize these larger systems and use them along with material medicines, broader opportunities for healing may be realized.

This is particularly the case when one uses imagery within a comprehensive pain management strategy. Individuals are not aware of their inner doctors, their beliefs, expectations, and other imaginary processes pertaining to broader mind–body–spirit integrity (Baer et al., 2003). A shift in attention inward, toward pain-related and healing images, may assist in connecting an individual's consciousness with these largely unconscious processes. With access to these images, opportunities for transformation arise: "Critical in promoting one's health is to know you are the expert on what hurts or heals you, to trust your inner instincts, and to honor your beliefs and emotions" (Baer et al., 2003, p. 148). Consciously through acts of will or automatically through natural momentums, the imaginary flows of information involved in building our sense of ourselves and ourselves in the world may be shifted when we become immersed in the imagination.

Epstein (1986) was among the first to describe with specificity the role of systems of cause in allowing for the healing power of the imagination. He suggests that imagery carries the natural potential to induce coherence or integrity in body–mind systems because images exist outside of the limitations of space and time and because images may be transformed through will. Damaged flesh, for example, exists within actual space and time and may not be transformed directly through the power of will. When one focuses attention on tissue damage, what one experiences is just that: tissue damage, right there, right now. On the contrary, damaged flesh within the imagination may be transformed beyond the bounds of time, space, and willful action. One may stretch the flesh to an infinite length or press it into a dot so small that it vanishes. Or one may travel into the past, before the injury occurred or into the future where it already has healed. The brain experiences and reacts to the imagery either way, whether one is having this experience within the boundaries of the physical universe or in the imagination. Beyond the shackles of space and time, the imagination allows one to transform images in the direction of healing: "The present instant is the stilling of time, and imagination is the presence of the present displayed, permitting the human being to move toward order" (Epstein, 1986, p. 27).

The reason that the will is more capable within the imagination is because it is beyond physical time and space and the imagination does not contain the same cause and effect dynamics as the physical world.

Similarly, within the mind, imagery is an inductive process, which works in an opposite manner from deductive verbal reasoning. Epstein (1986, pp. 27–28) provides an apt description of the inductive and creative nature of the imagination:

> Just as gravity is a given in the physical world, a given of the imaginal process is the image's attribute that it is a part containing the whole .... All non-logical systems share the property of the part containing the whole. These systems are based on the inductive process, which moves from the particular to the general, in contrast to propositional systems that are based...on deductive logic and tend to go from the general to the specific .... Etymologically, "heal" is derived from a word meaning whole.

This is a description of the natural tendency of imaginary processes to go find their missing parts, to return wholeness, and thus to bring about healing. For example, try to imagine just a part of your leg, like your ankle, alone and isolated. You will find that this is nearly impossible to do. Your ankle image will repeatedly attempt to grow a foot on its bottom and a body on its top. This is the nature of image-based, experiential thought. Similarly, try to imagine a father alone. This does not make sense in the imagination. An image of a father involves other family members, children, along with those other aspects most associated with fatherhood (e.g., a pipe and slippers, a lawn mower). This is what Epstein means when he says that the part contains the whole. The ankle is a portion of the leg. The father is a portion of a family.

In our divergent, inductive reasoning, concepts are inherently fuzzy (Kosko, 1993), as opposed to dichotomous (e.g., black–white, true–false). In the divergent imagination, an ankle may or may not have a sock, or hair, or a particular shade of skin that covers it. In the divergent imagination, a father may smoke a pipe and wear slippers, he may mow the lawn in his robe, or he may care for his children. The image of father brings with it an infinite range of possibilities. Verbal, deductive logic works in the opposite direction: If it has a whole leg, it must have an ankle; if it is a male who is caring for his children, he must be a father. The end conclusion in deductive reasoning is clear, end of story, ankle or nonankle, father or nonfather. The end conclusion within the inductive realm of the imagination is never completely reached or completed. Rather, the imagination is always seeking resolution, conclusion, wholeness, and, thus, healing.

Let us return to the original question posed at the beginning of this section: How does imagery work? Our general answer was: Through the interaction of systems. At this point we may offer a more specific answer: Imagery allows for integration and adaptation in the flows of information within the consciousness of the body–mind. Admittedly, this is a very abstract suggestion. Flows of information? Consciousness of the body–mind? Integration and adaptation? To understand this suggestion concerning how imagery works, we will need to explore the nature of systems in greater detail. Epstein's (1986) suggestions about the systemic operations of the imagination were not based on scientific principles. Indeed, Epstein argues vigorously against the use of empirical evidence in the study of the imagination. Given his suggestions about the inherently nonmechanistic manner in which the imagination works, and the limitations of science in the mid 1980s, this standpoint appears quite valid for the time in which he was writing. However, a great deal of powerful systemic theory has been developed and tested in the last 20 years or so. Thus, taking along the wisdom of the inner doctor of the imagination, it will be useful to explore even further into the systemic operations of the body–mind to obtain an even deeper sense of how the imagination may restore body–mind integrity, flexibility, healing, and pain relief.

Self-Organizing Biopsychosocial Systems: The Operating Room of the Inner Physician

The operating room of the inner physician is a complex adaptive system. All sources of knowledge point toward this conclusion: The wisdom of the ancient healing traditions, the modern medical heroes Albert Schweitzer and Herbert Benson, and also the data of recent empirical investigations. Specifically, the extreme variability in analgesic responses to imagery, the idiosyncratic nature of individual healing images, and the large array of individual causal factors in pain suggest that imagery impacts pain in complex ways. As practitioners, we must be mindful not just of the unique set of causes that underlie each patient's pain experiences but also of the relations among those causes as they unfold over time.

Melzack's seminal *gate-control theory* of pain (Melzack & Wall, 1965, 1996) opened the theoretical gate to the impact of numerous psychosocial factors on pain perception (e.g., attention, beliefs, coping behaviors, personality, social relations). Imagery may impact each of these interactive factors and thus may impact pain in complex and unique ways across individuals. However, studies investigating more complex models of treatment that incorporate this idea have not been forthcoming.

As was outlined previously, many studies have demonstrated the pain-reducing impacts of guided imagery both in lab-based efficacy studies on analogue pain and in effectiveness studies of clinical pain. Nevertheless, answers to the process-related treatment questions of how, how much, which types, and for whom have remained elusive. The most consistent result (besides general effectiveness) has been pronounced within-subject variability in response to imagery, with some participants showing large benefits and some very little or none (Fernandez & Turk, 1989; Hackett & Horan, 1980; Holroyd & Penzien, 1986; Mannix et al., 1999; Stevens, 1985; Stevens et al., 1987; Tan, 1982; Turner & Chapman, 1982; Worthington & Shumate, 1981). These results appear to be a product of the use of linear research tools to study a decidedly nonlinear phenomenon. From a systems perspective, the magnification of individual differences that has occurred in these experimental investigations suggests that imagery treatments are having complex, multifaceted impacts on the participants, a potentially interesting result in its own light (Pincus, 2006).

This interpretation is suggested even more strongly due to the gross simplicity of most experimental imagery treatments, most of which involve 2 minutes or less of imagery training (Pincus et al., 2003). Indeed, simple interventions are necessary within traditional experimental designs. They are a hallmark of good experimental research and are not expected to result in increased error in dependent variables. Nevertheless, study after study has demonstrated the splintering of well-controlled imagery interventions into complex, multifaceted, and idiosyncratic reactions by participants, like white light that is refracted through a prism. Far from "error" (as it is usually treated in linear statistics procedures), this type of effect serves as a sign that imagery impacts pain by way of a complex system. Moreover, it is even more impressive that these rather simple interventions have shown such consistent efficacy. It is therefore logical to conclude that deeper, more individually tailored image therapies may hold even greater potential for treating pain. Yet the limitations of customary research practices impede the empirical investigation of interventions that are more ecologically valid, multifaceted, and tailored to unique patient presentations.

Gradually, the clinical research is going to catch up with theoreticians and practitioners who are using multimodal and individually tailored treatments. As in other sciences (e.g., mathematical physics), psychological theory often outpaces empirical verification. In the area of systems theory applied to pain and imagery, this is clearly the case. We are not suggesting that there is anything intrinsically wrong with empirical research or superior about theory. On the contrary, the slow pace of empirical verification is a testament to the fact that we lay more trust in empirical results, as they are more carefully derived than expert theory, no matter how logical or brilliant a particular theory may seem. Nevertheless, it will be useful to examine the development of the latest systems approaches to understanding pain and imagery and to consider them along with strong clinical judgment as we await empirical verifications and refinements.

Classical Systems Theories

Despite the focus on simple treatments and simple causes, theoreticians have been mindful of the systemic nature of pain and imagery since the beginning of clinical research in this area (Tan, 1982; Weisenberg, 1979). Within these early systemic models, the individual factors underlying pain are conceptualized as parts of a larger pathogenic system, and the keys to therapeutic change are considered to reside within the relationships among causal factors rather than within a single independent cause.

Following from this *general systems* tradition, Melzack (1999) proposes an updated version of the original gate-control theory referred to as the *neuromatrix* theory. This model centers on a homeostatic general systems framework (Engel, 1977; Von Bertalanffy, 1968) in which pain and stress work together in an adaptive manner, acting as a kind of emergency brake to prevent dangerous fluctuations in regulatory body processes, such as temperature or blood sugar.

During the 30-year period between the gate-control and neuromatrix theories, a variety of similar *biopsychosocial* models have been proposed (Dworkin, Von Korff, & LeResche, 1992; Engel, 1977; Turk & Flor, 1999). Each model has attempted to integrate biological, psychological, and social factors, again primarily from the viewpoint of traditional general systems theory, which despite its more promising epistemology has been hindered by a lack of theoretical precision and empirical methodology (Pincus, 2006). Indeed, some of the best ideas about the workings of general systems underlying imagery have been limited due to their antiresearch perspective (i.e., Epstein, 1986). Just as linear research designs should not pretend that simple causes are the only possible causes, systems theory need not dispense with research altogether. With respect to understanding imagery, the former is myopic to the point of near blindness, whereas the latter throws the baby out with the bathwater and begs the question of why we would use an antiempirical "theory" instead of just returning to the shamanist healing traditions of the past.

Chapman, Nakamura, and Flores (1999) are among the first to take a balanced approach to understanding pain, allowing for complex causes while developing a theory that is testable. They begin by nesting pain within the context of consciousness. They then describe consciousness as an *emergent* and *self-organizing* system (p. 35). The concepts of emergence and self-organization belong to a broader class of models existing under the umbrella of nonlinear dynamical systems (NDS) theory, which is an updated and more empirically oriented version of the general systems theory of the 1960s (for a review of NDS research in psychology, see Guastello, 2004). Each of the specific modeling strategies within NDS has in common the ability to account for disproportional and complex causes that unfold over time. The dynamics of emergence and self-organization more specifically refer to the spontaneous order that has been observed to emerge in systems once a sufficient number of causal agents become involved in the exchange of matter, energy, or (in the case of psychological systems) information (Bak, 1996; Haken, 1984; Kauffman, 1993, 1995; Prigogine & Stengers, 1984). The spontaneous order of anthill creation, flocking behavior, and neural networks are well-established examples of self-organizing emergence from biological systems, whereas the therapeutic bond (Tschacher, Scheier, & Grawe, 1998), coordination in small-group problem solving (Guastello, Hyde, & Odak, 1998), and family dynamics (Pincus, 2001) represent a few examples observed within psychological systems.

In addition to emergence and self-organization, a number of other concepts from NDS may become helpful in guiding the research and practice of imagery treatment for pain. Because of its inherently systemic outlook, NDS theory is able to cross disciplinary boundaries from physics and chemistry through biology and into psychology. Thus, it opens the door to a search for general principles that apply across scientific disciplines and across scales of measurement (from small to large and back), a search that moves in the opposite direction from traditional, linear, and reductionist research in psychology (Guastello, 1997). Furthermore, in perhaps a more practical sense, NDS methodology would not be hindered to the same extent by problems such as the error variance of the outcome research just described. Therefore, the following concepts have the advantage of accounting for complex explanations of healing imagery that are more consistent with ancient healing traditions while remaining empirically testable.

Complexity, Overdetermination, and Fractal Geometry

The theoretical concepts that may be most helpful in future research and therapy for pain fall under the umbrella of *complexity theory*, which is related to self-organization and theories of complex adaptive systems. Complexity theory (Kauffman, 1993, 1995) examines the processes through which systems emerge, self-organize, and change adaptively over time. According to complexity theory, pain syndromes would be expected to emerge through the complex coupling of many causal factors as they *inform* one another over time. For example, when a patient feels pain and withdraws and lies in bed all day, the patient is informing a negative self-concept. This information may inform the person to feel bad, which informs hopeless thoughts, all of which may feed back on the original pain to make the experience more noxious and debilitating. Complex information feedforward and feedback mechanisms lead to general coherence and self-regulation within a patient's pain system. Quite literally, the pain system emerges and then gains a life of its own.

Like other living systems, the pain becomes *overdetermined*, meaning that there are more than sufficient causes to generate and sustain the pain syndrome over time, even if one or more of the individual causal factors is improved through treatment. For example, if withdrawal to bed is stopped through sheer willpower, the negative self-concept, affect, and thoughts could fill even the healthiest activities with pain. As such, overdetermination within pain systems makes them robust against treatment effects. On the other hand, this overdetermination may assist clinicians if they focus their interventions on key systemic processes within the pain system. For example, if the negative self-concept occupies the most central role as a conduit of unhealthy information for the other factors, imagery targeting one's sense of self may be the most efficient intervention. This common-sense idea is similar to the misguided search for *magic bullets* in traditional clinical trials from biomedical research (Engel, 1977). However the NDS approach is different in that it identifies its targets based on its relationship with other causes rather than on its independence from them, and it allows for a unique set of targets to exist for each patient. Furthermore, complex adaptive systems display some characteristic structural features that may provide clues about the location of these key targets of intervention for both clinicians and researchers.

Specifically, if pain systems are self-organizing, they likely will display *fractal* characteristics. In other words, they will be self-similar or isomorphic across scales. Self-similarity across scales means that if you were to enlarge a small part of the pattern it will look similar to the whole pattern. For example, a branch, up close, looks like the whole tree. Fractal patterning provides a clue that the underlying process is an open, self-organized system (Bak, 1996), and, indeed, fractals are ubiquitous in natural systems that generate branching patterns across space or time, such as plants, geological fault lines, earthquake magnitudes, heartbeat intervals, snowflakes, and rivers (Kauffman, 1995; West & Deering, 1995); they are like the fingerprint of Mother Nature.

Hypothetically, fractal geometry may help to explain how similar patterns may be found in pain phenomena across life domains and across scales, such as common stereotypic/rigid patterning in interpersonal dynamics, pain behavior, pain cognition, and physical processes at the site of pain. One rather striking example of fractal patterning may be found in clinical accounts of specific symptoms that are represented symbolically within images (Sheikh, 1986), such as images of burning, tearing, or blockage. In these instances, the pain images and physical symptoms may be considered to be different branches from the same systemic tree. As such, fractal geometry could help to provide a deeper theoretical grounding for the clinical wisdom that has led to a focus on such images in treatment.

Self-Regulation

Prior to formal NDS theory, the self-regulation central to complex adaptive systems was referred to as positive feedback within cybernetic models (DeAngelis, Post, & Travis, 1986; Wiener, 1948). Again, circular cause means that either directly or through a chain of intervening events, a variable regulates itself or the system in which it is embedded. The result is a kind of snowballing process, whereby changes in the variable at a starting point self-amplify, leading to increasing change over time. Eventually, a ceiling or floor is reached within these processes of exponential change, like a snowball rolling downhill that reaches some critical size. One well-studied example of positive feedback in neurophysiological pain processes is the killing of cells in the hippocampus (a brain region associated with the consolidation of memory as well as the processing of emotion) by high cortisol levels that are released in response to chronic negative affect (e.g., stress). As the hippocampus is destroyed, an individual hypothetically becomes less able to cope with negative emotions, which increases cortisol levels, causing further damage to the hippocampus and so on (Melzack, 1999). In a psychological example, one's expectation of pain may lead one to search for pain until it emerges to a mild extent, leading to catastrophic thinking, negative affect, a search for sympathy, a more intense focus on the pain, and so on, cascading to the point where the pain reaches its maximum.

Yet living open systems are not truly cybernetic or homeostatic, and this fact leads NDS researchers to question the notion of set points and simple feedback relationships within the life sciences (Bak, 1996; Prigogine & Stengers, 1984). The primary reason for this revised thinking is the fact that living systems have the ability to break down and reorganize in more complex and functionally adaptive ways in response to internal or external crises. Although it would be advantageous to design car engines that could reassemble following breakdowns, mechanical systems lag behind natural systems in this respect (at least so far). Self-regulating mechanisms can govern the behavior of the *entire* system and even invoke a systemic reorganization. Thus, self-organizing systems have the potential to exhibit metafeedback, global self-regulation. This global self-regulation inherent in living systems is a technical description of the more intuitively appealing inner physician described by Albert Schweitzer and others. The system seeks to find the most adaptive global response to challenge and to heal in response to damage. When imagery is done correctly, the patient and practitioner join with and provide assistance to this self-regulating process.

Once identified, the self-regulating mechanism of pain may be used therapeutically in a couple of complementary ways. First, a clinician may try to break the causal chain at some *singular point* (Prigogine & Stengers, 1984), which is a fragile point in the system that is critical for overall systemic tuning, like the first domino in a systemic row. For example, imagine one finds the causal chain: pain signals → increased somatic focus → negative expectation → negative affect → pain signals. Various imagery techniques may be aimed at one or more of the causal links, such as transforming the pain signals, distracting from the increasing somatic focus, blocking the negative affect through positive emotive imagery, changing the negative expectations through covert coping practice, reinforcing a nonpain schema, or resolving symbolic imaginal conflicts associated with the pain. Within a fractal structure, these singular points would likely involve the clinical factor occupying the most central role within the information exchange process of the pain system, like the trunk of the systemic tree. Hypothetically, images occupy such a position for many patients. The complement to this sort of regulatory chain breaking at the system's information crossroads is to reinforce the healthy self-regulation processes that run counter to the pain processes, such as the continued practice of switching from pain images to healthy images over time (Ahsen, 1984), which will lead to positive feedback between self-efficacy regarding pain and the decreased severity and chronicity of pain experiences. In other words, therapists need to help patients find things that work and to encourage them to do more of those things, living the prescriptions of the inner physician.

Homeostasis and Far-from-Equilibrium Dynamics

Much of Melzack's (1999) neuromatrix theory of pain was based on the somewhat antiquated cybernetic notion that living systems seek homeostasis or equilibrium (Prigogine & Stengers, 1984). This position is based on the idea that biological systems are mechanistic and closed, meaning that the boundaries of the system are sharp and clear, again like the engine in a car. It is now commonly understood that living, natural systems are open and that they constantly exchange matter, energy, and information with other systems (Bak, 1996). This ability for open systems to exchange information is the primary distinction that allows open, living systems to self-organize from a chaotic state and, in a related fashion to reorganize in a more complex form in response to a challenge without breaking the second law of thermodynamics (which states that entropy increases invariably over time; Prigogine & Stengers, 1984). In living systems, equilibrium is equivalent to death because once equilibrium is achieved, change becomes impossible, precluding systemic adaptation.

However, pieces of the old homeostatic notions are correct. Though a system as a whole does not seek homeostasis, certain systemic parameters (e.g., brain temperature; Melzack, 1999) may require careful tuning to keep them from crossing critical thresholds, which would lead to some unfortunate systemic reorganization (Kauffman, 1993), such as the transformation from being alive (far from equilibrium) to being dead (homeostatic). Research in NDS has demonstrated that often multiple and complex changes in systemic variables serve to maintain these critical set points for other areas. For example, tightrope walkers may flail their arms wildly to stay balanced on one foot when falling would constitute a major threat to the entire system. So, a system may display far-from-equilibrium dynamics (Prigogine & Stengers, 1984) in one aspect while maintaining relatively narrow set points in one or more other systemic parameters.

With this in mind, Melzack's (1999) notion of pain as a quasi-adaptive response within physiological systems may be expanded to pain's relationships with psychosocial set points. An obvious theoretical candidate for many pain patients would be bottled-up emotions, particularly anger. If one's sense of self, interpersonal domain, or early learning history has taught one that anger must be constrained to a relatively low critical threshold, physical pain may become a functional means of constraint through a variety of processes, such as distraction. At the same time, pain could be a consequence of affective constraint through physiological processes such as muscular tension. Theoretically, imagery may allow an individual to cross these emotional boundaries in an as-if state, which, due to its decreased threat and increased freedom, may be more therapeutic than the actual expression of anger. Or, less directly, imagery may serve as good practice for more assertive expressions of anger in the future.

Bifurcation Theory

The existence of nonlinear relationships within systems by definition indicates that changes to some parameters, even large changes, will make no difference within the overall system whereas other, even minuscule, changes will alter the overall phenomenon drastically. As in the previous example, a change in the expression of negative affect, such as anger, may lead to the emergence of new coping responses within the self-system, removing the need for a pain syndrome to maintain a dysfunctional emotional range. A *bifurcation point* is simply a value for a parameter in a system, which, if crossed, will reorganize the system in some qualitative sense (Kauffman, 1993). It is a threshold that acts like a dynamical key, unlocking a new systemic organization, for example, between illness and health. Bifurcation points are a more general class of the singular points (Prigogine & Stengers, 1984) previously described and thus may unshackle self-regulatory dynamics when they are crossed.

For pain patients, bifurcation theory helps to explain why there is so much variability in the responses of different individuals to the same treatment: Everyone's pain systems ought to contain unique arrangements of bifurcation points. Furthermore, the related difficulty in treating and assessing pain within a single individual at different points in time may be explained by the idea that people's *bifurcation space* (a mapping of the threshold structure of a system in theoretical space; Kauffman, 1993) can have dynamic qualities itself. This means that people's systemic relationships change over time such that the thresholds may be continually reshuffled. The most extreme example of differential treatment response occurs when patients respond strongly to placebo treatments (Spanos et al., 1993). One explanation is that these individuals have extracted the necessary information from the placebo to activate a bifurcation. In other words, people fit themselves into therapies to some degree, and not simply the other way around, analogous to a lightning bolt that seems to move only downward from a cloud but actually arises from ground points to meet the cloud charge partway up.

Again, imagery can help patients cross bifurcation points within the safety of a covert world, where consequences will be relatively immaterial and thus less damaging. Bifurcation theory assists therapists in seeking out and crossing imaginary boundaries with patients. It allows therapists to reasonably expect that these points will exist for some patients. Therefore, therapists may assume from the outset that large changes at a single point in therapeutic time-space may have little impact whereas some small change at another point may have a huge impact; this would be an illogical anomaly to be ignored or explained away within biomedical models (Engel, 1977).

Once therapists' eyes are opened to possible bifurcation points within patients' imaginal landscapes, they may focus their searches on points of resistance, difficulty in imagining, or incomplete images (Ahsen, 1984; Sheikh, 1986). For example, most people can imagine themselves in a hostile state given a hostility-evoking imaginal context. The inability to do so or the presence of other defenses in the form of rigidity, strain, and overcompensation may point to a relatively shallow bifurcation point. Finally, once a bifurcation is crossed, the patient can be assisted in developing a sense of control and efficacy over its future management. In other words, if a particular healthy image is uncovered that removes the pain phenomenon from its ecological niche within the pain system, this image and the extended range of possible systemic vector states that goes with it can be reinforced and integrated into a patient's everyday life.

Information Entropy, the Edge of Chaos, and Health

For some individuals at a given point in time, a bifurcation point may exist within a schematic location that is not readily accessible to the current self. For example, there may be an unsolved problem within some specific episodic memory, which has been buried under layers of subsequent experience (Ahsen, 1973). This idea is similar to psychodynamic notions of the unconscious effects of early trauma but may be updated through an appreciation for cognitive research viewed from an NDS perspective. Children are less able than mature adults to respond with flexibility to different challenges. One reason for this rigidity may be the relative immaturity of self, other, and world schemata in children. To maintain these relatively fragile representations, children respond in rather stereotypic, predictable, and inflexible ways to various challenges. For instance, cognition ideally progresses from simple object-based reasoning, to concrete representative thinking and on to abstract reasoning (Piaget, 1972). Similarly, behavioral sets evolve from rather simple and predictable patterns to more sophisticated and complex (varied) sets of responses as one matures. For example, a young child who is being teased may have only the options of fighting back or running away. An older child may have the previous options and, in addition, may entertain the possibilities of telling an adult or of enlisting a coalition of other children against the bully. An adult ideally would have even more available options.

In regard to pain and imagery, this evolutionary progression toward increasing complexity and flexibility may suggest that inflexibility or rigidity in pain-related imagery would underlie the systemic causes of clinical pain. In other words, rigidity, stereotypy, and predictability would be the soil from which chronic and recurrent pain syndromes would be expected to grow. Research in the area of complexity is coming to an increasingly clear view that systems poised at the edge of chaos (EOC) (Kauffman, 1993, 1995)—also known as the point of self-organized criticality (SOC) (Bak, 1996)—are the most functional and adaptive. A technical description of the EOC–SOC boundary region is beyond the bounds of the current discussion. Metaphorically, however, it is a sort of transition region between frozen, relatively static systemic behavior in which small changes in one part of the system do not do much to the rest of the system and a boiling, turbulent system in which even small changes are amplified in wild, relatively unpredictable ways. At the SOC–EOC boundary, the best of both worlds exists: a coherence that keeps system parameters from fluctuating wildly and a flexibility that allows parameters to change in adaptive ways over time based on internal and external challenges to the system. These varied lines of interdisciplinary research may help to explain the progression from simple and rigid to complex and flexible in the development of psychological systems.

In the case of clinical pain, one may reasonably argue that some aspect of the self-system has been stalled in this progression, residing at the rigid, static end of the continuum due to a loss of information complexity. In the short run, the rigid information boundaries that limit information within patients' psyches may help to maintain integrity, to keep them from coming unglued so to speak. The notion is similar to homeostatic models of pain where some significant parameter, such as expressed anger, must be maintained around a set point. However, within the psychological systems related to pain, it may be more accurate to suggest that a number of information boundaries exist that keep critical thresholds from being crossed, such as the expression of ego-dystonic anger or the experience of a traumatic memory. The self is maintained, albeit in a more rigid, more primitive, and less adaptive state.

Living systems are open and interactive, exchanging information complexity both horizontally among classes and vertically across scales (Prigogine & Stengers, 1984). In some cases, synergetic attunement occurs among neighboring systems, leading to broad synchrony and coherence (Haken, 1984). Thus, it is possible that especially insidious cases of clinical pain may enslave other biological and psychological systems pertaining to the person. The most extreme clinical example of this is when pain invades a patient's sense of self and social domains so that the person becomes rigidly cast in a sick role (Weisenberg & Keefe, 2002). In other words, a rigid and stereotyped response to nociception at the physiological level may reach out and grab hold of the person's self-schema, interpersonal schema, and affective range, rendering them all relatively static, predictable, inflexible, and thus less adaptive over time. The pain system creates a degraded fractal structure within the person's biopsychosocial system. Just as a tree with only one branch will have trouble thriving in a forest, a person with one painful mode of interacting may not fare well socially.

Another possibility is that self-organizing pain systems sap the complexity from neighboring systems by draining them of information. Again, open systems must interact with other open systems, importing and exporting information as systemic behavior becomes more or less complex respectively (Prigogine & Stengers, 1984). Thus, the systems that interact most proximally with a pain system could theoretically become more rigid, inflexible, and information deprived as the pain system feeds of their complexity, like a parasite that drains nutrients from a host. Conversely, if the information and flexibility can be restored to these neighboring systems, such as through the imaginal traversing of bifurcation points within those systems, then this life-giving entropy is reclaimed from the pain system and given back to a person's psyche.

This last bit of theory is admittedly very abstract. A more down-to-earth example is a medical doctor's test for physical rigidities in pain assessment and treatment, such as pressure checks on tender spots (Albright & Fischer, 1990; Okifuji & Turk, 1999; Weisenberg, 1979) or assessing one's range of motion in painful injuries. Imagery psychotherapists may seek out tender and inflexible spots of the person's representational system that are attached to the pain phenomenon (e.g., an episodic memory of a trauma preceding the onset of symptoms). These spots may be transformed theoretically by crossing a bifurcation point, leading to increased complexity and flexibility in the images, choking the information supply to the parasitic pain system, just as newer cancer treatments (e.g., angiogenesis) aim to stop the growth of the blood supplies to cancerous tumors (Cooke, 2001).

This comparison between rigid psychosocial dynamics and rigid physiological dynamics at pain sites may in fact be literal as opposed to metaphoric: Rigid isomorphic phenomena may cross scalar boundaries from consciousness to physiology and back up within a fractal, branching causal structure. For example, Flor, Birbaumer, Schugens, and Lutzenberger (1992) found that patients with chronic back pain showed stereotypic muscle responses at their specific injury sites in response to stressful imagery, just like a plant that shakes all over when one small branch is moved. In addition, they found significant relationships among measures of coping styles, pain chronicity, physiological arousal, and subjective ratings of stress. Even though their results were not interpreted from an NDS perspective, they suggest the possibility that rigidity may branch from cognition, through physiology, and on to specific muscles at pain sites.

If these insights are correct, the specific causes of psychogenic pain may not matter as much as the discovery of the rigid systems in which the pain is nested, followed by a therapeutic journey across the bifurcation points within one or more of those systems. The expected therapeutic results within the representational and physiological systems would be increasing and more flexible information flows among these systems, washing out the rigid, painful processes.

Imagery as Shadow Experience

Imagery is generally considered to be a set of techniques rather than a theory of psychotherapy per se, and imagery work is compatible with virtually any theory of psychotherapy, from cognitive-behavioral to psychodynamic (McMahon & Sheikh, 1986). When viewed within the context of the systems concepts outlined herein, this often overlooked ubiquity of imagery across the schools of psychotherapy may become clearer.

Bandura's (1977, 1986) social-learning theory represents the most mainstream scientific view of imagery; it is a shadow to experience. Bandura improved on mechanistic radical behavioral views of human learning by stressing the role of information as opposed to learning history in guiding behavior. His highly influential theory of social learning describes four sources of information ranging in strength from largest to smallest: actual experience, vicarious experience, physiological information, and verbal persuasion. Vicarious experience means observational learning, which includes self-imagery as a relatively potent form of vicarious experience due to the obvious similarity (unity) between the subject and object.

Many of the tests of imagery on pain rely either implicitly or explicitly on images as social-learning experiences, in which a person may learn to cope better with pain through covert rehearsal of coping techniques to be used later during a pain episode (e.g., Achterberg et al., 1988) or by providing imaginal coping strategies that give a person actual coping experiences. Though these techniques have been shown to be helpful in reducing the impact of pain, they may be seen as somewhat palliative, improving self-efficacy in a person's ability to manage pain rather than transforming consciousness to a state in which pain is no longer welcome. We would suggest here that Bandura's theory has moved our understanding of imagery in the correct direction but that a deeper and more central understanding of imagery may help to make better sense of both empirical and also clinical observations.

The Triple Code Theory

Each of the foregoing NDS concepts is consistent with and in some cases equivalent (albeit with different vocabulary) to the ideas within the triple-code model (Ahsen, 1972, 1984, 2000; Sheikh, 1986) of imagery therapy. According to the model, images (I), somatic responses (S), and meaning (M), together known as ISM, are linked codes within images that Ahsen (1972) refers to as *eidetics* (the term as used by Ahsen is not to be confused with eidetic memories from cognitive psychology; for a review of this distinction see Richardson, 1983). When the imaginal system is integrated, activation of any of the three codes leads to the emergence of the other two states in any variety of orders depending on a number of clinically relevant factors (Hochman, 2002).

The triple-code model (Ahsen, 1984, 2000) is a modern theory of imagery that may fit well within an NDS understanding of pain. The ISM model suggests that activation of any of the three codes (image, somatic, or meaning) will invariably lead to the emergence of the other two states to which it is linked. So if someone holds a specific image in consciousness, a specific somatic response and meaning structure will emerge; conversely, a change to any of the coded states will lead to a change in the others. Also, any of the codes may be primary in invoking the other two. For example, meaning may invoke syntonic images, which then invoke syntonic somatic states. This theory of imagery closely parallels independent lines of empirical work in cognitive psychology known as neoassociationism (Berkowitz, 1993), which again describes the connections of emotional states, episodic memories, sensations, thought processes, and meaning structures (schema) through the activation of theoretical nodes, which are connected in a complex, associationistic network. Achterberg et al. (1988, p. 84) describe this theoretical process as it relates to the effectiveness of imagery treatment for reducing the intense pain associated with burn treatments:

> Image, somatic response, and meaning become linked in an infinite number of complex ways and predetermine behavior, attitudes, and all manner of human functions…. Interpretation of the situation has drawn its power from the somatic-image bond…. The current protocol [imaginal coping] apparently served to unyoke physiological and verbal expressions of fear and pain associated with burn treatment. And hence, reactions to the actual treatment were somewhat ameliorated.

Within the triple-code model, images, sensations, and meaning enter consciousness in tandem and may be pulled into consciousness through a change to any of the individual pieces. Thus, states of consciousness emerge like patterns of string in a game of cat's cradle (the children's game in which a string is wrapped in complicated ways around the upturned fingers of both hands). Changing the way a single segment of string is wrapped around even one finger invokes the emergence of a whole new pattern in the strings across both hands.

Hochman (2002) suggests that the triple-code model might serve as a more general theoretical model (beyond the narrow context of pain imagery) that might be useful for updating analytic personality theory in a manner that is more consistent with modern biological science, is more ecologically valid, and is more amenable to scientific inquiry. Indeed, she even makes some rare references to NDS in her discussions of the approach: "His [Ahsen's] system runs parallel with the new chaos or dynamical systems theory" (p. 129). Furthermore, Ahsen (2000) introduces constructs such as *ISM strings* that are described as dynamic process structures involving image, soma, and meaning. These structured yet dynamic strings may be thought to act like information vectors, providing direction and velocity within the flows of consciousness.

When considered from an NDS perspective, each aspect of the triple code may be conceptualized as a channel of information. Therefore, the disintegration of the eidetic (disconnection of Image, Sensation, or Meaning) hypothetically involves a decrease of information entropy at the site of (biopsychosocial) injury. If this is the case, eidetic psychotherapy may work by restoring integrity and biopsychosocial flexibility that is lifeblood to a wounded system. These ideas have remained central within the applied eidetic imagery texts from the theory's inception (e.g., Ahsen, 1972) up to more contemporary practice (e.g., Dolan, 1997).

While it is centrally relevant to imagery, Ahsen's work lies outside of the mainstream of psychotherapy. Furthermore, although the triple-code theory began with a close alliance to behavior therapy (Ahsen & Lazarus, 1972), it has evolved away from incorporating behavioral principles toward the more esoteric, nonempirical clinical traditions associated with psychoanalysis. Recently, behavior therapies have been evolving toward similar abstract ideas emphasizing the importance of subjective realities of individuals and the ways language representations may hinder learning by closing off individuals to experiential awareness (Hayes, 2004). However, these developments have focused more on verbal language relations and logic rather than on broader imagery processes proposed in similar work by Ahsen and others. Still, it appears that the trend in psychotherapy toward integration will involve unifying concepts such as flexibility, integrity, and openness to information.

The Imagery-Sensory Lexicon of Experience

Ahsen (1984) argues against Bandura's (1977) view of imagery as an epiphenomenon or shadow experience and assigns it a more central position in guiding meaning-making processes and somatic responses in a nonsequential and nonlinear manner. Furthermore, this central position is maintained whether the person is currently attending to the image. From this perspective, Bandura's (1977) sources of confidence building information may be considered to exert their influence by changing the dynamic flow of images, which continually underlie people's experiences. Actual experiences would then be expected to enhance efficacy expectations simply because they are the most vivid and absorbing, which gives them greater image shifting impact. Bandura's (1986) own research results may be reinterpreted to support the view that images are a central factor in guiding such aspects of consciousness as behavioral sets, affect, and somatic responses. For example, Bandura (1986) found that snake phobics' ability to handle boa constrictors was better predicted by efficacy expectations than by actual past experiences. This suggests that the current imaginal states of individuals with respect to snake handling were the best predictors for their snake-related behaviors whether or not they were focusing on the images per se. In other words, their state-specific snake-handler slide shows were rolling somewhere in their consciousness whether they were consciously watching them or not. This idea is not very different from the mainstream notion of self-talk from cognitive therapy, which aims to identify unconscious (i.e., automatic) self-talk that is believed to underlie anxiety and depression (Beck, 1991). In fact, people's preference for imagery-based interventions over self-talk in response to painful stimulation would suggest that self-talk may in fact represent a running commentary on the content of images as opposed to independent cognition relating to sensory input. Contrasting the differential levels of attention required to attend to images versus self-talk in a controlled experiment could serve as a rather simple test of this hypothesis.

Furthermore, this running slide show interpretation may help to explain the comparable therapeutic efficacy of hypnotic analgesic suggestions with and without imagery (Hargadon et al., 1995) and some nonimaginal placebo treatments for pain. For example, Spanos et al. (1993) had an especially strong and unanticipated placebo effect in pain reduction, larger than the impact of a self-monitoring control condition and even somewhat larger than their experimental imagery-hypnosis intervention designed for chronic headache sufferers. Their placebo condition involved looking at four slides of random dots, flashed for 0.5 seconds at 15-second intervals, a flashing rate that made the stimulus sufficiently ambiguous. Participants were told that the slides contained hidden messages designed to ameliorate pain by changing their unconscious autonomic processes. Finally, a specific key word was paired with the treatment to be used as a mnemonic cue during periods of stress or headache to trigger calmness and healing. Furthermore, the positive results of this rather sophisticated placebo were not related to expectations of treatment efficacy, which tended to be low at the outset of treatment. So it is unlikely that the results were based on expectation biases. One reasonable explanation for their results is that the participants projected their own healing images on the ambiguous slides and invoked them later to modify unhealthy images associated with their headaches, all without conscious attention to the images. If this was in fact the case, the hoax may have been on the experimenters, who designed a bogus intervention and therapeutic rationale, which in fact worked just as they said it would.

The role of images as central guiding factors in current reality-making processes is also in line with research on the role of top-down processes on perception described in Chapter 1. The overall picture that emerges is that states of consciousness are continually constructed through the self-organized mixing of bottom-up sensory process and top-down imaginal process. Each experience emerges from the backdrop of an imagery-sensory lexicon of possible states of consciousness, and with each comes a limited range of affective, sensory, cognitive, and somatic vectors of change over time. As such, if the imagery-based factors involved in pain consciousness can be ameliorated through the direct transformation of the associative network in which they are nested, the experience of certain pain disorders will no longer be possible after successful treatment. This explanation is in line with empirical studies that have found relationships between absorption in but not vividness of images and therapeutic efficacy (Kwekkeboom, Huseby-Moore, & Ward, 1998; Marino et al., 1989; Spanos & O'Hara,

1990). This idea is also in line with the rigidity/flexibility hypothesis supported by NDS theory, which suggests that a pain system may dissipate if the consciousness making processes attached to it are infused with adaptive flexibility. On the grandest scale, this line of thinking helps to bring the ancient and more clinically satisfying theories of imagery closer to empirical testability.

Imagery as a Schema Portal

Ultimately, the most efficient and effective use of imagery for pain that has a dominant psychogenic causal component is to transform the actual associative networks in which pain lives, be they schema, the neuromatrix (Melzack, 1999), consciousness (Chapman et al., 1999), the ISM (Ahsen, 1984) or neoassociationistic networks (Berkowitz, 1993). For convenience, and because all of these theoretical lines are essentially describing the same process structures, the term *schema* will be used to suggest that imagery may be viewed as a schema portal, through which people can gain access to their own consciousness-making structures. Once one has entered the schema portal, one experiences images with the same multidimensional flavor as actual experience (e.g., sights, sounds, touch). As a doorway to the abstract interconnections of consciousness, imagery therapy may provide the unique opportunity to experience one's own experience-making system and thus to modify it.

In imagery work, pain patients may be seen as astronauts who move through this schema portal into the experiential vacuum of inner space to work on the life support systems of the self. The imagery therapist may be seen as ground control, attempting to guide the astronaut through the often complicated procedures that must be carried out in the unique environment of the imagination, where time and space may be warped, where the will is enhanced, and where anything is possible. It is clear that a variety of therapeutic imagery techniques may be helpful in facilitating the process of self-discovery and self-modification of pain within this imaginal realm. The use of systems science in describing pain processes may provide a first step for practitioners, a sort of general orientation for the selection of specific procedures for specific patients.

Pain and Imagery: How It Works

The research results from the past 30 to 40 years are clear thus far: Imagery is a highly effective approach to pain management. These findings are consistent with the wisdom gleaned from more than 20,000 years of healing practices within the shamanic traditions. That is, imagery is an ancient art, which can now be studied through scientific means. Investigators and clinicians must take into account, however, the fact that both imagery and pain do not lend themselves readily to research methods that have traditionally been used to study material processes. Since imagery lies outside the bounds of time, space, and finite content, it has posed a challenge to researchers interested in understanding the broader and deeper role of the imagination in human experience. Similarly, the complex and highly variable causal systems underlying people's experiences with pain have contributed to a split between the available data of the scientist and the clinical knowledge of the practitioner.

The experimental and clinical research on imagery for pain each points to the same conclusion: Imagery is highly effective in the treatment of pain. Nevertheless, the research also suggests that people are prone to idiosyncratic responses to imagery. Furthermore, deep and individually tailored treatments and questions about how imagery works are still largely unaddressed. In these areas, practice remains well ahead of science.

The conflict created by this science-versus-practice distinction may be resolved through the use of concepts and methods from NDS. By focusing on the processes involved in pain imagery (rather than the content), these concepts allow for controlled examination of treatment effects without oversimplifying patients or interventions. Despite the infinite variety of pain images and treatment response seen in clinical practice, great similarities may exist in the processes of pain etiology and the structure of pain-related images. The most general prediction from NDS would be that pain-related images are more rigid and stereotypic than health-related images. Complexity theory further suggests that these rigid images may be systemically tied to rigid physiological processes across different scales (from material to emergent mental structures) of reality. This connection may exist within a fractal (branching) structure, which could be empirically identified and quantified with respect to complexity. If such a structure exists, it would suggest that pain systems are maintained through self-regulating information flows, which could be altered by crossing bifurcation boundaries (critical thresholds) within the pain system. Hypothetically, the experience of such a crossing of boundaries may act to return information flexibility, complexity, and integrity to pain-related eidetics.

Yet until these questions are examined empirically, therapists will continue to use deep, transformational imagery procedures to treat pain. A number of these procedures are described in Chapter 7. These approaches help clinicians to locate key pain-related images from episodic memory and to provide some heuristics for processing those images. Yet the specifics of where to go when and how are left to the creative sensibilities of the patient and therapist.

The various concepts from NDS may help practitioners as they wait for research to catch up with practice. NDS theory may also provide a rational that support the use of deep, comprehensive, and individually tailored interventions in treating pain. Indeed, most therapists are not waiting for science to tell them what to do during imagery therapy. The fact that imagery has shown such consistent efficacy in the treatment of pain may be more than enough evidence for most. Yet NDS may provide a language and a means to recognize the dynamics that occur during sessions, opening therapist's eyes to directions to search for therapeutic change in the imaginal realm and to ways to understand these changes as they occur spontaneously during treatment.

Metaphorically, the practitioners assume the role of ground control, assisting patients in making an inner voyage into the unbounded and infinite realms of their imaginations. Far more than make-believe or shadow to experience, these realms can be considered to be the central arena in which phenomenological meaning is created. Clinicians can thus feel more confident in targeting rigid images within this realm and in using dynamic (over imaginary time) and structural (over imaginary space) flexibility as a sign of positive treatment response. They may expect disproportionate change to occur when critical thresholds are crossed. They may expect rigidity to spread to neighboring systems, such as the self-systems and the interpersonal systems, and even across the "gate" to the physiological systems of patients in pain. Therapists may conceptualize imagery as a means to unlock trapped reservoirs of information that can rejuvenate these areas of biopsychosocial stagnation.

CHAPTER 4

The Process of Image Therapy

I can give you nothing that has not already its origins within your-self. I can throw open no picture gallery but your own. I can help make your own world visible. That is all.

Hermann Hesse
(Quoted in Sheikh, 2003, p. iii)

The following information is intended to help you to understand the process of image therapy and the ways that it will vary from patient to patient. It is helpful to have a road map of sorts and also a set of tools as you move through the treatment processes. This map will allow you to move more smoothly from the assessment and planning tasks of the first session to completion of the active phase of treatment. A set of general tools and principles will assist you in making any necessary detours you may need to take along the way.

There are so many things to remember and to accomplish during ther-apy that we are always at risk of losing track of the patient. We continu-ally assess all factors from the medical to psychosocial to make decisions regarding coordination with other colleagues on the treatment team and to consider adjunctive treatments that will be used along with imagery. We evaluate attitudes toward treatment, medical history, psychosocial history, and the specific dynamics of the patient's pain. We seek to form a strong working alliance, to develop a collaborative treatment plan, and to convey confidence. All the while, empathy is at the top of our list as well, as we try to gain a deeper and more detailed understanding of our patients' worlds. The list may go on and on, and the first session potentially can become a hurried and pressured experience.

We suggest instead that you approach each session in a patient-centered manner rather than an information-centered manner. Specifically, two things are crucial. First, ask your patients to tell you their stories. What brought them in to see you, where did it all begin, and what has happened along the way? Second, develop empathy. To empathize means to understand your patients' worldview in an *as-if* manner (Rogers, 1951). Sympathy, feeling your own emotional reaction based on your patients' experiences, may be fine. However, it is no substitute for empathy. The same may be said for advice, no matter how good that advice may be. There is no substitute for empathy, because empathy brings you into your patients' worlds. Empathy is far more than a technique or something that makes for a good working relationship. Empathy is the starting point for everything else you will do: assessment, treatment planning, rapport building, and intervention. The accuracy with which you are able to understand your patients' world will determine the quality of every other aspect of treatment. Everything depends on empathy. Furthermore, if your patients are able to bring you into their worlds, they will experience increases in their own self-understanding and insight as well as a release from the demoralizing isolation of being in pain. This will improve their sense of control and mastery over pain. Finally, empathy will allow you to dispense with working from a list of questions or being concerned about knowing what to ask. If you actively work at understanding your patients' worldviews, you will ask all the correct questions spontaneously based on the information you need to *get it*. How will you know when you get it? Your imagination will tell you. When you can imagine your patient's worldview, when you see it in your own mind, then you will be in a process of empathy, where the best treatment occurs.

Indeed, in the first sessions of therapy the emphasis is on entering a process of empathy, and this process will continue to guide your therapy from the beginning, through the middle, and to your final session. The use of image therapy for pain always will involve the imaginations of both the patient and the therapist. It is within the common ground of your co-imaginations that relief will come. Accept that this will be the case, and you will be able to focus more on your patient-guided imagination than the forms and questionnaires that always accompany our modern health-care environments. You will be more effective, and your patients will be appreciative.

The First Session

Fortunately, most of your patients will arrive to the first session wanting to tell you all about their pain, because most of the other people in their lives will be actively avoiding the topic. They typically will tell you about the pain in the form of a pain narrative—stories about them and their pain. Most of the information that you will want to gather during your first session will be covered spontaneously within the patient's pain narrative, and your follow-up questions may be based on attempts to acquire deeper empathy. Nevertheless, a few details will generally be overlooked. It is important to keep in mind that different pain patients will require different styles of assessments during the first session. For example, if you are treating an individual for fairly simple procedural pain (e.g., surgery), then a relatively quick assessment may be obtained to rule out complicating factors and to select imagery techniques (Syrjala & Abrams, 2002). More complex cases, such as chronic pain with possible personality disorders or trauma, will require more complex and detailed assessments. Furthermore, complex cases involving high levels of demoralization and difficulties in expressing relevant information may require a much slower process of assessment and treatment planning.

Within your patients' pain narratives, you should pay particular attention to their relationships with pain as well as to the cycles that occur within these relationships. The following is an example of a segment of a pain narrative from a patient with fibromyalgia:

> I can tell pretty much right away when I wake up if it's gonna be a good day or a bad day, so I start out wondering "what's the point?" To be honest I just wish I was dead. I know for sure, I'm not getting out of bed today, no matter what the doctors tell me, it's not gonna work. And I'm glad no one is in the house in the morning, because if they were they'd just piss me off anyway, because I can tell they're sick of it too, so they ignore me or try to get out of the house quicker so they don't have to deal with me. So I wake up with a mild ache all over, and my whole body, the muscles, the joints, they all seem like they're sort of screaming. Not like loud screaming, when the pain hits. More like they can hear it coming, you know like that sound of a missile about to hit, how it whistles? And they don't know what to do, like it's gonna hit 'em and they know they don't have anywhere they can hide. So I lie there waiting, and sure enough about five minutes later it always hits. It starts in my legs, around the knees; feels like the joints are swelling up like balloons about to "pop" and like my knee is just going to explode into tiny pieces of glass. Then usually my back starts to ache, and then it just sort of spreads like through my whole body. It's like a dull ache under my skin, and it sort of goes whomp … whomp … whomp … whomp, in a steady rhythm. But my joints are the worst. There it's like a sharp pain, and a feeling of swelling. Like that balloon feeling, you know?

This patient's pain narrative is rich with imagery as well as with information about her sense of coping style, identity, relationships with others, her relationship with treatment, and her relationship with the pain as well. This patient's dominant sense modality appears to be auditory, since a number of her spontaneous images were described in terms of sound (e.g., screaming muscles, whistling missile, popping joints). These images are potential targets for intervention, such as the anthropomorphized muscles that scream while waiting for pain and have no place to hide, the pain that first comes in the form of a missile strike, the balloon-like swelling of joints, the rhythmic aching of muscles, and the glass inside the joints when there is a pending explosion that never comes. For the image therapist, the details of these images are as important as the physical details conveyed by an x-ray. For this reason, the most important task of the first session is to listen with care to the narrative of the patient.

Determining your patients' dominant coping style will be helpful to you in designing a course of treatment and selecting specific techniques. For example, people who cope with pain in an active manner will more readily use imagery techniques in which they can participate. These patients will tend to want more involvement in guiding the treatment process and will move more quickly toward using imagery independently. Similarly, they will tend to be more active within their imaginations, conjuring up imaginary scenarios in which they play an active role in making transformations. These patients more likely will come from populations seeking treatment for acute or procedural pain rather than chronic pain.

The previously given narrative reflects a more typical, passive, and avoidant coping style, which has evolved over years of coping with the chronic discomfort of fibromyalgia pain. Such patients tend to respond best to a more directive treatment relationship and also to more directive and prescriptive imagery scenarios. They also tend to require more interaction with their treatment providers and more support toward becoming more autonomous and self-directing within their imaginations, until they eventually take over the direction of their own treatments. Finally, it is important to assess your patients' flexibility in coping, the ability to be more active or more passive across situations. Generally speaking, your treatment process will be easier with patients who are more flexible in their relations with pain as well as in their general relational and coping styles.

In addition to coping styles, you will need to assess the impacts of pain on your patients' relationships, particularly to family members. The previous narrative clearly suggests hurt and angry feelings toward family members who failed to understand her situation and who, she believes, are actually trying to avoid her. Beneath this hurt and anger, there probably is a deep sense of sadness, loneliness, and vulnerability. These feelings underscore her sense of hopelessness in the face of the pain as well as her thoughts of dying. It is clear as well that she is experiencing herself as a captive of the pain, which comes reportedly in the morning and takes away her entire day. Consequently, the morning will be a critical time on which to focus treatment so that she can gain a sense of control, allowing her to go out into her life and begin to build a healthier sense of identity.

A person's self-images are central to this sense of identity, and self-images are created within the context of relationships. For example, if your patient has become dependent upon family members as a result of her medical condition, then her self-images will involve dependency, and her identity will come to involve a sense of dependence as well. The more dependent she becomes, the more central will be dependence within her self-images and her sense of identity. Similarly, her self-images and identity will be negatively impacted by high levels of interpersonal rejection, conflict, and isolation as well. In many cases, family members will be actively involved in the treatment process, either within the office or within the home as your patients practice imagery techniques between sessions, and family involvement even may be as subtle as discussing the treatment with your patient. Even if you never meet these individuals, their beliefs and feedback to your patient may inform your patient's identity and relationship to treatment. As a result, it will be important to listen for the reactions of friends and family within your patients' pain narratives and to address any negative reactions at the outset of the treatment process.

Another key theme within your patients' pain narratives will be their relationships with your therapy process. The previous narrative mentions a distrust of the doctors' advice (e.g., I'm not getting out of bed today, no matter what the doctors tell me, it's not gonna work). Thus, we can assume that this patient will come to the treatment relationship expecting to be left short of options that she can count on in her daily experience. She is likely to come to the first session feeling misunderstood, vulnerable, angry, and generally distrustful of you and your interventions. Since your patients' relationships with treatment will impact every aspect of it from beginning to end, it is important to correct any distortion or misinformation at the outset and to help them develop more accurate and positive understanding of imagery and how it may be helpful to them. To address past treatment failures, attend with empathy to your patients' experience with other treatment providers and then work toward creating a more open, honest, and collaborative relationship with them, one that will be seen as distinct from past failures.

The most common problem you probably will encounter in the first session will be the demoralization that accompanies the idea that image therapy implies that their pain is not real—that it is all in their heads (Barber, 1996; Syrjala & Abrahams, 2002). The information presented in Chapters 1 to 3 was intended to provide you with an understanding of where this "all in your head" myth originated and why it is false. However, most of your patients will not appreciate this level of depth and detail presented in these chapters. Therefore, you may be more persuasive if you understand your patients' beliefs, however mistaken they may be, and address these particular beliefs with persuasive examples. These examples include the use of imagery by college athletes to promote quicker and less painful recovery from knee surgeries (Cupal & Brewer, 2001), the effectiveness of imagery in treating phantom limb pain, and the fact that the brain is the central location for pain perception, not the body. You then could describe imagery as the best possible way to impact neurological structures and functions. If you find yourself arguing, step back, and stop. Arguing will be nonproductive, no matter how correct your arguments may be. Instead, respond to arguments by attempting to develop deeper empathy with your patient. In this manner, you both may arrive at a deeper understanding of the particular resistance to imagery.

As you continue to introduce the topic of imagery with your patients, you will want to help them to develop their own simple conceptual models that will help them to understand how imagery works. Similarly, you will want to help them to understand how real pain can be treated with the imagination. One rather clear way of doing this is to explain the gate-control theory (Melzack & Wall, 1965) to your patients (Syrjala & Abrams, 1996):

> Pain is most often signaled by nerves in the body, which are trying to alert you to tissue damage so that you will be motivated to take some type of self-protective action. As these signals move up to the brain, they pass through an area at the base of the brain called the Substantia Gelatinosa, which researchers have found to act as a sort of a gate. If the gate is open wide, then the pain signals move from body to brain quickly and smoothly, signaling pain. When we close the gate, however, pain signals decrease. Some pain medications act to turn down the volume on those messages coming from the body, while some act to shut this gate. In a sense, medications pull the gate shut from the bottom, from the body, so that the brain doesn't get the signals. In imagery, we use the brain to do the same thing, naturally. In a sense, we are using your brain activity to push the gate shut from the top, shifting the mental activity that adds fuel to the fire. In this way, imagery works in the same way as pain medications, but from the opposite direction. Pain medications are more targeted and direct; so when they are working well, they tend to shut the gate tight. In addition to chemicals, the pain gate may open or close based on the emotions and the meaning that goes along with pain: the ways that the brain is interpreting and making sense out of the pain signals. So when we use imagery, we are changing the way your brain will react to these signals. This closes the gate, which low-

ers the intensity of your pain. Tell me, does this make sense? What questions do you have about what I just explained?

It is important to stress to patients who have pain syndromes in which physical causes of pain are not observable (e.g., fibromyaligia) that imagination as a treatment does not imply that imagination is the cause of their pain. One way to confront these assumptions is to point out how common it is for effective treatments to have little to do with causes of illness. For example:

> One thing I want to make clear is that your pain is real, absolutely real. No one would want to experience the discomfort you have been having. Believe me, I know this. So it is important for me to explain to you that our use of the imagination to decrease your pain does not in any way imply that the pain is simply in your imagination. Think instead of the imagination as the medicine. Many forms of medicine are effective and yet have little to do with the causes of illness. For example, colds are caused by a virus, correct? Yet rest, balanced meals, and liquids are the primary treatment for the common cold. A cold is caused by a virus, not by a deficiency in chicken soup and orange juice. And yet, balanced nutrition and rest help the body to fight the virus and to heal. By using imagery, we will help you find ways to find balance and calm mentally, so that your brain and body can better fight these pain signals, find a balance, and heal.

For many patients it will be helpful to go beyond verbal information and to provide experiential evidence that will demonstrate how imagery may be helpful with their pain. This may be accomplished rather simply during the natural flow of the consultation. For example, patients may be asked to rate their pain from 1 to 10 at the start of the consultation. Later, they may be asked to rate the pain they felt during a period in the consultation process in which they were engaged in the discussion. For a more directive approach, you may ask patients to rate their pain and then describe the happiest moment in their lives, obtaining full details about the event and the way they felt. Nearly every patient will report a decrease in pain following this narrative. Then you can compare these decreases in pain with the decreases in pain that you will be aiming to achieve by conjuring up soothing imagery.

Yet no matter how skilled you become in providing examples and explanations, it is vital to ascertain if they make sense to each patient. This is particularly true for patients with personality disorders and related conditions, which have led them to become significantly dysregulated, demoralized, or conflicted. Such individuals may be prone to misunderstand the information you are trying to convey, due to negative biases, concentration problems, or distrust. In these cases, it even may be helpful to ask patients to repeat the explanations back in their own words or to come up with their own examples of times when their pain improves along with changes in stress or mindset. You should explore any distortions in an open and nondefensive manner, with the goal of understanding your patient's perspective. Once you have that understanding, you may begin to have an open dialogue about imagery but not a moment before. Once again, everything in treatment begins with empathy.

At the outset of treatment, you also should assist your patients in understanding the particular strengths that imagery has in impacting physiological processes. You can explain to them that the research is clear and unequivocal in demonstrating that the brain's reaction to imaginary experience is equivalent to those of actual experience. A simple demonstration may be carried out by directing your patients to imagine that they are sucking on lemons while attending to the physiological reactions and taste sensations that they experience:

> Find a comfortable position in your seat there, allowing your arms and legs to feel the pull of gravity upon them. Close your eyes, and shift your attention to your breathing: in through your nose ... out through your mouth [stated in time with actual breaths] ... in ... out ... and allow your breathing to grow deeper, slower, and calmer. With each new breath, feel the weight of your limbs, pulled toward the ground. With each breath, allow yourself to grow more and more relaxed. Imagine the space in your mind as a blank screen, dark and empty. And now see a lemon, bright, yellow, and round. Focus on the skin of the lemon, see the texture of that yellow skin and reach out and hold the lemon in your hand. Notice the weight of the lemon, the coolness of its skin; feel its texture on your fingers and in your palm. Hold the lemon below your nose and breathe in deeply, inhaling its scent. Experience the freshness of this ripe, beautiful lemon. Now take the lemon and place it on a cutting board in front of you. Pick up a sharp knife and cut the lemon in half. Notice the juice of the lemon, the firm yellow pulp inside. Notice the scent of this pulp, rising up from below your nose. Now take your knife and make another cut, making a quarter of a lemon. Hold this large, juicy yellow wedge up in front of your mouth. Touch it with your tongue. And when you are ready, bite into your lemon. Taste the flavor of its juices filling your mouth. Now tell me, what did you experience?

At this point, assist your patients in describing all of the sensory experiences they have had: visual, tactile, olfactory, and gustatory. Help them to recognize the salivation and puckering that has occurred as well as the relaxation that they feel from being immersed in a pleasant scene. Finally, help them to recognize that relaxation, concentration, and attention to all the sensory aspects of their imagery made the imagery stronger and more potent. These will be skills that you will be building in your work together to change the body's physiology and perceptions of pain:

> Now close your eyes again, and imagine the tree from which your lemon came. Picture it in your mind as clearly as you can. See the leaves, the branches, the colors, and especially the bright yellow lemons hanging from the tree. Walk up to the tree and pick a good lemon. Again, hold the lemon in your hand as you did before; feel its weight, the coolness of the skin upon your hand. Now this time I want you to focus your concentration upon the lemon. We are going to make it sweet, like lemonade. Without cutting the lemon, I want you to focus on the lemon becoming sweeter and sweeter. Picture the granules of natural sugar, increasing within the flesh of the lemon. See the crystals forming, overtaking the tartness, making the fruit sweeter and sweeter. Now cut this sweet lemon in half with your sharp knife. Now cut again and raise this quarter up to your face. Examine the pulp to discover the delicious sweet sugar inside this lemon. Taste the grainy sugar with your tongue. Now bite into the wedge and notice that it tastes just like sweet lemonade. Still tart, but delicious.

After this second lemon image, you can explain to your patients one of the particular strengths of working within the imagination. Though the imagination provides you access to the brain and body, which you can influence by exposure to experiences within the imagination, the imagination does not have the same physical limitations as the physical world. Not only can you turn a lemon from sour to sweet simply through concentration, but you also could have shrunk the lemon, grown the lemon to the size of a watermelon, or shrunk yourself down to take a trip inside the lemon. You can explain to your patient that the unlimited possibilities of the imagination allow you the flexibility to expose your brain and to prompt the body to react in many more ways than you could in the physical world. You also should encourage your patients to view their treatment with you as a playful process. Encourage them to give free rein to their imaginations, as they did when they were children. The medicine you will be using with them need not be sterile or uniform—quite the opposite. You will be exploring their imaginations for those unique experiences that will be helpful in reducing their pain. Within the imagination, the possibilities are limitless.

Some patients will arrive at the first session in significant pain or will experience a pain flare-up during the initial assessment process. The emergence of pain during the first session may be interpreted as a good opportunity for introducing imagery and establishing a positive working relationship (Barber, 1996). If pain emerges during an initial setting, an ideal strategy is to assist your patient in helping you to understand the pain. Rather than distracting them from the pain, help them to gradually lean into the pain, telling you how it feels. The better they can help you to understand the unique sensory aspects of their pain, their various reactions to the pain, and the metaphors that naturally emerge as they are experiencing the pain, the better you will be able to build your own accurate images of your patients' pain experience.

Furthermore, reacting to the pain experience in a sensitive yet open manner will begin a process of shifting your patients' relationship to the pain, to you, and to the treatment. Specifically, you will be demonstrating the power of acceptance and the fact that imagery treatment will not involve avoidance of pain or quick symptom relief. You will be demonstrating your professional role and willingness to hear all about their pain and pain reactions, in great detail, which will probably differ from your patients' typical experiences; particularly, your patients with chronic pain will have learned by the time they come to see you that people generally do not want to hear about their discomfort. Furthermore, you will establish a collaborative relationship, in which the patients are the experts on their own experience and collaborators in generating solutions. This role of the therapist as partner may be different from that of other health practitioners, who assume direct control to take steps to get rid of the pain immediately or to express sympathy (i.e., pity) rather than empathy (i.e., understanding). Imagery does not work in that manner. You also will help to establish realistic expectations for treatment. Although the available images and the range of transformations to those images within the minds of your patients are virtually limitless, your patients should not be led to expect that imagery is a panacea. In most cases, some degree of pain will remain after treatment is complete. In this regard, the role of imagery treatment for pain is distinct from other forms of modern medicine, which tend to foster expectations of quick and complete symptom relief.

During the first session, prior to the use of any formal imagery techniques, patients typically will describe pain-related imagery spontaneously, as in the example at the start of this chapter. Patients may describe pain as burning, stabbing, heavy, sharp, dull, and so on. Indeed, such descriptions are so common that you may not have recognized that these are descriptions of pain images. Virtually any physical description will contain some sensory aspect, and therein lies the spontaneous imagery. It will be helpful to take note of these images. Not only will you be able to bring these images up later to use in your treatment, but attention to spontaneous images will help your patients feel listened to and understood and will help them join you within the process of image-focused treatment.

Similarly, to become an image therapist you will need to become more aware of the imagery that you and those around you are using in your metaphoric descriptions of pain and treatment. For example, a practitioner may describe medications as "fighting" pain or some other intervention as "building" pain resistance. The imagery evoked by the word *fighting* may come in a number of varieties, each with different levels of effectiveness. Is the medication a small boxer, up against the ropes with a larger opponent with the name *PAIN* printed across the top of his trunks? Or is the medication the dominant fighter, beating pain regularly to the punch? Is the "building" of pain resistance made out of straw, out of brick, or out of steel?

Along these lines, McCaffery and Beebe (1989) develop useful guidelines for using these language-based images in pain treatment. First, after choosing a particular pain relief measure, one should attempt to explain how it works in a language that paints a mental picture. For example, while administering an analgesic one could say:

> The medication you just took is a strong pain blocker, working to close calcium channels that signal unnecessary pain. As you begin to notice relief, you may picture the medicine filling these channels, like a key that fits perfectly into a lock, the medicine locks these channels up, shutting them down. As these channels shut down, many thousands at a time, the tiny signals for pain gradually will become extinguished.

Second, employ simple words and sensory phrases that are likely to arouse comfort in your patients. Such words include *floating, dissolving, quieting, releasing, loosening, soothing, healing, smaller, softer, smooth, cool* or *warm*, and *release*. It is important to remember that the use of language will typically evoke an image automatically. It is unfortunate, for example, that there is no word that is the direct opposite of *pain*. The use of the phrase *pain relief* automatically will evoke a patient's image for pain. The same may be said for words like *agony, suffering*, and *discomfort*. Coupling with any of these words positive terms like *relief* or *reduction* does not remove the image of the negative word from the mind of the listener.

Finally, if patients are offered images of the cause of their pain, they also should be provided with images of pain relief. Language is like the scalpel of the imagination. If you open up a negative image through language, you should be sure to close it up with language as well. For example, if a patient is told that the physician will make an incision during surgery that is likely to trigger a pain response and prolonged pain during the healing process, the patient also should be informed of comforting events that will be involved in the procedure, such as a soft dressing, a soothing cold pack, medication flowing to the area to soothe it, and rest and nutrients that will assist in repairing and healing the wound. Within traditional Western medicine, aftercare has become an afterthought. Discussion of cutting flesh, removing tissue, and sewing a patient back up will evoke clear pain-enhancing images. Therefore, the countermeasures should be described as well to provide the imagination with a more balanced view of what is going to occur.

One of the final tasks of your initial session or sessions is to begin to build a collaborative case conceptualization with your patient. A case conceptualization is a working model of your patient's pain and of the way imagery may be helpful. This working model must be created collaboratively, because your patients maintain expertise on their pain and imagination, whereas you are the specialist in using imagery for pain relief. Neither you nor your patients have direct access to the other's information, so you must work together to understand what is going on (the clients' knowledge) and what can be done (your knowledge).

An infinite variety of working models is possible to understand each patient's pain, and similarly there is no limit to the potential healing impacts that imagery may bring. In Chapter 1 we learned that pain is influenced at a minimum by attention, perception, conditioning, beliefs, schema, affect, coping behaviors, identity, and the relational dynamics between the patient and the various aspects of the patient's world. In Chapters 2 and 3 we learned that imagery has the potential to bring novel flows of information and change within these various aspects of the patient's life, washing out the rigid biopsychosocial processes that surround a patient's experiences with pain. Case conceptualization involves taking all of this information and boiling it down into a plan of treatment.

Perhaps the simplest way to begin to capture these dynamics in an understandable way with your patients is to focus on the cycles involved in their experiences with pain over time. Again, in nearly every case, this information will be conveyed to you in your patients' spontaneous pain narrative, and there will be no need for extra assessments or structured interviews. For example, one patient described being injured on a construction site where he was a top foreman with more than 20 years of experience. At the end of a particularly long and draining day, a steel beam broke loose, shattering his face and skull. Following successful reconstructive surgery, he has continued to experience intense headaches that come out of nowhere. He has been out of work for many months and is desperate to return to his job, but at the same time he is afraid that he could cause an accident at work should one of the headaches hit him unexpectedly. Consequently, he is ambivalent about returning to work, and this reaction has created conflict with his employers and stress and conflict within his marriage. By attending to key aspects of your patient's pain narrative, you can identify a pain cycle initiated by a traumatic accident involving loss of control, ongoing pain that is similarly unpredictable and uncontrollable, high levels of identity-discrepant fear and impotence, identity-discrepant ambivalence about work, and stress and conflict in his most important life relationships.

Headaches are driving this process and to some extent result from this process, in which this patient's former sense of identity has been shattered, leaving him stuck in rigid cycles involving pain, fear, loss of control, loss of identity, conflict, stress, and more pain. Imagery potentially may be helpful to this patient within each of these primary cyclical factors—for example, in addressing the pain directly, in desensitization to the traumatic memory of the accident, in establishing control, in identity repair, in creating interpersonal harmony, and in promoting relaxation.

In developing a conceptualization of this patient's pain, you will want to collaborate with the patient as you explore the specific nature of these cycles, which aspects of the cycle are dominant, which aspects are prone to triggering headaches most directly, which aspects may be left out, and which aspects, if any, were not included in the original pain narrative. Once you and your patients have identified the most important cyclical aspects within their particular pain process, you can discuss the ways imagery may be helpful in softening any of these aspects. Just as you needed your patient to clarify the most important aspects in the pain cycle, you will need to be clear in conveying the possible benefits of imagery and the best likely first target. For example, for the previous patient, you could explain that the original traumatic memories appear to be closely associated with his pain as well as with every other aspect within his pain cycle. However, you may want to begin with some simple relaxation imagery before you head into the trauma-related imagery, because the relaxation imagery has a high potential for some initial benefits, which will be encouraging and facilitate the subsequent work of exploring more sensitive image content.

The collaboration process around targets for treatment should also include the role of other procedures and adjunctive treatments (Achterberg, Dossey, & Kolkmeier, 1994). Some common adjunctive treatments include the use of antidepressants, exercise, touch therapies (e.g., acupuncture, acupressure, massage), psychoeducation, assertiveness training, problem-solving skills training, conjoint relationship therapies (e.g., couples counseling), and various forms of behavior therapy (e.g., changing coping habits). In the previous case, treatment could involve working with the prescribing physician to identify pain medications that would be least likely to interfere with the demands of construction work, consulting a marital therapist to improve marital communication, asking the patient to begin keeping a pain journal to identify more specific pain triggers and patterns of headache frequency and intensity, or perhaps vocational counseling to explore career options should he wish to transition away from working on construction sites.

The specific conceptualization and ways imagery may be helpful are unlimited, yet the discrete list of psychological factors will assist you in narrowing the possible relevant aspects in patients' pain conceptualization.

Furthermore, understanding patients' pain always follows from the information they include within the pain narrative, particularly the dynamics described within patients' pain-generating cycles. The most beneficial impacts of treatment are likely to be seen when the transformation of pain-related images leads to an opening up of information regarding patients' identity and the relationships that serve to inform those identities. Yet even simple relaxation may lead to a cascade in causally linked factors, resulting over time in a shift to the identity that is better able to manage pain. For example, relaxation may assist our construction worker in making sense out of his accident, leading to decreased guilt, more openness to his wife's concerns, and the ability to put pride aside and take a less demanding job if necessary. Alternatively, relaxation only may set the stage for more direct imagery involving symbolic representations of the original traumatic injury. Perhaps the steel beam that hit him will become a monster to be slayed, or perhaps his headaches are trying to tell him to spend more time building his life outside of work. There is no way to know for sure. Again, patients are the expert on the contents of their own imagination, whereas you are the experts in the processes that may be used to get into the imaginations and work toward healing.

A final task to complete during the initial assessment phase, prior to the active phase of treatment, is to develop a sense of your patients' goals. Generally speaking, goals should be as specific and realistic as possible. Goals may be directly related to pain reduction, such as percentage reductions in pain intensity, increases in pain tolerance, or reductions in pain frequency in the case of episodic pain. For example, "My average pain intensity [or tolerance] rating will decrease by at least 30% for three weeks in a row," would be a realistic goal to record and use as a way of measuring success. These types of goals will require that your patients make daily recordings of their pain experiences. This record is beneficial in a number of other ways: For example, it allows patients to turn and face their pain, it increases mindfulness in their pain episodes, and it decreases overreliance on avoidance and distraction strategies. Goals also may be set with respect to functional outcomes: for example, the ability to resume athletic activities, the ability to resume some enjoyable hobby that pain has interrupted, or the ability to return to employment. Ideally, you should record and track progress on a short list of goals, including both direct and functional goals.

While it is important to have an optimistic outlook during the first session of image therapy, it is also important to remain realistic, particularly in making goals. Imagery is of course not always effective in pain management. Even the best medical treatments are about 70% to 80% effective on average. Furthermore, outcome studies suggest that although the average positive effects of imagery are going to be quite good, they typically are not going to lead to the complete eradication of pain.

Finally, it will be useful to address some specific issues that tend to interfere with image therapy at the outset of treatment, such as limited abilities to use mental imagery due to severe mental illness or poorly developed imagery abilities. Some patients may hold unshakable views that the use of imagery is an indication that others see their pain as merely being all in their heads, thus hindering motivation and expectations. Success may be hampered by factors that interfere with motivation or trust in the therapeutic relationship, such as the presence of severe personality disorders. In the worst scenarios, imagery techniques actually may lead to increases in pain. This may occur, for example, if patients are pushed toward uncovering intense emotional issues with which they are not yet able to cope effectively. For these reasons the therapeutic process should be open and collaborative, and the stance of the image therapist should reflect balance between optimistic creativity and pragmatic caution.

In certain situations, it will be useful to slow the treatment process down during or immediately following the intake assessment. Factors that may indicate a need to delay the active phase of treatment are numerous. Some patients may have limited time and energy to devote to image therapy. Medical conditions may create obstacles. Financial considerations may be important, or other more pressing emotional issues may need to take priority over pain management. In the next two sections, we discuss two of the most frequent obstacles: (1) problems with motivation; and (2) problems with imagination skills. Fortunately there are some guidelines for remediating these issues; often just a few additional preparatory sessions prior to entering the active phase of imagery treatment will prepare patients for imagery work.

Motivation Enhancement

You will need to assess your patients' motivation for treatment near the beginning of image therapy. Maddux (1991) describes a set of three simple questions that are very helpful in this regard, which have been modified here to assess motivation for imagery therapy. On a scale from 1 to 10 (1 is low; 10 is high), ask your patients:

1. How confident are you in the ability to use guided imagery in managing your pain?
2. How confident are you that your pain will become more manageable when our treatment is completed?
3. How important is it for you to get relief from your pain?

As a rule of thumb, ratings of less than 7 in any of these areas warrant some exploration and remedial intervention before you begin the active phase of treatment.

The first question assesses *efficacy expectations* (Bandura, 1986). Do patients believe that they have the ability to follow through with treatment procedures? Low scores in this area may be related to obstacles in getting to the clinic, difficulties with relaxation or concentration, or generally low levels of personal efficacy or self-worth. Overcoming these obstacles may require a range of interventions, from simple problem solving to referral to treatment for depression. Regardless, it is advantageous to know about any barriers related to patient self-confidence before embarking on a treatment program.

The second question provides an assessment of *outcome expectations*, patients' confidence in treatment. If they do what is asked, is the outcome likely to be beneficial? Low numbers in this area generally require some further discussion about how imagery is likely to work, finding an explanatory model that makes sense to patients. If common ground can not be found and disbelief is pervasive, even after some experiences with imagery in the session or after the use of motivation enhancement techniques, then it may be best not to continue with treatment. Patients will not be motivated to do the tasks of treatment if they do not have sufficient expectations of positive outcomes.

The third question assesses *outcome value*. Patients may believe in their ability to do the procedures of imagery and may expect positive outcomes to arise from these efforts; however, if these positive outcomes do not hold a high value for patients, motivation for treatment will falter. It is unlikely that many of your patients will provide low ratings for outcome value. Pain does hurt, after all. However, you may encounter patients who have adjusted to a chronic pain condition and will have some misgivings about the changes that may come if they are better able to manage their pain. For example, they may have ambivalence about returning to work, becoming more active, or branching out socially outside of the medical and pain communities into which they may have settled. Any ambivalence about ostensibly positive outcomes of treatment should be fully explored at the outset so that these conflicted motivations do not interfere with treatment.

If patients score low in one or more area and if you find that their barriers to motivation are rather strong, you may wish to try motivational interviewing, an approach aimed at increasing motivation for change (Jensen, 2002; Miller, Benefield, & Tongigan, 1993; Miller & Rollnick, 1991). Motivational interviewing is based on the transtheoretical model of psychotherapy (Prochaska, DiClemente, & Norcross, 1992), which outlines five stages of change depending on the level of patient motivation:

1. *Precontemplation* is characterized by a lack of conscious understanding of the need for change or will to change.
2. *Contemplation* is characterized by some rudimentary attention to the problem and the possibility of change still without the activation of the will.
3. *Preparation* is characterized by mental planning for change and the initial activation of the will.
4. *Action* is characterized by the initiation of novel behavior.
5. *Maintenance* involves ongoing self-reinforcement, continued improvement, and relapse prevention.

Within this model, improvement is conceptualized as a cyclical spiral, in which patients move through each of the five stages repeatedly over time as they reach healthier and healthier plateaus with respect to the targeted behavior change. For example, a patient with chronic pain may move through the contemplation phase, engage in a multimodal treatment plan moving through the action and maintenance phases, and then return to the clinic to make further gains. This model is compatible with the assessment of motivational beliefs (e.g., self-efficacy) previously outlined, so it may be used together toward the goal of increasing motivation for therapy.

The essential assessment task in motivation enhancement therapy is to recognize patients' location within the stages of change. Patients in the precontemplation to the early preparation stages will require more insight-oriented approaches. For example, they may need to explore the aspects of their lives that would be pushing them toward engaging in treatment and the factors that are creating barriers. Within the active phase of imagery treatment, these individuals may benefit more from exploration strategies such as *in-body travel* or anthropomorphic techniques (i.e., making the pain into a creature that can be queried for insights) rather than strategies aimed at a specific goal, such as relaxation or strategic pain reduction procedures. Patients in the latter stages of change, from preparation to maintenance, probably will benefit more from specific structured imagery techniques presented within a prescriptive and structured treatment plan.

To facilitate the movement from the earlier stages of change into the action phase, you can use motivational-interviewing strategies (Jensen, 2002). The aim of these strategies is to use the therapeutic relationship to facilitate the growth of insight, will, and planning for change. It is important to remember, however, that motivational interviewing does not rest on principles of direct persuasion or selling the patient on the need for change. As Jensen explains:

Although an assumption of MI [motivational interviewing] is that clinician behavior plays a key role in the development and maintenance of patient motivation, the approach paradoxically argues that the ultimate responsibility for change lies within the patient. In short, the clinician's task is to enhance motivation; the patient's task is to take action. (p. 74)

A persuasive message is persuasive only if it is heard. Individuals who have been in chronic pain and who have arrived at your office still in the state of precontemplation likely have encountered many of the arguments that you would propose for the benefits of lifestyle and alternative medicine approaches in managing their pain. But, motivational interviewing focuses instead on interpersonal neutrality and listening. If you question your patients in a neutral tone with respect to the possible benefits and liabilities of using imagery for pain, then you will be most likely to engage them in an open and honest dialogue. Within this open dialogue, your patients will be more likely to generate their own reasons for joining you in taking the necessary steps toward change. The messages will be more motivating if they come from your patients themselves.

Furthermore, taking a power-oriented and prescriptive stance with patients who are lacking intrinsic motivation for change is likely to engender resistance or passivity in the therapeutic relationship. With patients low in motivation, it will be more effective to take a step back from persuasive strategies and to avoid giving advice. The step back provides the interpersonal space for the patients themselves to step forward and to move toward contemplation and preparation under their own motivational steam.

On the other hand, motivational interviewing is not effective if the clinician is simply passive or disengaged. In this regard, Miller and Rollnick (1991) suggest five key principles that describe what the therapist should do instead of convincing or advising. First, *express empathy*. With empathy, your patient will be more open to exploring the problems associated with pain and the barriers to engaging actively in treatment.

Next, *develop discrepancy*. This means that in a nonconfrontational manner you should actively listen for discrepancies between your patients' goals and their pain conditions. When discrepancies are identified, reflect them back to patients from a neutral yet engaged interpersonal stance— for example, "It sounds as if your pain has been leading you to become increasingly unhappy with your life, yet you have mixed feelings about doing the imagery exercises at home? Help me understand these mixed feelings." In discussing discrepancies, your aim is to help them to become clearer and more elaborated so that they will become more recognizable to your patients over time.

A third strategy is to *avoid arguing*. Arguments with your patients can lead only to losses on both sides. Even if you appear to win the argument and you convince your patients to make a change, you have put them in a one-down position, and they are unlikely to continue to follow through with the change process without your ongoing pushing. You may have won the short-term argument, but in the longer-term interpersonal process you have lost. If you find yourself entering an argument over a specific change that you feel needs to be made, switch instead to empathy seeking. If you can understand your patients' resistances, then the resistances will be more salient to both of you. This is the first step toward moving out of the precontemplation stage toward helping your patients to make a reasonable choice to either change or to keep things as they are.

The fourth strategy is to *roll with resistance*. While resistance is the enemy of change, it must be honored as a worthy enemy. If you discount resistances, you communicate to your patients that they are unimportant and that they should not be held up by such things. You run the risk of judging your patients for their resistances or entering into a conflict with respect to the relative size of their obstacles from your perspective rather than from theirs. On the other hand, if your initial reaction is to acknowledge and explore the patients' resistances without bias, then you will join with them in a collaborative process of understanding the obstacles and of finding ways to remove them.

Finally, motivational interviewing involves the *support of your patients' self-efficacy*. Again, confidence in the ability to do treatment, positive outcome expectations, and outcome value is essential. A number of strategies may be used to enhance efficacy, but all essentially are aimed at helping patients first to succeed and second to attend to these successes. If patients are failing, no amount of persuasion will make them feel confident. The experiences of failure will override any relatively superficial verbal encouragements. Some patients genuinely will be lacking in competence and therefore will have justifiably low-efficacy expectations. Other patients will be more successful than they think, but they will have biased efficacy expectations because they fail to notice their successes. For the first group, acknowledging their general lack of success in an accepting manner will provide a first step toward building success. Once they are able to forgive and accept themselves as flawed yet typical human beings, then you can begin to help them to build up their skill levels. For example, if they have tried in the past to use imagery but found that they repeatedly became distracted, you could assist them in doing simple imagery exercises to increase the time of engagement. Once some success is being generated, you can model reinforcement of success by providing constructive and enthusiastic feedback and by prescribing the same to your patients within themselves. This type of supportive feedback is also the intervention of choice for patients with low confidence due to negative self-distortion or bias. For these patients, it will be best to simply direct them to begin the process of increasing attention to success.

Imagery Skills Training

A small subset of your patients will admit to low confidence in their imagination skills. For most, this lack of confidence arises due to a misunderstanding of the level of imagination ability required to effectively use imagery for pain management. Although image clarity and detail are helpful, immersion within the imagery is more central to impacting one's physiology. Thus, it is helpful to remind certain patients that their imagery need not be as clear and detailed as are images in a movie, for example.

However, with those who continue to speak of low confidence in their imagination, one can use experiential exercises again. For example, nearly all can imagine familiar places, such as their bedroom. You could ask them to close their eyes and describe it, obtaining details about colors of walls, bedspreads, and other objects around the room (Samuels & Samuels, 1975), along with information from the other sense and experiential dimensions. For example, you could assist self-doubting imaginers in conjuring up images associated with their first homes, encouraging them to move from detailed visual objects to sounds, smells, temperature, emotion, thoughts, and other experiential aspects that may be associated with these well-represented images.

The exercise of imagining one's bedroom or other familiar locations also may be used to illustrate the ease with which centrally relevant and repeated experience becomes better represented within the imagination. This realization may help patients to understand that the imagery that emerges in association with their pain will be the most centrally relevant and meaningful material and that the process of treatment is one of uncovering and discovering rather than creating or conjuring up.

Some individuals who actually are low in imagination skills will benefit from relaxation training, concentration training, or image clarity and control training prior to the active phase of treatment (see Sheikh, Sheikh, & Moleski, 1985, for detailed accounts of such training). Relaxation training helps individuals learn to tune out external stimuli, to disengage from internal verbal chatter, and to decrease muscular tension, all of which may interfere with immersion in sensory images.

Concentration training works from the opposite direction, enabling individuals to willfully pull themselves more deeply into imagery. A number of concentration activities may be used, such as counting breaths and then increasing mindfulness of breathing with each additional count, focusing one's attention on a detail within the visual field and examining this detail in depth, closing one's eyes and imagining each thought contained within a cloud that is floating by on a summer's day. The goal is mindfulness, a state in which one is focused on the desired set of internal or external stimuli from a position of detached interest. One is fully engaged in concentration on a target yet is fully disengaged from willful action on that target. One is in a state of intense focus balanced with radical acceptance. Though formal training in meditation is not necessary to do imagery, it may be helpful in this regard.

For patients who are more verbally than perceptually oriented, practice in manipulating shapes within the imagination may be helpful prior to or along with the active phase of treatment. For example, McKim (1980) describes an exercise in which patients visualize a red cube that is sliced into 27 smaller cubes. They then are asked to visualize the number of cubes that have red on three, two, and one side, respectively. In a similar exercise, individuals are asked to mentally fold a two-dimensional design to create a new three-dimensional design, which they then describe within the imagination.

Less abstract exercises involve examining naturally occurring scenes from patients' lives and directing them to conduct transformations to the perspective or features within these scenes. For example, patients may be asked to engage in imagery of a river from the level of the water and then to slowly rise up to take an aerial view, noting the snakelike shape of the river from this perspective. From here, they may be guided to make the river become an actual snake, which may then curl up and go to sleep. When viewed from the side, the snake may resemble a soft-serve ice cream cone, which patients may proceed to eat and enjoy. These types of exercises also serve as practice runs, whereby patients and the therapist become accustomed to working together as a team within patients' imagination.

Lazarus (1977) describes a number of more advanced techniques for improving clarity within the imagination, such as the blackboard exercise, in which patients imagine themselves writing letters on a blackboard until the entire alphabet is produced. When imagination skills are at an advanced level, individuals should be able to report seeing the entire alphabet without fading and be able to report back the alphabet backward, every third letter, and so on. Similar techniques include imagining a room with a dimming light bulb, where objects within the room become clear and then fade into darkness at will. Finally, one can examine an actual object in the treatment room, such as a piece of art, and then recreate it within the imagination, describing each of its salient features. Then the object can be reexamined in the actual room again and again, adding features that had been missed with each new round of imagery until the image increasingly resembles the actual object. The exercise resembles painting the image of a model on the canvas of the imagination.

Some patients, particularly those with trauma histories and significant psychopathology, will be fearful of internal focus at the outset of treatment; some may even fear closing their eyes in your presence. For these individuals, it will be helpful to fully explore their fears. Subsequently, if imagery is still considered to be a potentially beneficial form of intervention, you could assist these patients by having them focus their attention on a central object, approximately 3 to 4 feet in front of their faces. Such concentration will tend to fatigue their eyes and may prompt them to close their eyes naturally (Dossey, Keegan, Kolkmeier, & Guzzetta, 1989). If fear persists, they should be assisted in gradually lengthening the amount of time they are able to keep their eyes closed. For these individuals, as well as for those who report a lack of detail in their images, sensory training may be helpful (Samuels & Samuels, 1975). Essentially, sensory training involves the development of the skill of sensory awareness in people's everyday lives. You can assign specific exercises, such as focusing on visual aspects of certain objects within your treatment setting or in patients' lives, between sessions. These visual aspects of focus can include colors, degrees of shadow and light, size of features, textures, and perspectives.

Similarly, one can assist patients through the creative exercise of decontextualizing everyday objects. Decontextualizing objects means attempting to experience objects in a raw fashion, without reaction, meaning, or association, as if one were viewing the object for the first time. For example, patients can be asked to examine a book and take note of its spatial qualities, such as the relative thickness of the binder, the thinness of the pages, and the patterns of shapes created by the text on each page. You can instruct patients to adopt different experiential roles in their observations, such as seeing an apple from the perspective of a starving person, an agricultural worker, an artist, and a grocer, to attend to the sensory aspects of the apple which become more salient from each perspective (Sommer, 1978).

The Active Phase of Treatment

The active phase of treatment begins following assessment, treatment planning, goal setting, and the completion of any remedial interventions that may be necessary, such as motivation enhancement or skills training. This phase of treatment may begin as soon as the end of the first visit or after several months of preliminary work, depending on the situation of your patient and the procedures of your clinic. The duration of this active phase also will vary, from one- or two-session brief therapy for simple procedural pain to a year or more for complex personality dynamics or trauma that may be contributing to a chronic pain syndrome. It is important to remember that large clinically meaningful benefits have been observed in the research for procedural pain, experimental pain, and chronic conditions with relatively short and simple imagery interventions, typically running twice per month for as few as six sessions. Thus, clinicians using image therapy can plan their typical treatment frequency and durations around these relatively brief and infrequent parameters. Also, most experts in the use of imagery for pain management suggest that practitioners approach the therapeutic process from a collaborative stance, with high expectations for patient involvement (e.g., Syrjala & Abrams, 2002). This will be particularly crucial if the plan is to use a short, biweekly treatment frequency that will emphasize regular practice by patients between sessions and the acquisition of skills that eventually lead to self-guided imagery patients can do on their own.

It will be important to keep in mind that many of your patients will display resistance to doing practice exercises between sessions. These resistances do not necessarily signal low motivation, and they definitely should be interpreted as normal, rational, and even expected responses to the treatment process to be explored in an atmosphere of complete acceptance. Resistance to doing imagery exercises between sessions probably will arise from your patients' fears of being out of control in the face of the pain. When identified and understood, this fear can be channeled into motivation, because exercises are specifically intended to increase patients' control in the face of pain.

Some discussion of the varying approaches to control may be helpful in this regard. For example, you may wish to frame control for your patients in terms of primary versus secondary control (see Hayes & Duckworth, 2006, for a complete discussion of control strategies applied to pain). Primary control means direct control, imposing your will on another entity to make it change its behavior. Primary control is particularly emphasized within individualistic Western cultures, as reflected by common phrases such as, "grabbing the bull by the horns." Direct control works well in psychology when applied to behavior and other simple applications involving willpower. However, when direct-control strategies are overused or applied to situations that are not responsive to willpower, one may encounter negative paradoxical effects. Imagine for a moment what would happen to most individuals if they were to actually try to grab a bull by its horns. Generally speaking, the overuse of direct-control strategies in attempting to manage internal experiences results in paradoxical responses, whereby noxious internal experiences increase rather than decrease and patients end up feeling even more out of control. For example, trying to force an image out of consciousness is likely to bring it more sharply into focus, trying not to feel anxious typically increases levels of anxiety, and trying to force pain to decrease will probably increase the pain. Repeated encounters with failures in direct control such as these are likely to drive the rigid movement in the opposite direction toward the overuse of avoidance and distraction in many of the pain patients.

Secondary-control strategies, on the other hand, involve release and acceptance. These strategies are emphasized in collectivist cultures and

Eastern philosophical traditions, particularly Taoism. For example, a traditional Taoist allegory describes the paradoxical strength of water in the face of stone, which resides in the ability of water to flow around stone. When encountering an angry bull, secondary-control strategies would emphasize keeping a close eye on the bull and carefully stepping out of its path. This approach is reflected by the rodeo clown rather than by the cowboy. It is important to note that secondary control is not the same as avoidance or distraction, which are analogous to running wildly from the bull or pretending that it is not there.

In home exercises as well as imagery within session, the aim is to assist patients in the combined use of primary- and secondary-control strategies. For example, Achterberg et al., (1994) suggest that patients approach exercises each day with the intent of checking in with their pain, *softening* and *opening* themselves to it. You cannot begin to address pain through imagery if you are always running away from it. Nor can you address it if you are wrapped up in an all-out wrestling match. Remind your patients that the goal is not complete control over pain. Rather, encourage them to *lean into* the pain just a bit and see what might be done for its management.

It will be helpful to structure imagery done within and between sessions so that the exercises can become ritualized and routine. At home, patients should attach their imagery exercises to a routine positive daily event or activity—for example, a meal, time spent reading, or a few moments in bed in the morning upon waking. Once a set time for practice is established, the steps in carrying out an imagery exercise will be consistent across techniques and may be taught as five simple steps (Syrjala & Abrams, 2002):

1. Start with a concentration activity, for example, focusing on breathing, staring at an object in the room (e.g., candle flame) until eyes close, or focusing on a mental object in the imagination.
2. Increase relaxation, for example, by deepening breaths, tensing and releasing muscle groups, or simply allowing yourself to become more fully immersed in concentration and focus.
3. Enter into the imagery exercise and follow it through to completion.
4. Reflect within the imagination for a moment on how the exercise went.
5. Return to alertness for further reflection on ways that any benefits may be applied throughout the rest of the day.

Making these steps routine through practice will allow your patients to build habits for the use of imagery that will be long lasting and self-sustaining after the treatment is completed.

As you begin to do imagery in session with your patients, it will be helpful to use their primary sense modalities as the gateway to specific images. The primary sense modality for most patients will be visual, followed by auditory, but a few will prefer the other senses. You can discern the primary sense modality from your patients by attending to the language they choose, such as, "I see what you're saying," as opposed to, "I hear you." If it is unclear what their primary modality is, you can simply ask them their opinion on the matter, or you can experiment with them within an imaginary scene to discover which modality contains the most salient features. Once you establish the primary sense modality for each patient, you should provide guidance and suggestions to bring as many of the other senses into the experience as possible, one by one.

As you do imagery, it also will be helpful to provide suggestion about what to expect and how to react in regard to the content of internal experiences and about the ways you will be interacting in your roles of imaginer and guide. Specifically, patients should be encouraged to be open, creative, and ultimately in charge within the therapeutic relationship. By encouraging them not to self-censure any of their imagery, you may provide the reassurance that everyone's imagery is unique and that all images are to be accepted and valued for the information they may convey. Let your patients know that if you suggest some aspect of experience that does not correspond to what is happening internally, they should let you know and go along with their internal flows rather than your suggestions. The patients' experience should always take precedence, and patients should feel free to modify and adapt around anything you are suggesting.

In the same vein, it may be helpful to begin with basic imagery for beginners and to keep your narratives as open and nonspecific as possible (Dossey et al., 1989). As you and your patients become more familiar with their typical imagination scenes and processes, you may be able to be more specific, for example, by asking if a familiar character has arrived yet or if the pain is still blue and cold as it was the last time it was imagined. This rule of thumb about starting vague and then following your patients' feedback as you become more specific is essential within each imagery session. It may be helpful to follow general scripts when you begin to use imagery. Over time, you will capture the general process and become more comfortable with improvisation. Essentially, you are directing your patients to experience something and to engage each of the senses, but you are relying on them to describe back to you the specific content of those internal scenes.

In general, negative images and conflict motifs within imagery scenes will be particularly important to attend to, even if you are using relatively simple image techniques where such narrative themes may not be expected to emerge. Shifting the relationships with these images (e.g., speaking to them instead of running from them) and other transformations of such images will usually bring about improvements in health and wellness, particularly if they are elaborated and processed for meaning after the imagery procedure is completed. Nevertheless, it is also important to emphasize to patients when such images emerge that they are in control of their use of the imagination and ultimately the session. You should make clear to your patients that they may let go of the image or, if necessary, open their eyes to end the current scenario if material becomes upsetting or otherwise threatening. Also, it may also be helpful in such situations to remind patients that their thoughts cannot hurt them and that this is one of the benefits of battling such demons within the imagination. Creative measures may be taken as well, such as supplying patients with armor, growing them into a larger or more powerful people, or providing them with a magical shield when faced with the threat of monsters.

In addition to regular verbal reports from your patients about their internal experiences, you also should attend to their nonverbal reactions to imagery—for example, their posture, muscle tension, facial expressions, eyelid movements, and respiration. If you have any questions about what they are experiencing, simply check in with them, asking them, for example, if they are sufficiently relaxed and immersed. If they describe a situation that calls for increased relaxation or immersion, suggest some maneuvers that may lead to that state and direct them to report back to you.

As you interact in this manner, you will need to keep in mind that things move more slowly in the imagination than in the physical world. Thus, you will need to speak at a slower-than-normal pace, taking short pauses between each new suggestion. Again, it may be useful to have patients let you know when the suggestion has become manifest, because each patient will have his or her own characteristic pace (Syrjala & Abrams, 2002).

The natural laws of the imaginary world are distinct from the physical world in a number of other ways in addition to timing and limitless possibility. Understanding these peculiar laws will assist you in making successful journeys into the imagination, just as an understanding of gravity and other laws of the physical world are helpful on a physical journey. Akhter Ahsen (see Sheikh, 1978, for a description) categorizes these principles into four *laws of the imaginary world* that he calls *magical laws of the psyche*: (1) part is whole; (2) contact is unification; (3) wish is action; and (4) imitation is reality. The first law, part is whole, describes the imagination's automatic process of completing partial images. The whole-seeking process may occur in images of physical objects in space, such as imagining numbing in part of a finger, which will then naturally spread to the rest of the hand. Part is whole is useful because the imagination's own momentum toward the completion of images (i.e., completion momentum) rounds out that would be more difficult to conjure up one at a time. For example, if a patient's pain is represented as a dragon and the patient wishes to become a knight, this transformation may be most efficient if the patient simply imagines himself or herself in a suit of armor, which will bring along with it a lance, a steed, and a courageous attitude. In addition to objects in imaginary space, part is whole may be applied to time as well, since the imagination's completion momentum will tend to work toward finishing script-like scenarios to their end. For example, once the battle with the dragon has begun, the scene will tend to continue until completion under its own momentum without the clinician suggestion or patient's will.

The second law, contact is unification, describes the special quality of imaginary touch, which allows an individual to meld with an object. For example, a patient in pain may imagine the most comfortable blanket imaginable, made of the finest, softest silk. By making contact with this material in the imagination, the patient may absorb its qualities, experiencing that sense of softness and comfort internally. Through the process of completion momentum, again, the imagination naturally will seek to unite things that could conceivably go together. Therefore, whenever aspects of the imagination may benefit your patients through unification, you simply can bring them into contact with one another in the imagination. For example, if pain is represented as fire and your patient sees a block of ice, you could ask if he or she would like the ice to go to the fire. If the answer is yes, the unification process will begin spontaneously.

This example also illustrates the third law, wish is action. This law describes the fact that the imagination is not passive but automatically triggers activity. For example, if your patient is battling the pain dragon and wishes that the dragon would get a sore throat and become unable to breathe fire, the simple wish automatically will bring this about within the scene. Similarly, your patient could wish for a smaller dragon, a longer lance, or an army of helper knights to assist in the battle. While imagery often moves at a slower pace than physical reality, wishes in the imagination move at the speed of neurons firing, approximately 50 times per second, which is fast indeed. The wish is action law is particularly useful during times of imaginary emergency.

The final law, imitation is reality, describes the fact that personal transformations occur more easily in the imaginary world than in the physical world. If the patient wishes to shift identity in the imagination, he or she needs only to imitate the desired identity. If your patient wishes to become brave in fighting the dragon, then puffing out the chest and making bold proclamations should do the trick. If your patient identifies role models who are brave, assertive, or strong, then he or she will need only to act like those individuals to incorporate their attributes into his or her own identities. Imitation is reality may be considered to be equivalent to wish is action, except that it works in the opposite direction. In wish is action, the thought becomes the action, and in imitation is reality, the action brings about a different outlook. In applying each of these laws, it is useful to recognize that they tend to work together; for example, by simply desiring to touch the picture of a role model in the imagination, a patient may obtain an entire role model's identity, combining the laws of contact is unification, part is whole, wish is action, and imitation is reality in a single step.

These general rules presented here are intended to assist you in being comfortable and confident in your work with patients in their imaginations. It may be helpful to refresh your memory concerning the general principles of the treatment process. In summary, here is a list of the top 10 tips to guide you in the active phase of imagery treatment:

1. Assess motivation and commitment to carry out regular practice between sessions and intervene as appropriate.
2. Assess pain intensity and tolerance (i.e., 1–10 scale) before and after the use of imagery.
3. Try to determine the patient's dominant sense (e.g., visual) and experiential (e.g., thinking) modalities, and then emphasize those modalities in the imagination.
4. Be aware of your choice of words, such as the use of the word *pain*. Words probably will trigger the image and, in the short term, lead to increased intensity of those images. For example, say, "Your arm is becoming more comfortable and relaxed," rather than, "The pain is diminishing."
5. Language used by the therapist in imagery work must be action oriented rather than passive. Patients can imagine that they are doing something, but it is impossible for them to imagine themselves not doing something.
6. Make sure your patients are sufficiently relaxed before beginning imagery and that relaxation is reintroduced as needed before using specific imagery interventions.
7. Speak more slowly than you would during typical conversation to allow time for images to emerge and to become clear. It may be helpful to imagine along with the patient to maintain a comfortable pace.
8. Do not try to force the image on the patient; simply offer it using phrases such as, "If you wish, you may …" or "You might like to …." Keep track of what your patient is experiencing and modify your guidance as needed.
9. Remember that although it is very helpful if the image is vivid and lifelike, it is more important for patients to be absorbed and engaged within the imagery. Querying multiple sense (e.g., sight, sound, touch, taste) and experiential (e.g., temperature, feelings, thoughts, physical sensations) modalities will bring your patients deeper into the imagination.

10. When appropriate, use the open and creative aspects of the imagination to your advantage, asking your patients for creative solutions to imaginary scenarios (e.g., "What would you like to do with those sharp little needles?") and using the laws of the imaginary world to emphasize your patients' power and control within the imagination.

CHAPTER 5

Pain Management

Simple Techniques

However interesting, plausible, and appealing a theory may be, it is techniques not theories, that are actually used on people. Study of the effects of psychotherapy, therefore, is always the study of the effectiveness of techniques.

London
(1964, p. 33)

The specific imagery techniques presented in the next three chapters have been arranged in three parts according to their depth and complexity: Simple techniques are presented herein; deeper techniques are described in Chapter 6; and deepest techniques are in Chapter 7. Simple techniques tend to be brief, easy, and focused directly on pain rather than broader issues. These techniques are desirable for patients with procedural pain (e.g., those who have had a planned surgical procedure), for patients who have high levels of functioning, for patients who are just beginning treatment, or in treatment settings with limited scope of care.

The techniques presented in this chapter begin with simple conversational imagery and a variety of relaxation scenarios. Next, a variety of techniques derived from the cognitive-behavioral traditions are described, beginning with simple rehearsal techniques for procedural pain. These techniques provide a slightly more complex theoretical grounding to the use of imagery than relaxation alone. Here the focus is on decreasing fear and other negative emotional reactions to pain and on increasing levels of self-efficacy in the ability to manage pain. Finally, a number of simple transformational techniques are covered. Once represented, these symbolic pain images are manipulated in simple ways to shift the perception of pain, typically toward reduced intensity. Simple techniques tend to have relatively simple theoretical rationales as well; for example, they may involve gate-control theory to reduce sensory or emotional inputs to the pain experience. These techniques can be practiced easily by patients at home, and the inductions and imaging procedures are more or less scripted.

There is no clear line that distinguishes these different levels of depth in technique. Nor should you consider each technique to be fully independent of others within or among the three chapters. There is significant overlap across categories and the specific techniques themselves. Furthermore, some patients will begin doing a simple technique and end up in a deeper technique by the time you are through, if you follow their lead. Once you have reached a comfort level in doing image therapy with a variety of patients, this type of open experimentation is desirable.

Each technique includes a description of the approach, an example of the general guidance provided to the patient that you may use as a model for your own work, and additional references should you desire further background on the approach. As you move along with your own comfort level and that of each particular patient, you may find it helpful to combine approaches. For example, you may want to select a simple relaxation procedure followed by a deeper technique. Feel free to combine approaches or to modify approaches along with your patients in the spirit of creative collaboration. The following procedures are starting lines for any number of imaginary journeys you will take. The variety of finish lines you may potentially encounter with each of your patients is limitless. Bon voyage!

Subtle Conversational Imagery

During routine verbal interactions with patients, healing images often emerge spontaneously. For example, patients might say that their medications "fight" their pain, or a therapist might say that regular exercise "builds" pain resistance. The use of positive imagery through language is not likely to be presented to patients as imagery treatment. Rather, the practice of these principles will occur during routine interactions with patients. It is important to be mindful of the language you are using to describe the treatment and healing process and, perhaps even more importantly, of the language your patients are using to describe their pains. Your patients will respond in healthier ways to your interactions if they rest on positive imagery that fits with their own internal representations.

For example, after selecting a pain relief intervention you should attempt to explain how it works in a language that paints a mental picture. For example, while administering an analgesic you could say, "This medication is designed to travel through your blood stream, seeking out sites of pain and shutting them down. Once those sites are closed down, the surrounding tissues will experience steadily increasing levels of comfort, which will promote healing." This short description conveys imagery in which the medication is seen as active (e.g., "travel" and "seeking out") and also dominant over pain (e.g., "shutting them down" and "closed"). Positive language involving increasing comfort and healing rather than decreasing pain is recommended: The word *pain* was used only one time, and in the image this pain was limited to specific sites that soon would close. A number of "good guy, bad guy" archetypes could be invoked through such a simple description, for example, of cops shutting down a rowdy party. Yet a patient's eyes remain open, and the language within the description is simple and transparent.

Generally speaking, you describe pain relief with words and phrases that are likely to arouse images of comfort (see also Chapter 4 for the use of positive language in pain treatment). Similarly, if the causes of pain are described then images of healing should be described as well. For example, if patients are told that they have inflammation, they should also be informed about the protective role that inflammation provides, as well as the conditions that will bring the inflammation down. In Western medicine, we typically are most focused on the intervention or procedure and less on the healing process. Yet the power of language spoken by the treatment providers and the images they connote should not be overlooked. A description of routine healing procedures will be activated following surgery and other interventions, and they will have the potential to increase levels of comfort and speed the healing process. McCaffery and Beebe (1989) are a good source for additional discussion and guidance on the topic of using language-based conversational images in the treatment of pain.

Relaxation

Relaxation is considered to be a state marked by a relative absence of anxiety and skeletal muscle tension. Most relaxation procedures include a mental device to block distracting thoughts, a passive attitude, a quiet environment, a comfortable position, and behaviors previously conditioned to result in relaxation, such as deep abdominal breathing and a focus on peaceful images (Benson & Stark, 1996; Korn, 1982, 1983; McCaffery & Beebe, 1989; Sheikh et al., 1985; Syrjala & Abrams, 2002).

Relaxation appears to be one of the most important prerequisites for the experience of vivid and absorbing imagery, because it seems to allow the process of becoming aware of internal states to begin. During relaxation, the noisy, hectic world is shut out, and the inner world, the realm of imaginal experience, has a chance to become the focus of attention (Bakan, 1980; Gendlin, 1981; Sheikh et al., 1985).

It follows that pain-relief imagery generally is preceded by relaxation techniques. Again, relaxation is believed to increase the effectiveness of pain-relief imagery by enhancing the vividness of one's images and thereby one's absorption within them. Recall that empirical studies have demonstrated consistent effects for relaxation alone in the treatment of pain. This therapeutic impact can be understood through a cyclic and systemic understanding of the pathogenesis of pain disorders: Pain perception is impacted in concert by factors such as attention, affect, coping responses, and beliefs. Each of these factors moderating the perception of pain can be affected by levels of anxiety. Numerous relaxation procedures have been developed over the years, and it is beyond the scope of the current discussion to review them all. A number of other sources contain additional information regarding relaxation procedures for pain management (Korn & Johnson, 1983; McCaffery & Beebe, 1989; Naparstek, 1994; Ost, 1987; Samuels & Samuels, 1975; Sheikh, 2002), and Miller (1983) produced an excellent audio recording of guided imagery vignettes for pain management (available at http://www.drmiller.com/products/body; see also Miller, 1997).

Favorite Place

One simple relaxation script that can be used following deep breathing or some other concentration-focusing induction (see Chapter 4) is imagery of a favorite place. An example follows from Syrjala and Abrams (1996, p. 252):

> As you enjoy this feeling of deep comfort and well-being, allow yourself to begin to create a special place of your choosing. A place where you feel safe and secure and content. It may be a place you have been before, it may be a place you would like to go now, or a place only in your imagination. All that matters is that you find a place for you right now. And begin to notice that place. Notice if it is indoors or out. Observe what is all around you. Take it in. Notice the colors, the different hues and tones of color. Perhaps there are reds or yellows … the light and the dark shades, the light around you …. Explore the shapes in your surroundings … perhaps you can reach out and touch things, notice what they feel like …. Are they soft or hard, rough or smooth, warm or cool? Making it all real for you now, enjoying being in this pleasant, safe place, experiencing it fully.

Once within a special place, patients may be instructed to select one salient object or aspect of the place, a word that may be used to represent the entire image. Have your patients repeat this key word several times within the imaginary scene to increase the association between the word and the special place. Then, between sessions your patients may be instructed to practice returning to their special place at a set time each day (e.g., upon waking in the morning is a good time). After several weeks of practice, they may begin to evoke the special-place imagery and the sense of relaxation that comes with it prior to or during a stressful or painful experience. The resulting relaxation may reduce pain directly or may simply allow them to better engage in effective problem solving or healthy coping responses.

Other Places: Beaches, Mountains, and Gardens

In addition to the more general relaxing imaginary voyage to a unique favorite place of patients' choosing, more directive imaginary excursions may be taken to specific destinations that most individuals find relaxing. Kroger and Fezler (1976) provide a menu of relaxation scripts, including the ubiquitous beach imagery, as well as less common destinations such as a mountain cabin and a garden scene. These scenes are described subsequently in the form of scripts adapted from the originals.

In each scene, it is important to engage, at a minimum, the dominant five senses of sight, hearing, touch, taste, and smell. Visual, auditory, and tactile senses are typically the easiest to engage, in that order, particularly within a beach scene. The mountain cabin scene is designed to help with the more difficult tactile senses such as hot and cold, along with olfaction and taste. The garden scene really highlights the olfactory senses.

The desirability of any of these modalities will depend on patients and their experience with pain. As always, you should feel free to improvise as needed and to actively collaborate with your patients in the generation of individualized imagery experiences from the following scripts.

A Trip to the Beach

Close your eyes and take two deep cleansing breaths, in through your nose, and out through your mouth … in … and out [in time with patient's breathing]. Continue to breath at your own pace … and with each new breath, allow yourself to become more and more relaxed. And when you have come to a state of calm and relaxation, tell me so [wait until the patient does so]. Okay, allow the images in front of you to dissolve away, so that there is darkness in front of you. In your imagination, your eyes are also closed. When I count to three, I want you to open your eyes within your imagination. And when you open them, you will find that you are on the most beautiful beach that can be imagined. The perfect beach. One … two … three. In your mind, open your eyes and find yourself at the beach. Look down. You see that you are wearing your favorite, your most comfortable beach clothing. Notice the color of your clothing, whether tan, white, or multicolored. Notice the fabric of the clothing against your skin: soft, cool, and comfortable, perfect for the weather which is warm against your skin. Walk onto the beach and feel the warm sand under your feet. Look up and see the ocean. Hear the waves rolling onto the shore in front of you. Look out over the cool water. Notice the ripples, extending out to the horizon ahead of you. See the colors of the sea— blue, green, hints of yellow dancing on the distant waves, as the sun glows overhead. Feel the warmth of that sun on your face. Close your eyes and soak it in, feeling the warmth on your face, your cheeks and lips. Feel the breeze washing over the warm rays of sun, keeping you warm and cool at the same time. Comfortable. Smell the warm clean sand in front of you, and taste the slight saltiness of the air on your tongue. Notice the sounds of the beach, the sea birds, children play- ing in the water, or the simple sound of silence and rolling waves and gentle breeze, if you find yourself alone. You are completely calm and at peace. Walk forward and find a comfortable spot: perhaps under the sun or under the shade of a sleepy tree—wherever you would like. Now lay down your blanket of relaxation and have a seat or lie down and close your eyes, if you like. Take some time to reflect on the magic of this place, this perfect beach. Listen to the sounds, see the sights, and allow yourself to find a place of calm reflection, away from the real world. Just be. I'll check back with you after a few minutes to see if you are ready to return. Enjoy and relax [wait 2–3 minutes]. Tell me now, if you are ready to leave this magic beach? [If not, allow 2–3 more minutes, otherwise say:] Then let's prepare to leave. First, take one long last look around. Look at the beach, all the sights—the sky, the sun, and the ocean waves in front of you, going out to the hori- zon. Hear the sounds, smell the salt, and soak in the relaxation one last time. Choose one word to remind you of your magic beach. This will be a word you may say to yourself that will bring you back here, immediately, to relive the experience just as fully and vividly as it is now. Your word may be *beach* or *tree* or *shell*—whatever fits for you, to remind you of this place, and the relaxation you have found here. When you have this word, tell me. Now count to three and when you reach three you will open your eyes, bringing with you your state of perfect relaxation, to carry you through the rest of your day.

A number of suggestions were used within this beach scene, sugges- tions that may be used as desired and in varying degrees in other imag- ery exercises as well. First, the vignette involved focused attention on the patient's clothing. Attention to clothing within an imaginary scene is a good strategy for increasing emersion within the scene. Clothing has direct contact with the body and so assists patients in becoming embodied within the scene. Each new sensory aspect of the beach scene began with visual information and then proceeded to involve other sensory information, including sound, touch, taste, and tactile aspects such as texture and temperature. In each case, a variety of options were used, and details were left as open-ended as possible. The patient was guided to generate a key word that could be used as a trigger to evoke the scene and associated feelings of relaxation to be accessed in everyday life. This strategy may be helpful in other imagery situations, where it is useful to assist patients in generating a positive sensory, affective, or state of meaning that has been harvested through imagery during times of stress or pain. Finally, the therapist allowed the patient to decide when to return and to count to three rather than doing the counting. This option for ending an imagery session is especially beneficial for enhancing patients' self-efficacy, giving them a boost in their sense of mastery and the ability to end the scene and bring whatever changes have occurred with them into their wakeful day. Such an exit may be particularly appropriate toward the end of treatment, for example, when patients are making the shift toward using imagery on their own.

A Night in the Mountains   A night in the mountains is a relaxation scenario that is designed to involve the more difficult senses, such as smell and temperature. It also simply provides an alternative to the beach for patients who would prefer a night in a mountain cabin to a day at the beach as a means of relaxation:

> [Provide standard brief focusing, breathing, and relaxing suggestions.] Find yourself in a comfortable wood cabin. You are high up in the mountains, and it is the dead of winter. A fire is burning in the great fireplace in the middle of the cabin. You can hear the crackling of the flames, feel the heat wafting out and filling the room with warmth. You can smell the light scent of smoke and burning logs as you watch the fire. You even can hear the air being consumed by the bright, pulsing flames: red, orange, yellow, and a hint of blue rising from its coals. It's a big hot fire, and you are sitting close enough, in your soft, comfortable chair, to feel its intense heat on your thighs, knees, and shins. Stand up and walk barefoot over the soft bearskin rug in front of the fire to the window to take a look at the mountains outside. It is dark, and you run your warm fingertips over the cold, hard glass of the windowpane. Look outside and see the moon, full and white, rising over a grand mountain in the distance. The moon is round and white, like the snow sparkling below, covering the branches of tall, green fir trees surrounding the cabin. The fire is throwing deep purple flickering shadows onto the

closest trees, while soft blue shadows are cast across the snow from the moon slowly climbing in the darkness of the mountain sky. Push the window open and breathe in the cool, crisp mountain air. With each cool breath, you become more and more calm, relaxed, and at peace with the world. Smell the soft scent of pine and with each deep breath you breathe …. When you are ready, pull the window closed and walk back to the big fur rug in front the of the fire. Lie down on the rug. Feel its softness against your skin, and feel the warmth and comfort of the fire, now that it has died down just a bit. Watch the flickering of the flames, red, orange, yellow, and the blue near the coals. Feel the warmth on your face, and shoulders and chest. Smell the light smokiness and the scent of wood of the cabin around you and just relax….

The Garden   A trip to the garden is another option for those who do not find the beach or a mountain cabin particularly relaxing. Gardens, for example, the Garden of Eden, are archetypal symbols of innocence, life, health, and vitality. Gardens are almost universally representative of feelings of peace, calm, and relaxation. They may also promote inner contemplation and are likely to engage the broader senses, such as smell through the inclusion of various scented flowers. Most individuals can easily conjure a full and detailed garden scene, even if they do not have a garden themselves:

When you are ready, place yourself at the start of a path that leads into the most beautiful garden one could imagine. Walk down the path of soft short grass. It is morning in the garden, and the temperature is perfect, with a soft breeze flowing through the garden, moving the petals of the larger trees and flowers ever so slightly. You are barefoot, and the soft grass feels slightly moist from the morning dew. There is some humidity in the air that pulls the gorgeous smells from the flowers into the air, in molecules of water, pouring into your nostrils. Breathe deeply, and feel the scent of the flowers fill you with peace and beauty. You hear the songs of birds overhead, as they enjoy the morning air and the sanctuary of the perfect garden. Your clothing is light, and comfortable; it hangs freely from your skin as you walk deeper into the garden. There you see larger fruit trees, filled with ripe lemons and oranges. You may pick a lemon or an orange to carry along. Select one that is large and juicy, hanging in front of your hand on a low branch. Feel the coolness of the skin of the fruit in your hand. As you walk further into the garden, you find a patch of hundreds of rose bushes, surrounding a natural pool. The roses are pink, red, yellow … all the colors of the rainbow and more …

and as you walk up to the pool you can see that the rose petals have fallen and are floating upon the surface of the water. As you decide to wade into the warm water of the pond, you look down and see that your clothing has shifted into bathing gear. Walk into the water ... the rose petals, in all the colors, part around you as you walk into the shallow water ... chest high. You float in the warm water among the petals...the smells are so beautiful. Look around and soak in the beauty of your perfect garden.

Mental Rehearsal

Mental rehearsal involves the imaginary experience of going through particular steps to attain a specific goal (Newshan & Balamuth, 1990–1991), such as the mental practice that professional athletes like gymnasts or football kickers include in their regimen. Mental rehearsal also has been applied to situations in which the goal is to reduce the pain associated with certain medical procedures, such as bone marrow aspirations (LeBaron & Zeltzer, 1996), surgeries (Meyer, 1992), burn treatment (Achterberg, Kenner, & Lawless, 1988; Patterson, 1996), or childbirth (Lindberg & Lawlis, 1988; Oster, 1994). For example, the following is a brief excerpt from mental-rehearsal imagery for burn treatment from Achterberg et al. (1988, p. 86):

> Just let the fear go. Imagine now as the time approaches for you to get your dressings taken off and go to the bath—picture this in your imagination. Just relax, feeling deeper and deeper, breathing deeply whenever you feel uncomfortable. The nurse comes in now and starts to cut your bandages off. Imagine this happening, whenever you feel uncomfortable, breathe, relax. Imagine this happening, feeling the nurse cut the bandages off and your skin feeling the coolness. Take a deep breath and let any discomfort go, feeling relaxed and calm now .... You begin to get out of your bed—maybe by yourself, relaxed and calm and feeling very good.

Burn treatment is perhaps the prototypic example of the need for rehearsal prior to treatment, because burn treatment involving return to movement and activity typically is invasive, frequent, and long lasting, involving daily sessions over the course of several months. These rehabilitation sessions can be incredibly painful in the short term yet vital to long-term recovery (Patterson, 1996). Tolerance of the procedure will be greatly enhanced by enacting imagery of both the pain and the benefits prior to each treatment session. Depending on the particular coping styles of each patient, rehearsal of burn treatments may involve the use of distraction for more avoidant types or of transformation of pain and enhanced sense of control and predictability for those who are more control oriented.

Achterberg, Dossey, and Kolkmeier (1994) wrote extensively on the use of therapeutic imagery for other types of procedural pain as well. This type of imagery aims to combine actual anatomical and lab-based assessment information with mental imagery and healing transformations. For example, x-ray results, scopes, or anatomical illustrations may be used to assist the patient to invoke images that are aligned with the body's physical healing processes. Such imagery was the primary intervention described in Cupal and Brewer's (2001) study of recovery responses of college athletes following anterior cruciate ligament (ACL) reconstruction. In this study, participants reviewed the video images from their orthoscopes to develop accurate images of their actual tissue being repaired during the surgical procedure. Healing of this tissue along with the reduction of surrounding inflammation was a target of subsequent imagery sessions.

When selecting rehearsal imagery for procedural pain, it is important to consider the potential negative impacts of painful medical procedures on an individual's self-concept and interpersonal style. Imagery is especially suited to mitigating these negative impacts. Specifically, painful medical procedures may lead to increased dependence, lost sense of control and life mastery, a sense of incompetence in the face of difficult medical jargon and procedural descriptions, and, in the worst scenarios, the adoption of a victim role, a view of the medical treatment as an enemy, and a general sense of passivity toward recovery. Imagery can be useful in shifting these mindsets toward active and informed involvement within the treatment and recovery process (Bejenke, 1996).

Furthermore, it is important to keep in mind that the patient role, when combined with anxiety and stress, may bring many patients into a highly suggestive state during interactions with physicians. Therefore, physicians and other practitioners should be mindful of the language they are using with patients and of the images they can invoke. Images should be realistic yet balanced in regard to the benefits of the intervention and inclusive of the specific processes involved in healing and pain management.

Other Behavioral Imagery Techniques

Several other imagery techniques have been developed from the behavioral perspective, in addition to rehearsal for procedural pain. These techniques essentially rest on a number of different overlapping behavioral and cognitive-behavioral theoretical frameworks. The simplest techniques are based on systematic desensitization (Wolpe, 1969) in which the negative emotions (e.g., fear) associated with pain are diminished by gradually exposing the patient to pain-related images. Once fear and other negative emotions are diminished through imaginal exposure, the perception of pain may be decreased directly, and rehabilitation may be enhanced by reducing any overreliance on avoidance-based coping responses (e.g., inactivity). Behavioral therapists not only encourage patients to face the stressor in the imagination but also guide them in the practice of skills that aid in coping with the pain. This aspect of treatment relies on both *self-efficacy theory* (Bandura, 1986) and *stress inoculation theory* as applied to pain (Turk, Meichenbaum, & Genest, 1983). Self-efficacy theory describes the increase in pain-coping confidence that may be gained as patients observe themselves practicing coping behaviors within the imagination. In a sense, the patient is receiving instruction from a role model, but this role model is also the patient. Due to the equivalence between patient and self-model, this form of modeling, referred to as *participant modeling*, is the strongest form of observational learning that can be used to improve confidence and gain skills.

The related theory of stress inoculation relies on the fact that anxiety and other negative emotions are intensified by being surprised by a stressor or by feeling that the stressful situation is out of control. Individuals with anxiety disorders are more likely to overuse avoidance and distraction as coping methods (Meichenbaum, 1977), which compounds the individuals difficulties in the long run as these coping methods do not facilitate the learning of coping skills. Therefore, stress inoculation emphasizes the importance of learning coping skills to handle a stressor, and it also assists individuals in looking forward to plan for an upcoming stressor, to reduce the sense that the stressor is unpredictable and out of control. The name *stress inoculation* is a metaphor of inoculation against a viral infection, in which a small amount of dormant virus is injected to build up a patient's natural resistances to that virus. Similarly, in stress inoculation training, the aim is to expose the patient to low levels of dormant stressor (i.e., within the imagination) to build up the individual's natural coping resources and to shift the conscious attention to signs that the stressor may be coming.

The detailed rationale has been provided to enable collaboration more effectively with your patients to achieve the goals of this type of therapy and to focus on the relevant changes that are desired through treatment. Consequently, you and your patient will be better able to understand the process of treatment, to discuss the relevant outcomes after each session, and to change your procedures as needed to improve each of the outcomes independently, be they negative emotion extinction, confidence building, or skill acquisition.

The procedure is rather simple and involves a natural combination of imaginal relaxation, desensitization, and the rehearsal of coping skills.

Treatment begins by developing a hierarchy of triggers for pain and of situations in which pain is most unpleasant. For example, patients may describe humidity, stress, or lack of sleep as triggers for pain, and they may describe being in pain at family gatherings, at work, or when they are alone as most unpleasant. If patients are not aware of triggers and of various stressful situations, they should be assigned a pain journal for a week or two to gather the necessary information. Once the information is gathered, the patient should develop a hierarchy in which each trigger and each situation is rated from 1 to 10 (or 1 to 100) in terms of severity. Incidentally, simply gathering the information and building the hierarchy are likely to be therapeutic, because unconscious images arise during this process. Thus begins the process of desensitization, which in turn reverses an overreliance on avoidance and distraction coping methods and allows alternate skill-based strategies to develop spontaneously.

Lueger (1986) identifies two types of coping rehearsal: (1) *mastery modeling*, involving flawless and easy performance in the face of pain; and (2) *coping modeling*, involving great struggle and setbacks in the face of pain, during which the patient practices self- and world acceptance and waits until the pain subsides on its own. These approaches rest on primary- and secondary-control strategies, respectively (as discussed in Chapter 4). One would expect coping modeling to be the most effective approach, since the patient is developing skills to facilitate acceptance along with the ability to cope with and to survive even the worst of setbacks (Bellissimo & Tunks, 1984; Lueger, 1986). Yet, mastery modeling may be desirable in situations where mastery reasonably may be achieved.

Once the scored hierarchy of pain triggers and situations is developed, the person is guided to imagine the lower-level contents of the hierarchy first, signaling to the therapist when things become tough. At this point, the therapist may lead the patient through a prearranging covert coping response that has been worked out in session prior to imagery. Alternatively, the therapist guides the images to discomfort and then instructs the patient to spontaneously imagine his or her own responses. Both procedures can be useful in any particular course of treatment; for example, patients can begin by identifying their own spontaneous strategies (the second method) and then can make plans to rehearse those strategies in subsequent imaginary scenarios. The following is an example script of coping-based imagery from Turk et al. (1983, p. 326):

> Now as you sit in the chair, relaxed, imagine the scene in which you are waking up in the middle of the night from pain. It is very quiet. You don't wish to disturb anyone, but you are in pain. You have feelings of becoming depressed. "Oh no, not again. I'll never be able to have a good night's sleep." As you begin to feel the tension building in

your body, you first rate the pain on your 6-point scale. It is severe—a 3, maybe a 4. "What can I do about it?" You can hear yourself saying, "Oh yes, my plan for such occasions; don't make the pain worse." See yourself taking a slow breath. Breathing easily and evenly, helping reduce the pain. "Now to shift my attention ... Good."

Within this approach, imagery scenes tend to be short, lasting between 30 seconds and a few minutes, followed by a discussion of the experience to work through any negative emotions that are aroused and to process the experience for new meaning and coping-related beliefs. Furthermore, Lueger (1986) suggests that it may be helpful to regard treatment as consisting of three phases: (1) the *educational phase*, in which patients learn the rationale for coping skills, how to monitor stress reactions, and the negative impact of avoidance and withdrawal; (2) the *rehearsal phase*, in which patients learn techniques to manage stress responses and coping responses to stressful stimuli; and (3) the *application phase*, in which patients practice the coping skills during exposure to imagined stressors.

A number of additional procedures may be added to the application phase, based on the fact that the rehearsal of coping skills is taking place within the realm of the imagination. For example, patients may be instructed to view the imagery as a film, which can be slowed, stopped, or rewound, to enhance the patient's sense of control and to allow for such things as "do-overs" in certain situations. Specific coping skills that may be used include the practice of progressive muscle relaxation, breathing exercises, or even imagining the use of imagery. They key in coping practice within the imagination is not to eliminate the stressor in any sort of nonrealistic sense. Rather, the patient is guided in practicing any realistic and active coping responses that may enhance the experience of mastery over pain. In this regard, reassuring self-statements may even be practiced within the imagination. Levels of self-statements will depend on the degree of pain and stress that the patient is encountering. For example, four exemplary self-statements, ranging from the beginning of a flare-up to the end follow (adapted from Lueger, 1986):

1. "I've prepared for this flare up. If I stay calm and active, it will eventually pass."
2. "Okay, the pain is increasing now, but my breathing is deep and steady. I am focused on my activity and letting the pain alone."
3. "I knew the pain would come back and test me and that sometimes it would be worse than others. I'm not going to let it ruin my activity; I am prepared."
4. "Okay, that was painful but I'm okay. In fact, it wasn't as bad as it could have been and I'm proud that I stayed calm and allowed it to pass."

Simple Transformational Imagery

Simple transformational imagery is used to change the sensory aspects or the contexts of pain in a relatively direct manner (Fernandez, 1986). Barber (1996) describes two primary goals of the use of such techniques in cases involving chronic pain. First, one may aim to transform pain sensations to such a degree as to render them benign enough to be incorporated into the patients' day-to-day lives, decreasing their tendency to rely on dysfunctional withdrawal and avoidance coping strategies. Second, one may assist patients in coming to the realization that suffering need not accompany pain. This may help to remove suffering from the sense of self and from the ways the patient relates to others and to the world in general. The life impacts of even the simplest transformational techniques may be far-reaching

When attempting to transform an imaginary context of pain, for example, the situation or setting in which pain occurs is the target for transformation. Fernandez (1986) describes the use of this type of imagery: Subjects experiencing forearm pain were asked to imagine that they were spies, shot in the arm by their enemies, and were now being chased by these enemies down a treacherous mountain road. One can also find an example of context transformation within each of the imaginary journeys during childbirth. Within these imaginary scenes, labor pain is transformed from a relatively detached and medically oriented experience into a rite of womanhood, represented as a journey to greet the yet unborn child.

Sensory transformation imagery is simple imagery aimed directly at transforming pain sensations. As mentioned previously, Melzack and Wall's (1996) gate-control theory of pain proposes three relatively independent dimensions of the pain experience: sensory-discriminative, motivational-affective, and cognitive-evaluative. These dimensions combine to determine, among other phenomena, pain intensity. As the term suggests, these types of imagery interventions aim at the most simple and obvious of these dimensions: the pain sensations themselves. Numerous examples of this type of imagery can be found within hypnosis literature under the label *sensory substitution* (Barber, 1996). Some examples of sensations that have been used for this type of imagery include relative numbness, itchiness, and pressure.

To use sensory-transformation techniques, patients must have good awareness of the sensory aspects of their pain and must be willing to apply attention to their pain without increasing worry about the need to seek medical attention for the pain experiences as they shift. For example, if numbness is experienced by some patients, they will fear that there is some further injury that is occurring, even if the imagery-induced numbness is effective in blocking out the pain. Furthermore, since the substitute sensation needs to be plausible to the patient, it must not be too pleasant (Barber, 1996). A sense of tickling, for example, is not likely to work as a replacement of a sharp stabbing pain.

Stimulus-transformative imagery may be viewed as a special case of sensory-transformation imagery, in which the cause (either manifest or imagined) of the pain is changed or transformed. For example, stomach pain can be envisioned as tight steel bands, which are then loosened in the imagination (Levendusky & Pankratz, 1975). The following case of a 42-year-old paraplegic patient experiencing burning in his legs illustrates the use of sensory-transformation imagery focused on the transformation of the stimulus:

> The feelings that you describe (needles stabbing into his thighs) can begin to change, very slightly. Oddly enough, it may begin to seem as if the needles are becoming more and more blunt ... broad ... almost as if they have become tiny, massaging fingers. What an interesting sensation you can begin to have: thousands of warm, buzzing fingers, massaging your legs. Not entirely pleas- ant, of course, but perhaps a welcome relief. (Barber, 1996, pp. 89–90)

You should not be surprised if your patients go deeper than anticipated during these simple transformation procedures. They may experience shifts within the motivation-affective or cognitive-evaluative dimensions as well, or they may make broader self and relational shifts following changes in pain sensations, particularly if the pain is complex and if the imagery is relatively open-ended rather than scripted. The sensory-discriminatory dimension is like an entranceway into the pain system. For some patients, the journey will stay near the entrance; for others, the imagery will carry them deeper into the system. Therefore, these techniques are very well suited to patients who prefer to focus directly on sensations, who are more concrete and literal in their thinking, or who have relatively uncompli- cated pain syndromes (e.g., procedural pain) that is less likely to require broader schematic transformation.

Syrjala and Abrams (2002) describe numerous transformational tech- niques aimed at context or sensations. For example, one can imagine ice melting across a painful area, absorbing pain sensation, inducing numb- ness, or leading to tingling sensations that are mixed with the pain. Favorite place imagery may be conceptualized beyond relaxation as a means to transform the context of pain, whereby patients still may experience pain but in an imaginary place of their choosing. This may be particularly help- ful in pain syndromes or procedures that involve discrete, time-limited pain flare-ups. Pain contexts may also be transformed in a more meta- phoric manner: Patients can be directed to fly above their pain or to move down a path or a stairway away from pain and toward relief. Patients may shift their sensations by imagining pain channels to the brain, which may be blocked, or switches that may be turned on and off, or dials in which the volume of pain may be turned down. Other techniques focus on exploring the sites of pain in the imagination, opening the channels of pain rather than decreasing them to enhance acceptance and secondary-control strategies, or moving pain from the original site to a more convenient location. The list of possibilities is endless, particularly with some patients who will be able to generate their own idiosyncratic transformations with less guidance. The following examples provide some specific techniques to organize your work—starting points from which to explore and experiment.

Glove Anesthesia

A variety of imagery techniques may be used to transform a pain response into numbness in a particular body part (Hilgard & Hilgard, 1994). One example is *glove anesthesia* (Bresler, 1984). Within this procedure, patients learn how to develop a numbing sensation in their hands, which helps to convince them that they can have some control over the intensity of their pain. When the feeling of numbness is achieved, they learn to transfer this numbness from the hand to the pain site by rubbing it with the anesthetized hand (Bresler, 1984; Hilgard & Hilgard, 1994), employing the principle of contact as unification. This technique is demonstrated in the following example:

> You are aware that you are unable to feel anything in your hand. It is as if your hand is numb, without sensation, and you can take your hand and move it to where you feel discomfort, gently rubbing your hand over the uncomfortable area. And as you rub this numb hand, this hand without feeling, over the uncomfortable place, you are aware that the numbness is moving, is being transferred to that place, as if you were rubbing Novocain over the affected area, making the uncomfortable sensation cease. (Meyer, 1992, pp. 229–230)

The glove anesthesia technique is especially helpful for patients who are experiencing occasional flare-ups of intense localized pain, such as arthritis, lower-back pain, or procedural pains. The first step of the process, induced numbness to the hand, is an easier transformation, from neutral to numbness. It enhances confidence before the numbness is applied to the pain site. In the second step, the numbness is transferred in an automatic manner, without much direct activation of the will. This process of rubbing the numbness in, like Novocain, allows the imagination to bypass any self-doubts or lapses in patient confidence. Yet the technique involves a process of direct control, which is likely to reduce secondary pain contributors, such as anxiety, perceived helplessness, and a sense of being ill.

This technique can be practiced until the patient becomes more proficient in the numbing of the hand and managing occasional flare-ups.

Displacement

Another technique that allows patients to better tolerate localized pain is to displace the pain from one area of the body to another (Hilgard & Hilgard, 1994). First, patients are guided to concentrate the pain into a smaller area and then to move it to another body part, such as the hand, where the pain may be easier to tolerate. Patients themselves should be allowed to choose the area to which they would like to move the pain. The following is an example of a suggestion within an imagery session used to induce the displacement of pain:

> You may have already noticed that the pain moves, ever so slightly, and you can begin to notice that the movement seems to be in an outwardly spiraling, circular direction. As you continue to attend to that movement, you may not notice until some time later that the pain has somehow moved out of your abdomen and seems to be staying in your left hand. It seems to be very much the same sensation … yet, for some reason, it seems less bothersome. (Barber, 1996, p. 90)

If the displacement technique is effective, patients may experience relief through a number of different experiential channels. The pain may be easier to tolerate in the new location. In addition, perceptions of control, hope, and confidence may increase with improved pain management. The experience of moving the pain may decrease a patient's sense that pain is monolithic, all powerful, or all consuming. This procedure may aid the patient to realize that pain is an experience like any other, which will change over time.

Direct Diminution of Sensations

One of the simplest techniques for directly reducing pain through imagery is to use the imagination to diminish the noxious sensory aspects of pain (Barber, 1996). Possible suggestions toward this effect include turning down the volume of pain to reduce pain intensity or cooling the pain to reduce burning sensations. To maximize effectiveness, the choice of the reduction metaphor should match the pain image of the patient. The following is an example of suggestive language used within this technique:

> You can continue to enjoy feeling increasingly well, with each breath you take … almost as if the discomfort is somehow gradually going away…as if, somehow, the feelings are getting smaller and smaller and smaller, or, perhaps, getting farther and farther and farther from your awareness. (Barber, 1996, p. 88)

In another common pain diminution technique, pain is decreased through the use of scaling of intensity:

> And now you can see the number seven, the number you have given to your pain. And as you see this number, you see that it is slowly, slowly changing. Now the number is six. And as you look at that number, at the number six, you are aware that your discomfort has lessened. And a six is very much like five. And as you watch, the six is changing into a five. And as you see the five, you begin to feel more comfortable. And a five is not much different from a four. And a four is very close to a three. The number is now a three. And with each change the number makes, each time the number changes into another number, your comfort becomes greater. And with only a small change, with very little effort, you can see the number three turn into a two. And as you see the two, as you experience the two, you are more and more comfortable. (Meyer, 1992, pp. 221–222)

It is noteworthy that although the numbers are decreasing along with pain, the guide focuses more attention on the positive process of increasing relief than on decreasing pain. Within direct-diminution techniques, as in other techniques, it is important to check in with the patients to ensure that your pacing is in step with theirs and that the obstacles have not appeared. Some patients, for example, will become stuck at a particular number: They can move to pain at a level four, for example, but cannot decrease the value to three. In these instances, the guide can explore the nature of the blockage, working toward deeper techniques, or can encourage the patient to go ahead and stop at four for the time being.

Ostrander, Schroeder, and Ostrander (1979) describe a slightly more complex variant of direct diminution involving the transfer of hot or cold to a site of pain. For example, one can repeatedly imagine immersing one's finger tips in a bucket of ice water, imagining them becoming colder and colder. Once the experience of the cold finger tips is achieved, the patient is guided to physically rub the cold sensations into a pain site to transfer the sense of numbness to provide temporary relief during flare-ups of conditions such as osteoarthritis. Ostrander et al. also describe a technique involving hand-warming, which other practitioners agree can be effective for preventing the onset and lessening the intensity of migraine headaches, perhaps due to associated changes in blood flow in the extremities (Achterberg et al., 1994). In this exercise, one simply warms the hands in front of an imaginary fire (or similar heat source) while practicing relaxation through breathing and calm imagery. One can apply the warm hands to the forehead if desired, but this is not a necessary step.

Each of these techniques has the advantage of reducing pain in an indirect manner, through cooling or warming of extremities, and may be helpful to patients who wish to establish a sense of control over intermittent pain without applying deeper or more direct techniques. As with all imagery techniques, these strategies should be practiced by patients during times when they are not in pain so that they will be able to follow through with the technique confidently during a flare-up.

Dissociation

Dissociation allows patients to separate themselves from their pain by directing their attention elsewhere. Dissociative techniques (Hilgard & Hilgard, 1994) allow patients to be aware of their pain without suffering from it (Barber, 1996). In one variety of dissociation, patients deny the existence of the part of the body that is feeling pain:

> Think that you have no left arm. Look down and see that there is no left arm there, only an empty sleeve. An arm that does not exist does not feel anything. Your arm is gone only temporarily; you will find it amusing, not alarming, that for a while you have no left arm. (Hilgard & Hilgard, 1994, p. 66)

Kelly and Kelly (1995) present another dissociation technique called *leaving your body behind*. The technique directs patients to become completely dissociated from their bodies by allowing their consciousness to float away:

> As you settle in, so peaceful, comfortable, relaxed, and at ease, you are going to allow yourself to have a curious sort of experience. You are going to allow yourself to leave your body behind. Just imagine yourself seeing your body sitting there or lying there, comfortably hypnotized, and imagine seeing a sort of translucent image of yourself stepping out from your body. (p. 280)

When using this technique, it is important to reassure patients that if there is any bodily information they need to know while in this state, they would be informed immediately. This assurance allows them to more fully engage in the imagery:

> You see yourself stepping away from your own body, feeling safe and secure. You are allowing your spirit, your mind, your psyche to become somewhat detached and removed from your body. You know that it's there. You know what's going on in it. It doesn't matter very much to you, however .... Where you are, it's comfortable and safe. It's peaceful. It's relaxed. Any sensations come to you only very slowly .... You get news of your body. You get information about it,

but only rather slowly and sort of after the fact. (Kelly & Kelly, 1995, p. 280)

Incompatible Imagery

Incompatible imagery may be broken down into two types: incompatible sensory imagery and incompatible emotive imagery (Fernandez, 1986). They work by blocking the sensory and the motivational-affective dimensions of pain, respectively (Melzack & Wall, 1965). Emotions that are incompatible with pain include happiness, confidence, and pride. Furthermore, the relaxation techniques described at the outset of this chapter could be categorized as the simplest of the incompatible emotive techniques, in which relaxing images (e.g., a day at the beach or in a favorite place) block or dull the experience of pain.

Incompatible sensory imagery involves the use of pure auditory, visual, or other sensations that are incompatible with pain but not necessarily tied to a person's emotions (Fernandez, 1986). Pleasant imagery, such as blue skies, gentle warmth, fluffy clouds, and grassy meadows, can be used to inhibit pain (Horan, 1973). Instructing patients to use these types of images when they are experiencing pain can aid in reducing discomfort. One of many examples of this type of imagery given by Ferrucci (1982, p. 123) involves imagining a burning flame:

> Imagine a burning flame. See it dancing, drawing ever-changing designs in the air. Look into it as it moves; seek to experience its fiery quality. As you keep visualizing this flame, think about fire and its manifestations in the psyche: personal warmth and radiance, flaming love or joy, fiery enthusiasm, ardor. Finally, as you keep the flame in front of your inner eye, slowly imagine that you are animated by that fire, that you are becoming that flame.

The use of deeper varieties of techniques will be determined by the specific imaginal manifestations of a patient's pain and will involve a transformation of the motivational-affective dimension of the pain rather than a simple blocking it by an imaginary scene that evokes positive feelings. These deeper techniques involve the transformation of key developmental memories and therefore would be better categorized as follows. However, these techniques often become necessary when one evokes the emotional information associated with a particular pain syndrome.

For example, following a relaxation script, a patient was asked to describe the sensory aspects of her migraine headaches. She was then queried in detail regarding the emotions that accompany these sensations. She described feeling helpless, vulnerable, weak, and angry. This patient connected these feelings to episodic memories of being teased by other children on the playground. The stress of this time in life probably triggered the onset of these migraines, since they began shortly thereafter, and they have reappeared occasionally, particularly during times of stress. Through deeper exploration of the patient's pain narrative, it became clear that feelings of helplessness, fear, and suppressed anger were particularly linked to the headaches, acting as triggers and also as pain intensifiers.

In this case, the aim was to transform this patient's negative feelings within specific episodic memories, which involved tormenting by a group of 5th-grade girls on the playground. These memories were the focus of guided imagery, and changes in affect were the targets for transformation. Specifically, this patient chose to confront her imaginary tormenters in a number of powerful imaginary scenes. In doing so, her feelings of helplessness, fear, and repressed anger were transformed into confidence, power, and expressed anger. By shifting these emotional responses to migraines within these imaginary scenes, the patient shifted her relationship with the migraines as well and experienced reduced frequency and intensity of subsequent headaches.

CHAPTER 6

Pain Management

Deeper Techniques

The first step to better times is to imagine them.

From a Chinese fortune cookie

The deeper techniques in this chapter involve a greater degree of the symbolic transformation of pain than do the simple techniques of Chapter 5. These deeper techniques also involve more active participation by patients in exploring their imaginations and engaging their creativity. A number of experiential approaches follow that involve greater active participation from patients in creating symbolic transformations of imagery—for example, collecting a variety of pains into a ball that may then be removed from the body, representing the body and its pain as sand draining out of a bag, or representing healing resources in the form of radiant light. The present chapter concludes with a number of imaginary voyages through the body to directly interact with physical structures involved with pain.

The Ball of Pain

The *ball-of-pain* technique (Achterberg, Dossey, & Kolkmeier, 1994) works with resistance rather than against it. It encourages the full experience of pain before it is diminished, by increasing the patients attention to pain and the perception of the pain as a noxious experience: "Give yourself some time to relax and let go of your tension .... Scan your body now for any aches, pains, tightness, or discomforts, both physical and emotional" (Achterberg et al., p. 125). The guide continues to work with the discomfort of all varieties of pain throughout the body, rolling them together into a big ball of pain within the patient's consciousness:

> Now begin to gather up the pain into a ball, ... a glowing, colored ball .... When you have the ball firmly in your mind's eye, begin to change the size of the ball, noticing how the shadings and intensity of the color change as you make the ball larger ... and then smaller .... Change the size of the ball several times, allowing it to become very large, larger than your entire body ... and then watch and feel it shrink down to a tiny dot of color .... Play with the possibilities of size, intensity, and color. (Achterberg et al., p. 125)

As patients improve in their ability to manipulate the size and brightness of their imaginary ball of pain, they increase their sense of mastery, control, and confidence in relation to the pain. At the same time, flexibility is brought to the pain system, as the pain is allowed to change in size and intensity with the ball image. Thus, the sensory transformations involved in the ball-of-pain technique may be particularly well suited for those patients who experience a good deal of rigidity and stereopathy in their pain experiences and who believe that their pain can only increase during imagery rather than decrease. The flexibility induced within the experience of pain during this technique sets the stage for a more complete transformation of a patient's relationship with the pain: The pain is detached from the physical body:

> Move the ball of pain up to the surface of your skin now, and as you do so let some or all of the ball move through your skin and feel it resting gently on the surface of your body .... Notice the size and color again as you imagine the ball beginning to float above the surface of your skin, floating up and away ... moving across the room, and even drifting through the window or wall. (Achterberg et al., 1994, p. 105)

Mind-Controlled Analgesia

Mind-controlled analgesia is a relatively simple technique that aims to transform the pain experience by activating the healing process at the level of the subconscious (Bresler, 1984). Initially, patients are asked to draw three pictures: (1) the pain at its worst; (2) the pain at its best; and (3) a picture that symbolizes the most intense pleasure they could ever experience. The imagery exercise, which is practiced a few times per day, begins with a relaxation segment, followed by an experience of the patient's pain at its worst (the first picture). The patient is guided through imagery to transform the experience into the scene when the pain is at its best. Eventually, patients are guided to transform their experiences even further into the image of extreme pleasure. Following several weeks of practice in the imagination, patients are encouraged to shift their mindsets during actual experiences with pain. When patients succeed, they recognize that their views of the world change along with their unconscious images.

Opening Around Pain

Another technique that can be used to help diminish the discomfort and pain suffered by patients is called *opening around pain* (Levine, 1982). This technique aims directly at the rigid and closed emotions, sensations, and physical reactions (e.g., muscle constriction) connected to the pain site. As the name suggests, the goal is to open up these areas so that the patient can face the pain sensations directly and can cope through the practice of acceptance and secondary-control strategies. If the technique is successful, self-efficacy, secondary self-control (i.e., letting go), and biopsychosocial flexibility are restored, as the person is exposed to the pain sensations without their stereotypic coping reactions at the physiological, cognitive, emotional, and relational levels. Ideally, the technique reverses some of the avoidance-based coping dynamics that may paradoxically maintain and intensify pain disorders over the long term. Naparstek (1994) wrote some outstanding scripts on applying imagery to a number of different physical complaints. The following is an example segment from her script for pain management (also see http://healthjourneys.com for a variety of audio recordings of similar vignettes):

> And breathing into the pain, you can feel the soft energy of the breath moving all around and through it … the warmth of the breath massaging and opening tight, trapped energy … and breathing it out … (pause) ….
>
> And again, breathing into the pain … with care and concern for that part of your body … soft and easy … letting the gentle energy of the breath caress and release some of the pain … and breathing it out … (pause) ….
>
> And again … breathing in … and perhaps this time, if it feels right, and you can, putting your hands over the place that hurts … letting the warmth of your hands move softly and easily into the pain … encouraging your body to open to it…to loosen around it … so it can move more freely … and again, breathing it out. (p. 179)

The following is a hypothetical example of an opening induction in guided imagery adapted from Levine (1982):

Allow yourself to relax and become comfortable. As you relax, focus your attention on your body until you find an area of discomfort or pain. Allow your attention to completely wash over that area and feel the sensations that grow there. Notice how your body reacts to the pain. Do the muscles tighten and squeeze around the pain ... like a fist that squeezes tighter and tighter? ... Allow yourself to feel the discomfort, the tightness, the squeezing of the pain, like a clenched fist closing tighter and tighter. Notice any negative emotions surrounding the pain ... fear ... helplessness ... anxiety ... guilt ... anger ... squeezing the pain ... like a tight fist with white knuckles. Feel the body squeeze around the pain until it is exhausted. Why does it try to squeeze so hard? Now, allow this fist to begin to relax and to open. Moment by moment it opens around the sensations. Allow the sensations to stay, to be, to lie there calmly in the palm of the opening hand. As the hand opens the fingers move gently. Allow your fear, anxiety, anger, and other negative feelings to fall away, like water flowing between the moving fingers. The final feelings melt across the open palm until the palm itself melts back into the soft, warm, open flesh. All that is left is sensation, pure sensations floating freely in an open, soft, relaxed body.

Emptying the Sandbag

In this technique, patients relax and then are instructed to imagine their bodies as empty bags that they are filling slowly with sand. Their bodies will feel heavier and heavier, until the bag is completely filled. Next, they are instructed to focus on a single area of discomfort. Once the patients have done this, they are instructed to make a small slit in the sandbag at that area and to imagine the sand slowly trickling out until the sandbag is completely emptied and weightless. This process is then repeated for each area of pain (McCaffery & Beebe, 1989). The following is an example vignette:

> Now that you are fully relaxed, imagine that you are an empty brown sack. You are lying on the ground, completely relaxed and empty, bunched up and crumpled. Slowly, see yourself being lifted, as if by the hands of an invisible worker. You are now floating just above the ground, the top of the sack is open and ready to be filled. Imagine a slow, steady stream of sand being poured from above, slowly and gradually filling you up. The sand is light tan in color, almost white, and very fine, with a soft grainy feel to it. As you fill, you grow heavier and heavier, until you must be placed upon the ground. You are halfway full now, and the sand is so heavy. Feel your body filling from the bottom, up through your middle, and slowly to the top. Now you

are completely filled with sand. Take a moment to feel the fullness, the heaviness, as the invisible worker's hands lift you up above the ground once again. There you float, filled to the top with beautiful healing sand. Now, find the location on the sack where your discomfort is the most intense. Notice the signals coming from this site, dulled as they move through the thick weight of packed sand. Now imagine a sharp knife that will cut the sack open just above the site of pain. On the count of three, you will make the cut, and all of the sand will be emptied from the hole you make. Ready? One … two … three, cut open the sack. Feel the soft white sand draining out of the hole, rushing out like sand from an hourglass. The sack gets emptier and emptier, as the healing sand rushes out throughout the site of discomfort, carrying any uncomfortable sensations with it. You are more than half empty now, as the sand continues to rush out, slowing, slowing, until you are once again an empty sack, laying on the ground, relaxed, comfortable, and at peace. Feel free to lie there, as an empty sack as long as you would like, until you are ready to return to this world.

Spreading the Pain

Spreading the pain simply involves guiding pain to expand outward from the pain site into the infinity of space. As pain expands in this manner, its intensity becomes more diffuse. Patients are guided to let go and allow pain to flow outward from the pain site to fill the entire body, then the room, then the world and so on off the planet and into space. Spreading the pain is similar to other "opening" techniques in its emphasis on transformation through a process of release. As with many of the other techniques already listed, spreading the pain works along with most resistances to direct imagery transformation rather than against them. The patient's will is engaged in a process of letting go rather than of attempting to control pain directly. The following script provides an example of guidance through this technique:

> And now that you are fully relaxed, allow your attention to center on your pain. Focus your attention on that spot. Experience the pain you have there. Now gradually, allow this pain to spread outward from this spot. Allow it to move to neighboring areas of your body. Slowly, allow the pain to move, and to spread … until it begins to fill your whole body. Like a container slowly filling, continue to allow the pain to fill your entire body …. And let me know when your body is completely full …. And now we will allow the pain to spread beyond your body. It will move outward, leaking out through your

pores, right through your skin, as it begins to fill the room. The room is large, so give it time to fill. Allow the pain just to leak right out of you, as it slowly fills the room. And let me know when the room is full …. Now we will allow the pain to spread throughout the building … beyond this room. It spreads and spreads outward, filling all the rooms, hallways, stairways, every space throughout the building is filling, filling, spreading, outward … outward and beyond this building, it continues to spread … Until it fills the entire city … spreading, outward, spreading…and it continues to spread outward, filling the entire state … the country … and our continent … outward, spreading, spreading … filling the entire planet, land, sea, mountains, valleys, deserts, outward it spreads, and spreads … moving outward from our planet, up into the surrounding atmosphere, filling the skies, moving through clouds, surrounding the planet, bigger and bigger, spreading, outward … into the vastness of space …. It moves, out into the darkness, out beyond planets, beyond stars, out beyond the galaxy, it spreads, and spreads, outward, forever ….

Radiant Light

Numerous contemporary approaches to imagery involve the use of radiant light to fill and cleanse the body, to rejuvenate sore areas, or for metaphoric cleansing. These light-oriented techniques have been practiced throughout the history of imagery, in traditional shamanist practices and also within the various religious traditions of the world (Achterberg, 1985; Ostrander, Schroeder, & Ostrander, 1979).

For example, Korn and Johnson (1983) describe a prototypic procedure involving the filling of the body with white radiant light that finds areas of tension and pain, dissolves them, and then removes the residue as the light dissipates from the body. The following is an example vignette applying radiant light imagery to pain:

> [following relaxation induction] Imagine your body as a clear container, filled with light. The light is liquid, filling you up, from head to toe. See the vibrations of the light, and notice that they are dull. This dullness is your fatigue, your stress, and your discomfort. See the areas that are the dimmest, the dullest …. These are the areas in your body that require rejuvenation, that have become worn down, and are involved in your stress and discomfort. Since the outline and the light is you, your body, as you can see the light, you can also simultaneously feel the dulled vibrations, those areas that are asking for attention and rejuvenation. Now imagine growing all around the outline of your body all the colored lights of the rainbow. From the

brightest, cleanest violet you could ever imagine, through the blues, the yellows, oranges and reds. Each color has its own vibration .... You can almost hear each one ... as a distinct hum. The light grows and fills in around your body, like the water in a bath tub that slowly fills around you. And see how the light within your body, especially in your target areas, is much duller and darker than the light which now surrounds you. Slowly allow the energy of all of these rainbows of light to grow, until your outline is completely surrounded, and see the dullness of your body outline, bathed in this fresh, new, radiant light. Now, when we count to three, together, we are going to open a small hole, somewhere in your body. Often it arises in the head, but not always. It may be in the back, your navel, or even in a toe. Your body is going to open a small hole, to allow the healing radiant rainbow of light to enter into your body, like water rushing into a submarine. Because the hole will be small, like a pinhole, the light will be squeezed together, becoming pure, white, radiant light ... containing all the colors of the rainbow packed together. And as each vibrating, healing band of energy enters it will shake free any tension, and flush out any toxins. It cleanses your body–mind completely, bringing relaxation, rejuvenation, comfort, and rest to those dull areas that are asking for assistance. Do you understand (when patient understands, continue)? Okay, ready? One ... two ... three .... Tell me, where is the opening, and what is happening [The patient should describe a pinhole somewhere in the body, where white radiant light rushes into the body, flushing out any dull areas. Assistance should be provided as needed, such as aid to open the hole wider, to provide a drain if there is too much dullness that requires an exit from the body, and so on]. Continue to allow the white radiant light to fill your body, and tell me when you are full. Good. Now allow the light to cleanse any last bits of dullness, to clear out any small bits of remaining tension or discomfort from your body. Your tired body systems are grateful for the cleansing, the rejuvenation. You may even hear whispers of "thank you" as these dull areas become shiny and new, filled with pure, radiant, white light, the mixture of all the radiant colors of the rainbow. Your body will continue to drink in this light in the coming weeks and months, to bring relaxation and calm to any body systems that are in need. Hold the light within you, and feel it seep into your tissues, your muscles, and even your bones. Your body is drinking in the white, healing, radiant light, and is quenched. Now take a moment to calmly reflect, before you open your eyes and return to the physical realm.

Inner Journeys

A number of different techniques involve taking journeys. Journeys within the imagination are outstanding methods for enhancing patient participation in the imagery process, because journeys are naturally engaging. Moreover, inner journeys engage a patient's narratives about procedures and pain. Narratives are story-like schemas, which like all good stories unfold over time, with a beginning, middle, and end. The brain is naturally primed to create narratives, and therefore such imagery experiences will work with the mind's own momentum and connect rather easily to long-term and also implicit (i.e., unconscious) memory systems. Such narratives will also include characters, like protagonist and villain, themes, morals, conflicts, and resolutions, each intrinsically related to an individual's ongoing meaning-making process of self and world. Any number of inner journeys for relief and healing may emerge naturally during the treatment process. Two categories of inner journey are (1) inner-body travel and (2) journey as metaphor. Each has numerous variant techniques that can be used as part of that journey.

Inner-Body Travel

Inner-body travel techniques allow the individual to have direct access to physiological processes within the imagined body by traveling in imagination within the body to visit pain sites. Once the patient has arrived at the pain site, any number of direct or metaphoric techniques can be applied to promote relief and healing. Many popular films and educational science programs have used the idea of shrinking down to microscopic size and traveling within the body, and perhaps there is some archetypal quality that facilitates scenarios within the collective imagination. Archetypal or not, these techniques usually begin with the instruction to step out of the body to leave the resting or sleeping body behind, like a shell. This technique uses an emanation: The imagined self emanates from the original imagined self, resulting in two or more self-images. Once the individual has left the body behind, the emanation is instructed to shrink and then to enter the body through some opening, such as the mouth, as in this example:

> As you see yourself resting calmly and relaxed, imagine a second you stepping out of the resting you, like a fully formed second you, stretching out of the first. The original you is left behind, still resting calmly, while the second you is standing over yourself. Now I want you to imagine your standing self shrinking, slowly getting smaller and smaller. We are going to take a trip into your resting body to see what is happening within. We are going to travel into your body to see if we can fix whatever is causing you pain, to bring some additional relief and promote the healing process.

From here, the individual is guided on a trip through the body to the site of pain. You can collaborate with your patient to experience the various sensory aspects of the inner body along the way, for example, making note of the texture, wetness, and sights within the mouth, if this is where the journey begins. Optional equipment may be used to enhance the voyage, such as headlamps for better visual information or vehicles for travel through different areas or the body. Generally speaking, it will be beneficial to experience the different body systems with anatomical correctness (Achterberg et al., 1994). Therefore, review of medical images (e.g., x-ray, sonogram, arthroscopic video) can be helpful in preparing for such journeys within the body. However, physical limitations can easily be overcome due to the fact that the voyage within is imaginary; for example, the patient can dissolve through flesh barriers or imagine body parts symbolically as necessary.

Once a pain site is identified, a number of different techniques can be used to represent the pain, to interact with it in the imagination, and then to bring new information to this interaction, transforming the representation. For example, Achterberg et al. (1994, p. 104) describe a technique in which the pain is represented as an object. The procedure involves directing your patient to imagine all the sensory aspects of the pain and to allow the pain to become a familiar object that resembles those sensory dimensions. For example, the pain may be round and white like a soccer ball. Pain in the lower back may be represented as cables that are tied in a knot. Pain in the stomach may elicit the image of a sharp kitchen knife. Once the sensory aspects of the pain object are clear, transformation of those images becomes clear-cut. For example, the soccer ball may be deflated or kicked into a goal outside of the body (where it belongs); knotted cables in the lower back may be loosened and untied; and a sharp knife may be dulled, filed down, or melted and turned into a necklace worn by the emanated self, who is taking the journey within.

In addition to the transformation of imagery content within a journey narrative, patients can use these techniques to identify people, emotions, situations, or memories that are connected to the rigidities associated with the pain site. The following is a hypothetical example involving the identification and transformation of rigid and constrained emotional information through imagery:

Guide: As you find yourself more and more relaxed, allow yourself to shrink down into your chest, shrinking smaller and smaller until you are small enough to enter the pain area. And now you are a tiny you, inside your chest cavity, small enough to walk around and look at the inside of your chest and find the painful spot. As you explore this new area, notice the sounds you hear. Can you hear your heart beating? It is a relaxing thump, thump. Notice your breaths, slow and deep. Can you feel them swirl around you as you look for the painful place. You can see large thick bones, like dinosaur bones, and tendons, like ropes stretching across your chest. And at last you find the site of the pain. Notice the colors and sounds that you see there. When the image becomes clear, you may describe what you see there?

Patient: I see a wall of muscle …. No, it is like a woven quilt that is stretched tight. It is pulling from its edges and in the center is a bright red bull's-eye where the pain is radiating. It is like a trampoline standing on its side, but it is stretched too tight. It is right in the center of my chest.

Guide: Now, I want you to walk up to this bright, red bull's-eye and touch it with your tiny finger. When you touch this bull's-eye I want you to describe any sensation, feelings, thoughts, or memories that come to you.

Patient: It feels hot, and when I push it, I feel like it will rip. It makes me feel angry and helpless.

Guide: Look around you to see what you can do to make the fabric looser and more flexible?

Patient: I can see a basket next to me full of fabric. I am weaving more fabric into the quilt so that it is larger and does not stretch so much.

Guide: And as you weave more and more fabric into the quilt, what happens to the bright red spot, to your feelings and your sensations?

Patient: The quilt is becoming looser and looser. The wind from my lungs is blowing it around, like a sheet on a clothesline. The red spot is cooling and softening. I feel calmer and the pain is decreasing.

In this example, the patient was able to quickly find a remedy in the basket of cloth. This type of healing resource may not be found as quickly in general practice. Furthermore, any number of possibilities for healing experiences could become possible once the person begins interacting with the pain site. For example, in the case just presented, the patient may have been asked to probe for specific memories of anger and helplessness that emerged when the bull's-eye was pushed. Unleashing repressed emotions or transforming these experiences in a meaningful way could result in a transformation of the imaginary landscape within the pain site.

For intractable pain, one can travel to the pain site and breathe into the pain: "The individual leans into and expands the pain with breath, rather than fights it, to enhance mindfulness and acceptance" (Achterberg et al., 1994, p. 110). One can massage the pain to transform it, can represent it in some manner, and then can make structural changes to the representation; one may strengthen areas around the pain or shield them from the impacts of the pain, one may imagine changes in blood flow, temperature, and so on. Again, the imagination is limitless, so the most important thing to do once one has found the pain is to identify its imaginary interface and then to work on various transformations that will fit for the patient.

After helping patients to determine whether primary (direct transformation) or secondary (acceptance and openness) control strategies are most appropriate for their particular pains, one should also feel free to follow the course of narratives that will emerge within the original journey to pain narrative of each patient (Zahourek, 1988). For example, metaphoric images of pain may emerge as lightning bolts, bringing about a narrative adventure involving survival and renewal after a storm. Tissue growth and rejuvenation may trigger narratives of plants or young animals that are nurtured and grown within the imagination. Along these subplots within narratives, pain may be transformed in an even deeper yet less direct manner, as flows of information within plot, characters, themes, morals, or resolutions shift along with representations of body within mind.

A common theme in the imagery literature is the transformation of pain images involving a pernicious creature. For example, Shone (1984) describes a detailed case study involving a patient who journeyed to the site of pain within the body and found a large black cat with huge teeth pulling at his spine. In this case, the patient was guided to begin a dialogue with the cat to find out what he was seeking. After several sessions, the cat became satisfied that his message had been heard and the cat died. Subsequent sessions were used to facilitate the healing process: Images of white birds (i.e., white blood cells), devoured the cat's remains, and a crew of tiny workers repaired the nerves.

A number of other practitioners have described imagery narratives involving travel into a pain site to interact and resolve conflicts with a symbolic creature (see Alexander, 1971, for another early example). Newshan and Balamuth (1990–1991) even modified this type of approach for use within a prescriptive, multitechnique, group-based imagery treatment for pain. Some examples of pain images they describe include a drummer, drumming on the back of a patient and laughing when she asked him to stop; a snowman who frustrated a patient by repeatedly insisting he was not a snowman; a ball of fire that refused to communicate; a bear giving a suffocating hug to a patient rendering the patient speechless; and a red devil stabbing at patient with a pitchfork. Each of these imaginary creatures was addressed in time by each patient, leading to a transformed relationship with the creature and ultimately to a transformed relationship with the pain. Specific questions that can be used to engage the pain creatures in a conflict resolution process include the following:

- "What do you need from me?"
- "What can I do to live with you?"
- "How can I get rid of you?"

Perhaps more important than the questions asked is the emphasis on listening to the creatures reactions and responses. A case study illustrating a symbolic representation of the pain follows:

> Patient A is a woman who suffered from low back and leg pain for twenty years. She had stopped working more than a year before joining the group. She is single, with no children, and is close to her eighty-five-year-old grandmother. At the time she entered the group, she was also investigating surgical interventions and had been through an outpatient physical therapy back program. Her initial pain creature image throughout the first two weeks of the program was of a mule facing away from her, kicking her with its hind legs. She reported suffering greatly during the first weeks….In the third imagery session, she reported seeing a red devil who was laughing at her and stabbing her with a pitchfork. She was trying to beat him off with her pocketbook but was unsuccessful. During this time, she was still in a struggle about having surgery. In the fourth imagery session, the red devil returned but she was able to hide from him behind pillows. The devil searched but did not find her and she laughed at him this time. Also, in the first weeks, the mule never responded to her attempts to speak with him but the devil told her he was there to "make your life miserable." At the point when she was able to hide from the devil, she decided not to have surgery and also felt less pain …. In the last week, no pain creature appeared. Rather, she imagined herself looking at the beach and feeling happy—she reported that she enjoyed the beach, but had not been there in many years, and planned that as one of her upcoming goals. Her progress, although initially difficult, was steady and she reported increased socialization and activities. In the second to last week, she announced that she had taken a part-time job. (Newshan & Balamuth, 1990–1991, p. 36)

In this example, the conflict was resolved by hiding from the pain creature. In other situations, direct confrontation might be a better option depending on the patient's inner wisdom, which will emerge as you interact collaboratively within your role as guide. The following is a modified transcript (i.e., edited for readability) from a patient who experienced itchiness and pain due to sensory integration difficulties (i.e., related to a pervasive developmental disorder). This patient was unable to wear pants, particularly thick pants, due to escalating discomfort that began with itchiness and built to leg pain that would then spread to other parts of the body, such as headaches. He had not been able to bring himself to wear pants for several years, wearing only shorts instead. Following the development of a full behavioral hierarchy ranking the difficulty of wearing various types of pants (e.g., jeans were rated as most uncomfortable) in different situations (e.g., hot conditions where escape would be difficult were worst) and after an introduction to the rationale for the use of imagery in sensory transformation and practice using favorite place guided imagery, the patient was directed to imagine himself wearing an uncomfortable pair of pants:

Guide: Tell me, what number from 1 to 10 would you give to your experience of discomfort with wearing these pants?

Patient: I would say a 2 or a 3. The discomfort would be worse if I were actually wearing the pants, but I am only wearing them in my imagination, so the sensations are not too intense actually.

Guide: Okay. I would like you to increase the intensity of the discomfort gradually in your imagination, until you get to a number between 5 and 7. Don't go above 7 if you can help it. You may need to imagine a different pair of pants, increase the temperature or something to increase the level of discomfort.

Patient: Okay, well I've turned the pants into jeans, new jeans in fact. And now I can feel much more discomfort. Yes, in fact it is getting much worse [patient begins to make jerking movements in his seat and his facial expression reveals itching sensations].

Guide: Not above a 7 right?

Patient: No, it's alright. It's at about a 6 now, and I don't think it will go any higher. It's just itching pretty bad, that's all; the pain has not set in yet, but it will shortly unless I remove these jeans.

Guide: Okay good. Now imagine that the itching has a size or a shape to it, perhaps a sound? What do you see or hear when you look down at the jeans?

Patient: Actually I see ants, millions of tiny army ants. Not the gentle black ants you may see, those I would hardly mind. These are red ants, the kind that bite [flinching and twitching increases]. Oh, yes they are biting me now in fact and stabbing me with tiny pitchforks.

Guide: Look closely at the ants and describe them to me. Hold your ground and look at them squarely.

Patient: Yes, it's kind of strange, because when I look at them directly I can see that they are ants, but they are also tiny devils, with pitchforks, and they are laughing at me in glee the more I itch [patient imitates their laughter]. They live to torment; this is where they get their power. They are truly evil.

As this session continued, this patient discovered that when he stood his ground, the ants became a bit disorganized and confused, losing some of their "evil" power. When he ran from them or retreated into wearing shorts again in his imagination, the ants fell back into his skin fully satisfied and still laughing at him, with the ability to return whenever they desired to further torment him. In additional sessions, the patient was able to identify a magic stream of fire that he could spray from a can. He carried the can with him in a sort of utility belt and laughed back at the ants as he watched them burn. In a few seconds of spraying, the ants were killed, and the patient expressed great joy at watching them squirm, writhe, and scream in their own discomfort. During subsequent sessions involving gradual exposure to longer and longer actual (not imagined) periods of time wearing pants, the patient was able to quickly return to this image of burning off the devil ants as he stood his ground in the face of any initial itching sensations.

This vignette is different from other inner-body travel experiences in a number of respects. It did not require travel into the body, as the itching and pain were taking place on the dermis. In addition, the interactions and subsequent conflict resolution with the pain creatures (i.e., devil ants) were rather simplistic and rudimentary. Many patients will have more extensive interactions with their metaphoric pain creatures, but this need not necessarily be the case. In this situation, simply facing the creatures rather than running from them and then using fire as a weapon were sufficient to change the power dynamics and to resolve the ongoing conflict.

In summary, most situations will call for the combination of the various inner-body journey techniques described thus far, either in a prescriptive or more spontaneous manner. For example, Epstein (1989) provides a good description of a prescriptive multilayered voyage into the body to interact with pain. This narrative begins by transforming the pain into an object. Next, the patient enters the body with a golden can of hot oil. When the oil is poured on the pain object, the pain dissolves into a single, golden point. The patient is guided to imagine bright, radiant light flowing from this point into all parts of the body and finally leaving the body, carrying the remnants of transformed pain along with it. As a practitioner, your job is to provide an array of options to your patient, either in a structured discussion or during your actual imagery work. Like any journey, both structure and flexibility are each important to get your patient to their proper destinations.

Journey as Metaphor

Some medical procedures (e.g., sex reassignment surgery, removal of a life-threatening tumor, childbirth) may represent a transformation for an individual. While the transformation within each of these examples is very different, the process is the same. The medical procedure the patient is going to experience is going to involve a major life transformation, from one sex to another, from being terminally ill to vital and healthy, and into parenthood, respectively. Procedures involving life transitions are particularly well suited for imagery involving metaphorical journeys.

Such journeys as metaphor may be prescribed or more spontaneous, involving each patient's unique imaginary content. Following are two examples dealing with childbirth pain: The first is prescribed and was practiced several times in the months leading up to the birth, and the other was developed in collaboration with a patient to be used in a more spontaneous manner with her birthing partner during labor:

> Imagine you are walking down a path through the woods, on a journey to your baby, who waits at the end of the path, wrapped in a soft blanket under a beautiful tree. As each contraction begins, you find yourself at a foot of a hill, about 30 steps high, starting gradually and growing steeper at the top. Before you begin your climb up "Contraction Hill," calm yourself with 2 deep breaths, breathing in with any discomfort and then pushing those sensations outward with each exhale. As the contraction builds, imagine yourself taking each step up the hill, counting as you go: 1 … 2 … 3 … 4. As you approach the top of the hill, the contraction tightens as the hill becomes steeper and steeper. You are coming closer to your baby, step by step. As you reach 30 steps at the top of the hill, you are able to see a view of the entire woods below. In the distance you see your baby, resting comfortably in the soft blanket, underneath the most beautiful tree in the forest. Walking down the hill at a comfortable pace, the contraction softens, and comfort returns, as you count those 30 steps back down the path. You can see the next hill several minutes down the path ahead and view it with confidence. With each hill, you gain a view of your child, waiting for you at the end of your walk, down your path. Each hill brings you closer and closer to your beautiful child, waiting for you at the end of the path.

The next dialogue is a summary of an imagery scenario that was generated through a more open-ended guided imagery process in collaboration with an expecting mother at around the 30th week of pregnancy. The imagery was open-ended, beginning with a slightly modified favorite place relaxation script. What emerged was a scene that was unique to this particular patient. The scene was then practiced with her birth partner on a weekly basis up until labor. At the beginning of the labor process, after admission to the hospital, the birth partner guided the mother through the process of making the imagery more salient and engaging by gradually querying each of the sensory and experiential details of the scene. The imagery was evoked during contractions to bestow strength and a sense of peace. Because the imagery was idiosyncratic and predominantly self-generated, this patient reported great ease at eliciting the imagery during labor, even in the back of her mind, while her eyes were opened and she was not under the guidance of her birth partner:

Guide: Begin with a few slow, deep, cleansing breaths. In … and out …. With each inhalation allow yourself to become more and more relaxed …. With each breath out, release any tension from the day … in … and out…. Once you are relaxed, imagine yourself in a peaceful place, a place where you can go during the birth process to feel safe and comfortable … to relax and to draw strength. When you begin to experience this place of strength, safety, and comfort, please describe it to me so that I can see it too.

Patient: Well I'm not in the place yet, but I am traveling there. I am walking down a path through the mountains in Montana. And I hope this is okay, but I'm not exactly me. I am a young Native American girl, and I am going to a sacred lake to give birth. It must be a few hundred years ago, because we are living naturally, not on a reservation or anything like that. I am very pregnant … big around my belly, so it is hard to walk. There are two other women traveling with me. They are helping me to get to the sacred lake and will also be helping me through the birth process.

Guide: That's fine, great in fact. Tell me how are you feeling about the birth process, the lake, and the women who are assisting you?

Patient: I am excited and a little nervous, but I have a deep sense of calm too. I trust these women, who are experienced with the birth process. I know they will stay with me and help me. And I know that all of the women in the tribe before me have given birth in these sacred waters. I am eager to get to the lake and to give birth in the water…. It just seems very safe there, and even though I am very young and inexperienced, I am tough, and I have a deep confidence, like I am a young Indian girl but I have an old soul.

Guide: Excellent. Can you describe what you see? What are you wearing?

Patient: We are wearing comfortable clothing made of soft animal skins, brown, and we have comfortable moccasins. Oh, and I have a beaded headband around my head, a special headband that is symbolic of childbirth and safety.

Guide: And what do the mountains and the path look like? What do you see around you?

Patient: It is beautiful. I'm pretty sure we are in Montana. It is morning, and I see tall peaks in the distance, with snow on them, tall evergreen trees, and the path is soft and made of dirt. There are wildflowers around the path as well.

Guide: Good. Continue down your path and enjoy the colors around you, the white of the snow-peaks, the green of the evergreens, the browns in the earth, and the colors of the flowers. See if you can smell the scents of the trees and the flowers as you walk by. Feel the coolness of the morning mountain air around you. It feels cool and clean inside you as you breathe it in along your walk. Please continue to describe the scene to me as you continue your journey.

Patient: I can tell we are coming closer. The older woman of the two who are helping me, has made this trip many times, and she is telling me that the lake is just over this next hill. We're at the top of the hill now, and I can see the lake below.

Guide: Describe the lake to me.

Patient: It is the most beautiful lake I've ever seen. The morning sun is just coming over the peaks in the distance, and it is shimmering on the surface of the lake. It looks like a million gold coins, shaking across its surface. I'm pulling the women now, waddling down the hill because I'm eager to get into the water and have this baby. Enough is enough.

Guide: What do you mean by "enough is enough"? How are you feeling about the lake and the baby?

Patient: I'm ready to have the baby, and I really can't wait to get into the water. It looks warm, and it will let me float, so that I can feel lighter and more comfortable after this long walk.

This patient produced a rich and detailed imaginary scene, which is not unusual. Questions by a guide should prompt the patient to add detail in several sensory modalities to allow the images to become more clear and salient. When you, as the guide, are able to fully imagine the scene yourself, you will know that your patients are experiencing their imagery with sufficient intensity. Then, the guide can simply ask about broader experiential aspects of the imagery, aspects that will serve to facilitate the patient's immersion within the imagery. The description of clothing is a useful strategy, since *contact is unification* within the imagination (see laws of the imaginary world in Chapter 4). When the mother made her clothing more salient, she fell more deeply into the role of a young Native American girl, taking on her attributes of courage and strength (i.e., *imitation is reality*). Furthermore, guidance toward breathing in the cool mountain air and focusing on the more experienced women who were assisting in the birth voyage to the sacred lake probably enhanced this patient's sense of engagement in the journey as well.

At the end of the imaginary scene (which ended just after the patient entered the lake and the birth process began), the guide prompted the patient to take a final look at the lake and the mountain scene and to think of a single word that would capture the entire experience. The guide then suggested that the word *lake* could be used as an invocation, to bring the scene back into her consciousness whenever she felt she needed it.

It is noteworthy that this scene provided a perfect symbolic scenario to satisfy the complex array of relational needs the woman was experiencing in relation to childbirth; all of these emerged automatically simply from imagery prompts aimed at finding a relaxing place for the birth process. In your role as a guide you should not be surprised when relaxation or any of the other simple techniques described lead you and your patient into an imaginary realm that is richer and deeper than you had anticipated. This will occur especially when you use a more open-ended approach, in which your patients will produce imagery that is perfectly suited to their current relational needs.

The previous scene involved needs for strength but also support from the older and more experienced women. In this sense, the scene also involved a sense of tradition: The wisdom of childbirth is something that is passed on from woman to woman, from generation to generation. In this sense, the patient also mentioned this girl possessed an old soul, from which she could draw inner calm and strength. Paradoxically, this patient feels naïve regarding the birth experience but also healthy, strong, and deeply confident. This patient was neither Native American nor a believer in reincarnation. Rather, these needs blended with her spontaneous symbolic imagination to produce a scene that would provide healing and balance to her during a time of potential stress. For these reasons, patients should always be given the "right of way," so to speak, in modifying scripted or more spontaneous imaginary scenes to fit their particular relational needs.

CHAPTER 7

Pain Management
Deepest Techniques

When I asked Dr. [Albert] Schweitzer how he accounted for the fact that anyone could possibly expect to become well after having been treated by a witch doctor, he said that I was asking him to divulge a secret that doctors have carried around inside them ever since Hippocrates.

"But I'll tell you anyway," he said, his face still illuminated by that half-smile. "The witch doctor succeeds for the same reason that all of us succeed. Each patient carries his own doctor inside of him. They come to us not knowing that truth. We are at our best when we give the doctor who resides within each patient a chance to go to work."

Cousins
(1980, pp. 68–69)

The deepest techniques described in this chapter involve rationales and specific imaginary contents that are more complex or esoteric (and thus less amenable to empirical testing). They involve the highest levels of patient participation in generating unique imaginary scenarios that will vary greatly across patients, and they have the broadest focus on imaginary transformation, potentially involving identity and meaning. These techniques are not necessarily more difficult to carry out, nor are they particularly time-consuming. However, they may be particularly well suited to patients with higher levels of motivation for positive change, patients with more chronic pain conditions, and patients with pain-relevant histories of trauma, personality disorder, or other sources of general demoralization.

Our understanding of pain from Chapter 3 suggests that information cutoffs within the body–mind system would be expected to exacerbate pain and that reopening such channels would tend to be reparative. The various systems of the body and the various systems of the mind, conscious and unconscious, are quasi-independent yet highly interactive subsystems within the patient. Self-regulation occurs within and among these systems through information exchange. Disease occurs when integrity and complexity decrease among these flows. Therefore, it stands to reason that opening up one subsystem to another, opening the body and the conscious mind to relatively unconscious information, would have the potential to provide renewed integrity and flexibility among these systems.

Each of the deep techniques to follow shares this theoretical grounding. These techniques simply allow the clinician and patient to move further out from the physiological systems at the pain site, deeper into the mental and emotional systems whose flexibility and flows of information may have been compromised.

Ericksonian Hypnotherapy

Ericksonian hypnotherapy is not an imagery-based approach. In fact, it is not based on any particular set of techniques. Nor is it based on theory, and it would be incorrect even to refer to it as a "type" of therapy or as an "approach" (Haley, 1994; Mathews, Lankton, & Lankton, 1993). As a result, Ericksonian hypnotherapy is not easily taught or even described, as Gilligan (1994, p. 79) points out:

> One of the most interesting things that could be said about Milton Erickson is that he did not practice Ericksonian psychotherapy. He rejected theory, frameworks, and set techniques. His writings usually emphasized a few generative principles, then concentrated on describing specific cases where these principles were creatively applied. The effectiveness of his work inspired many, though few of us seemed to take his atheoretical claims at face value, instead, we proceeded on the assumption that *of course* there was a theory or framework, it was just hidden or unstated. This assumption conveniently allowed many of his students, myself included, to … explain what Erickson was "really" doing. A whole new field of Ericksonian psychotherapy was born, as the intricacies of Erickson's patterns were written about and promulgated at a dizzying rate.

Nevertheless, we attempt to provide a practical introduction to the work of Milton Erickson. Finally, we present some of the theory proposed by his pupils, which they derived from his case examples and lectures. We conclude with an analysis of some of the core principles that may be most helpful in using guided imagery to treat pain.

Ericksonian therapy is best understood with some initial introduction to the biography of Milton Erickson, because his prior life experiences were a primary source for therapeutic material (Erickson & Rossi, 1980; Saudi, 2005). He was born to a poor, working family in 1901 in Nevada and, at the age of 5, moved to a rural farming community in Wisconsin. Young Erickson overcame numerous physical limitations throughout childhood and adolescence, including tone deafness, color-blindness, and severe dyslexia (Saudi, 2005). By overcoming these cognitive challenges, Erickson became an intensive self-learner in the subtleties of sensory information. Indeed, many have credited these early challenges with Erickson's legendary ability to attend to the rich subtleties of nonverbal information flowing within his clinical consultations, such as pauses, vocal tones, eye movements, and shifts in body posture (Mathews et al., 1993).

Erickson's most significant challenge was his diagnosis with polio myelitis at the age of 17 (Mathews et al., 1993; Rossi, 1994), which Erickson's physician believed would be terminal. Not only did he survive, but he overcame his paralysis gradually over a span of 10 years, developing many of the self-hypnotic, imagery strategies that he would later employ in his work with others. Erickson describes this experience:

> I had a polio attack when 17 years old and I lay in bed without a sense of body awareness. I couldn't even tell the position of my arms or legs in bed. So I spent hours trying to locate my hand or my foot or my toes by a sense of feeling and I became acutely aware of what these movements were. Later when I went into medicine I learned the nature of muscles. I gained the knowledge to develop an adequate use of the muscles polio had left me with, and to limp with the least possible strain; this took me ten years. I also became extremely aware of physical movements and this has been exceedingly useful. (quoted in Saudi, 2005, p. 41)

Erickson's strategy was to use the remembered images of movement and body awareness as a platform from which to reconstruct his physical abilities. It seemed as if he had an implicit understanding that any part of the original memory contained the seed of the whole of the experience. With repeated work, day after day, he cultivated these seeds of imagined bodily sensation and movement back into a functioning body:

> Erickson's personal development led him to an understanding of the essence of therapeutic hypnosis as the accessing and utilization of the patient's own lifetime of experiential learning for problem solving. This is in striking contrast to the diametrically opposite focus of

academic and experimental hypnosis that conceptualizes hypnosis as a form of suggestion, manipulation, and influence imposed on the patient from the outside. (Rossi, 1994, p. 47)

Indeed, the essence of Erickson's approach was to grow healthy or useful parts of an individual's consciousness toward the realization of therapeutic goals. It was this focus on each client's unique set of experiential potentials and the fit of these potentials with each client's idiosyncratic set of problems, outlooks, and life situations that made Erickson's approach to therapy so exquisitely unique and, thus, so difficult for others to replicate or to teach (Mathews et al., 1993).

Erickson's physical difficulties continued into middle age, when he gained an even deeper phenomenological appreciation for pain and the ways it could be modified: "At the age of 51 he developed Post-polio syndrome, which caused him further muscular weakness, severe pain and confined him to a wheelchair. His own intense pain taught him how to help others to overcome theirs" (Saudi, 2005, p. 41). In fact, pain management was one of the primary contributions of Milton Erickson, which is saying a lot, since he is regarded by many as the most influential psychotherapist of the modern era (Haley, 1994; Mathews et al., 1993; Rossi, 1987). Indeed, most of the general information about how to approach, connect, and relate to clients in a healing manner (see Chapter 4) could be tied either directly or indirectly to his influence.

Erickson was not simply indifferent to theory and technique, but he even considered theory as antithetical to good clinical practice, because theory limits the worldviews of both clients and therapists, creating inevitable problems of fit between the tenets of the theory and the particular healing experiences needed for a specific client to change for the better. He considered techniques following from theory to be even more limiting to the therapeutic process, because they constrained creativity and put limits on potential habit changes (Gilligan, 1994). When practicing too close to theoretical orthodoxy or overly technique-driven manner, one is serving the theory or the therapist often at the expense of the client or the client's needed change (Mathews et al., 1993).

In particular, Erickson challenged many of the Freudian psychoanalytic notions that were practically monolithic in clinical practice at the time, particularly the notions of long-term treatment, a passive role for the therapist, and a detailed exploration of the client's past in relation to general personality functioning. Rather, Erickson actively engaged his clients, focusing on their current life situations, and only to the level of detail required to most efficiently solve their current problems. He focused on strengths to move with a client's own momentum toward opening possibilities for new learning and with a focus on getting the ball rolling toward the client's desired future (Mathews et al., 1993).

Erickson radically revised the view of medical hypnosis at the time (Mathews et al., 1993), and he considered hypnosis to be on a continuum: There exists a common subtle form of hypnosis, such as the dissociation one experiences while driving home along a familiar route, to deeper hypnotic states that may be used in some therapeutic sessions. Erickson defines hypnosis as:

> ... a state of intensified attention and receptiveness and an increased responsiveness to an idea or to a set of ideas. There is nothing magical or mystical about it; it is attentiveness to, absorption in, and responsiveness to an idea or a whole group of ideas.... In medicine as well as in dentistry this normal everyday capacity for intensely directed attention can be employed to concentrate and direct a patient's attentiveness and responsiveness to selected stimuli. (Erickson & Rossi, 1980, p. 255)

Indeed, Erickson strove to dispel the notion that hypnosis was anything special or magical or that it laid extraordinary powers within the hands of the hypnotherapist. Rather, Erickson focused increasingly throughout his career on hypnosis as being a process of relative receptivity rather than a state of suggestibility. This distinction allows clients to become active participants within a dynamic process of hypnosis, open to new sources of information from the therapist but also from within themselves. He focused in particular on using hypnosis to make use of clients' own internal suggestions, helping them to become more open to relatively unconscious sources of wisdom (Mathews et al., 1993).

Thus, Erickson used hypnosis with some clients as a tool to help him carry out the essence of his therapeutic work: to grow healthy or useful parts of an individual's consciousness toward the achievement of therapeutic goals. Erickson used many of the "simple" and "deeper" techniques described in the previous sections, such as suggestions for numbness, sensory transformations, and simple distractions. Yet his keen ability to listen to the whole person, along with strategic suggestions for behavioral or experiential changes, allowed these simple techniques to quickly cascade toward more profound and permanent therapeutic benefits.

Theoretical Framework

Despite Erickson's disdain for the limiting impacts of theory and technique, for the purpose of learning, it is useful to attempt to glean the outlooks and heuristics that Erickson used in his work with pain. First, it is clear that Erickson had an enlightened understanding of pain considering the era in which he began to practice. He conveyed a commonsense understanding of modern theories of pain many years before even the earliest theoretical accounts (e.g., the gate-control theory) were developed (Erickson & Rossi,

1980). With patients and in teaching seminars, he used common examples of the subjective and contextual phenomenology of pain, such as the soldier in war who notices after the battle an injury and then feels pain, which is still less than the pain he would have had if he had seen the injury coming beforehand. Erickson writes:

> We know that pain originating from observable physical injury can be forgotten and even lost by the development of an intense, absorbing interest in something else, by the simple distraction of attention, or by the introduction either accidentally or intentionally of an irrelevant, confusing, or even amusing external stimulation ... [such as] the example of the patient with severe body burns, who was suffering extensive pain and was about to be transferred out of the general ward because of his continued low moaning. Suddenly, an illiterate 40-year-old man, totally unacquainted with and completely frightened by hospital procedures, began running wildly about the ward in an open-backed hospital gown, trailing an enema bag and pursued by a nurse and an orderly. The patient with severe burns burst into laughter and laughed, as he explained, until he "hurt all over." Then he asked with surprise what had happened to his burn pains, as the mere recall of that ludicrous sight proved to be analgesic. He was not the only patient on the ward who found that scene and its recollection a satisfying analgesic ... the hypnotherapist utilizes these naturalistic pathways to facilitate pain relief. (Erickon & Rossi, 1980, pp. 235–236)

Erickson's own life experiences along with his ability to pull apart the finest details of the phenomenological accounts of others allowed him to develop an exquisitely detailed understanding of the ways pain entered the lives of patients, the ways patients related to their pain, and the ways these relationships shaped their unfolding day-to-day lives:

> Pain is not a simple, uncomplicated noxious stimulus. It has certain temporal, emotional, psychological, and somatic significance. It is a compelling motivating force in a life's experience. It is a basic reason for seeking medical aid. Pain is a complex, a construct, composed of past remembered pain, of present pain experience, and of anticipated pain of the future. Thus, immediate pain is augmented by past pain and is enhanced by the future possibilities of pain. The immediate stimuli are only a central third of the entire experience. Because pain is a complex, a construct, it is more readily vulnerable to hypnosis as a modality of dealing successfully with it than it would be were it simply an experience of the present. (Erickson & Rossi, 1980, p. 238)

Erickson proceeds to describe how he uses the rich temporal, sensory, emotional, and existential aspects of pain in his therapeutic work (Rossi, 1994). The structural and temporal complexities of pain as well as the great significance of pain within the lives of his patients are seen not as obstacles but rather as rich opportunities toward shifting these experiences in the direction of relief. Within the subtleties of the multifaceted pain experiences of his patients, Erickson would seek out a fragile point. These points could exist within some aspect of the pain complex, within a structural aspect (e.g., an emotional or sensory facet), or within the meaning of pain. Or fragile points could exist within the temporal nature of pain, the patient's experience of time between bouts, the imagination of future bouts, or times when the patient naturally experienced the pain as more bearable. Because patients invariably tend to view pain in simpler terms, as simple, unchanging, and immutable, Erickson would use the hypnotic process to set off small changes within these fragile points and then would harness a patient's own awareness of these changes to grow them over phenomenological time and space. In this way, the patient's own limited and negative view of pain could be used to advantage, as small suggestions for change in the pain experience could incite radical changes in patients' views of their pain. Erickson describes this process as such:

> To understand pain further, one must think of it as a neuron-psycho-physiological complex characterized by various understandings of tremendous significance to the sufferer. One need only to ask the patient to describe his pain to hear it variously described as dull, heavy, dragging, sharp, cutting, twisting, burning, nagging, stabbing, lancinating, biting, cold, hard, grinding, throbbing, gnawing, and a wealth of other such adjectival terms. These various descriptive interpretations of the pain experience are of marked importance in the hypnotic approach to the patient…. To consider a total approach is possible, but more feasible is the utilization of hypnosis in relation first to minor aspects of the total pain complex and then to increasingly more severely distressing qualities. Thus, minor successes will lay a foundation for major successes in relation to the more distressing attributes of the neuron-psycho-physiological complex of pain, and the understanding and cooperation of the patient for hypnotic intervention are more readily elicited. Additionally, any posthypnotic alteration of any single interpretive quality of the pain sensation serves to effect an alteration of the total pain complex. (Erickson & Rossi, pp. 239–240)

Erickson viewed hypnosis as a process of opening up a client's receptiveness to information, such as the examples of distraction and humor.

In particular, he tried to open clients to their own internal information toward the goal of pain relief:

> To the average person in his thinking, pain is an immediate subjective experience, all-encompassing of his attention, distressing, and to the best of his belief and understanding, an experience uncontrollable by the person himself. Yet as a result of experiential events of his past life, there has been built up within his body—although all unrecognized—certain psychological, physiological, and neurological learnings, associations, and conditionings that render it possible for pain to be controlled and even abolished. (Erickson & Rossi, 1980, p. 237)

Erickson's pupils, particularly Rossi (see Rossi, 1993, 1997, 2002) have proposed sophisticated, systemic, theoretical accounts that overlap to some extent with the nonlinear dynamics accounts for imagery presented in Chapter 3. As early as 1980, Rossi described Erickson's view of "the entire mind–body as one vast system of cybernetic communication in psychotherapy" (Erickson & Rossi, 1980, p. 49). Rossi (1987) later used the latest research on state-dependent memory and the hypothalamic-pituitary-adrenal (HPA) responses, particularly hormonal (e.g., neuropeptide) shifts, to elucidate Erickson's ability to harness and grow therapeutic aspects of patients' sensory awareness.

Rossi essentially sought to develop a scientifically grounded understanding of the ways information flows within the body–mind could be opened and how such openings could be healing. This quest led him eventually to suggest the merits of nonlinear dynamical systems theory (Rossi, 1997), and one may consider the underlying theory of Erickson's work to be more or less equivalent to the theoretical account suggested in Chapter 3. Indeed, Rossi's (1987) theoretical accounts of Erickson's work focus on the goal of entering the client's biopsychosocial phenomenology to arouse the inner healing potential that always exists there, waiting for the right time or some assistance: "All effective 'suggestion' is this process of accessing and activating the mind/body state-dependent memory and learning systems that encode a problem so that the patient's inner resources can be mobilized to reframe and resolve it" (p. 383). Indeed, this notion of the "inner physician" goes back much further than Rossi or Erickson to the work of Albert Schweitzer, Hippocrates, and before him to the earliest collective wisdoms of the world's shamanic traditions (Achterberg, 1985). You will notice that each of the deeper approaches that follow this section on Erickson has in common the "conjuring" up of the pain experience at the outset of the imagery intervention and then the activation of new biopsychosocial flows of information to promote flexibility and healing.

Erickson was particularly good at doing this at a time prior to the modern rediscovery of such ancient wisdom in modern medicine.

Basic Principles

In the literature on Erickson's work, one finds numerous lists of principles, with varying degrees of overlap, specificity, and length. We have boiled these lists down to four teachable aspects that can guide your clinical work: (1) be efficient and pragmatic; (2) be open and receptive; (3) be symptom focused; and (4) engage the creative unconscious.

Be Efficient and Pragmatic   Each therapeutic relationship that Erickson formed was unique, as were the techniques that emerged therein. No one will replicate Erickson's work, but his guiding principles are simple to recreate in one's own work (Erickson, 1994), particularly the principle of efficiency (Saudi, 2005). Indeed, the techniques presented herein are organized according to this principle: Simple techniques are presented first as they should always be your first option for intervention. Erickson never did more than was necessary in terms of intervention. Although there are accounts of Erickson's creative interventions with difficult clients, many of his interventions were frankly quite boring as well (Erickson & Rossi, 1979, 1980). If someone had asked him the common question about his primary theory of therapy about what he tends to do in session, the answer would have been, "As little as possible."

Erickson's daughter (e.g., Erickson, 1994) uses the metaphor of a farmer helping a chick to hatch in describing her father's work. He would slowly pull away just enough shell in synchronous timing with the chick's own struggles to allow the chick to emerge more or less on its own. Erickson always was mindful of the fact that pulling away too much shell, too quickly, or with too much force could cause damage to the young chick.

Similarly, Erickson respected the boundaries imposed by physical reality (Mathews et al., 1993). Erickson's daughter writes:

> [An] important part of Ericksonian therapy is a firm adherence to reality.... Reality itself is unchanging, but perceptions of reality and reactions to it vary with both circumstances and time.... Recognizing and separating reality from fantasy, wishes, idealism, and hopes is basic. Being able to offer alternatives, options, and other perspectives in such an intriguing, appealing, and appetizing way that the patient is enabled to expand perceptions and reach legitimate goals more effectively in therapy. (Erickson, 1994, p. 151)

Some—in fact most—patients will remain in pain. For some, the pain will be terminal; the patient will die. The last thing Erickson would have relied on would have been some idealistic expectations on the part of his patients, some miracle, or some guru-like personification of him as "the" source of healing wisdom. Erickson personified the exact opposite of the common stereotype of the hypnotherapist of the time, some powerful Svengali or magician type, with long extending fingers reaching out from a piercing gaze. Rather, his work, particularly his hypnotic work, was folksy; it was at all times deeply "respectful, effective, creative, and ... wholesome" (Erickson, 1994, p. 147). If he had had any persona, it would likely have been the gentlemanly country doctor whom you invite to stay for supper after a routine house call.

The implication for therapeutic work for pain is that you would always first tackle the most immediate, solvable, practical problem your client brings to you. Furthermore, you would listen carefully to your client's complaints to select the most densely interwoven problem within your client's life space. Just as you would want to pull away at the shell near a chick's beak, which is already loose and at the hub of an emerging network of cracks, pulling away at the problems that are central to your clients' difficulties will maximize the chances that any small changes will spread and cascade among the momentums of their day-to-day lives.

For example, a young female patient arrived at our clinic complaining of pain due to repeated overexertion: She repeatedly lifted heavy objects despite chronic reinjury of her back. She appeared to have a deeply wounded self-concept, a stall in her development of adult identity, depression, conflicted life goals, and a borderline personality disorder as well. In the style of Erickson, our initial steps were simply to use imagery to explore and rehearse her scenarios for lifting objects. By exploring her imagined lifting, we were able not only to improve her mindfulness during potentially injurious activities but also to gain access to connected processes involved in her sense of self in the present and the future. The goal, however, was always efficiency and pragmatism. Yet one can have faith that when it comes to intervention, even the stillest of waters will run as deep as they need to, as long as one maintains a steady and receptive therapeutic gaze upon them.

In addition to his own dispositions and life experiences, the simple and practical focus that Erickson relied on may have helped him to be, exquisitely observant of the totality of his client's life situations, leading to the second basic principle from his work.

Be Open and Receptive   Everything within the Ericksonian therapy process emerges from actively attending to the whole of the patient's neuron-psycho-social life situation, always listening deeper and broader, striving for a more complete picture of the client's processes, one that will bring forth clarity with respect to all of the hidden potentials for healing that lie within those processes (Erickson, 1994).

This process reflects Carl Rogers's concept of "empathy" (Rogers, 1951), the process of entering your client's world in an "as-if" manner. Rogers (1975) was very clear that empathy is never achieved—that it is a process rather than a state. One never "arrives" at a state of empathy. Rather, empathy is always moving, bringing both you and the client together, layer by layer into the client's subjective world. Rogers (1975) also understood that at its core, empathy was a form of trance and that it also was best facilitated through a process of mindful attachment and congruence: flexible and accepting connection to oneself and also to one's client. At the deepest levels, empathy will bring to the forefront the healing resources within the unconscious processes of your patient. Erickson's central achievement was the cultivation of this skill of entering empathic trance states with his clients.

To be like Erickson, then, you must first move theory and technique to the side. When doing imagery, you need not try to create therapeutic opportunities for your patients. Such opportunities will arise repeatedly, in a natural and ephemeral manner. You need only to keep careful watch for these opportunities as they emerge through the process of empathy and, most importantly, to take full advantage of them when they do arise. Simply, when all else fails or when you are lost as to what to do next, simply open up and listen. Everything else follows from this basic principle of listening.

Be Symptom Focused Listening and empathy should not be hodgepodge or willy-nilly. Symptoms are focal points for your patients for good reason. Symptoms and the suffering that they bring tell you all about who your clients are, what they value, what they need, and what they can imagine at the current time. As we discussed in Chapter 3, symptoms are "sticky"; they form connections through association with other aspects of our day-to-day life experience (i.e., through classical conditioning). Because of this stickiness, symptoms and suffering will increasingly find a home within a client's day-to-day life, particularly in situations where pain is chronic, intense, and recurrent. Just as any member of a household, troublemaking or not, pain and suffering will increasingly take on roles therein.

Pain may be serving some critical need for your client, such as allowing for the avoidance of intimacy, allowing for an external source of blame for a life that is no longer moving in a fulfilling direction. More simply, pain may be acting as a warning sign for careless overexertion. In any case, listening carefully to the role of pain within the larger life space will be important. Indeed, if you are flexible in your outlooks, symptoms may become your ally at times rather than your enemy (Saudi, 2005). This is a point that we explore in greater depth later when we discuss Erickson's use of paradoxical intervention. Once you begin to know how the pain fits into a set of relationships with the client and the other agents of your client's life, you will gain a better understanding of where healing will need to occur to fill in the gaps once the pain is diminished. On the most basic level, the focus on the symptom will help you to remain practical and efficient.

Finally, as you move toward a more comprehensive understanding of your clients, their symptoms, and their roles within day-to-day life, don't simply engage your *clients* in the process of empathy.

Engage the Creative Unconscious   Just as the term *empathy* tends to arouse mistaken notions in therapists of a simple act of reflective listening (Rogers, 1975), the term *unconscious* may arouse similar superficial misconceptions. Engaging the unconscious in an Ericksonian sense does not imply a form of insight making, as in classical psychoanalysis. Erickson focused instead on forming an interactive connection with those unconscious processes of his clients, often purposefully avoiding any conscious insights that would tend to disrupt such a connection.

Connecting with the creative unconscious processes of a client allows you to work with their natural momentums to facilitate the release of intrinsic healing potentials, new flows of biopsychosocial information. Imagine again the metaphor of the chick emerging from the egg. You need not understand on a conscious level the entirety of the chick's situation therein; rather, you need only join along in its struggles to break free. Erickson's daughter (Erickson, 1994) describes the manner in which the principles of practicality and being observant converged through the hypnotic process to allow for one's unconscious resources to be better used: "He couldn't define exactly where hypnosis began and other communication ended.... Part of a trance state is accessing unconscious resources. The wisdom that each of us has gained from living and experiencing life that is stored in the unconscious can be elicited with self-hypnosis" (p. 150). Indeed, her use of the term *self-hypnosis* is meaningful here, because on the broadest level, Erickson's approach to hypnosis was completely collaborative and democratic, not prescriptive or authoritarian:

> Erickson had respect, appreciation, and a genuine liking for his students and patients. This free-will offering was given without constraints and could therefore be accepted. This sense of value and appreciation was a part of his therapy as surely as were his creative interventions. Hypnosis can help build this sense of appreciation and respect. (Erickson, 1994, p. 151)

We suggest that you need not have any formal training in hypnosis to use hypnotic trance in your imagery work in the example of Erickson. When you do a typical imagery induction, even a simple breathing relaxation, you will be altering the states of consciousness of your client and also yourself. To work with the unconscious, you simply work along with these altered states, attend to them, and remain open to healing opportunities that may arise from their natural rhythms. As you enter into deeper states of "trance," along with your clients, you will naturally find deeper processes of awareness, which will open up pathways to greater creativity.

Again, you need not resort to magic or even spirituality (Rossi, 1987), unless your client finds a spiritual focus helpful. Rather, the healing potential of the unconscious may simply be regarded to lie dormant within the infinite reservoir of your patients' past experiences, their "experiential learnings" (Erickson & Rossi, 1979). Inasmuch as memory, conscious or otherwise, is a creative and constructive process that frames our imaginations of present circumstances and future potentials, the unconscious may be considered to be equivalent to the patient's most creative processes of imagination.

Basic Techniques

An endless array of specific techniques flow from the four core principles of practicality, receptiveness, symptom focus, and engaging of the unconscious. Indeed, many dedicated followers have spent the better parts of their careers in an attempt to catalogue Erickson's case examples and glean some taxonomy of Ericksonian technique. Yet each would readily admit that Erickson never actually repeated the same exact technique with two different clients. Therefore, in keeping with the principle of practicality, and with respect to this idiographic spirit of Erickson's work, we have grouped the techniques into three very broad categories here: (1) indirect suggestion; (2) the use of momentum and timing; and (3) the use of metaphor.

Indirect Suggestion   Direct suggestion within hypnosis is clear and simple: You instruct the subject to exhibit some behavior or to experience some specific form of imagery. Indirect suggestion is more open-ended, allowing the patient to become more actively involved in coming up with the particular response to a suggestion by the clinician (Erickson & Rossi, 1980). When one examines the contrast between direct suggestion, which is closed and specific, versus indirect suggestion, which is open, it should be apparent that there is room for a great variety of different indirect suggestions. One way of differentiating the varieties of indirect-suggestion techniques, for example, would be based simply on the degree to which they are open-ended or collaborative. "Allow something to come into your imagination" is very open-ended, whereas "Allow some new feeling or sensation to enter your arm" is less open-ended.

Another way to understand indirect suggestion is to separate out the two contexts that exist within interpersonal information exchanges: content and process. The *content* of a message is the message itself, the specific suggestion you give, whereas the *process* component is what that message conveys about the relationship between interactants (Erickson & Rogers, 1973), particularly with respect to power. If you instruct a client during imagery to gradually turn down the volume on pain as you count backward from 10, then the directive to "turn down the volume" is the primary content of the message, whereas the process of the message connotes that you are in control because you have given a directive. The metaphoric image comes from the outside of the client, from your suggestion, and the client will become relatively passive within this process.

This is not necessarily bad, especially if the metaphoric suggestion is effective and the client's pain turns down. However, Erickson and his pupils believe that indirect suggestions usually are preferable because they tend to provide a better fit for the client's need, they are less likely to provoke resistances (i.e., due to a healthy desire to remain in control), they are more likely to activate a client's healing sources of creativity from unconscious experiential learnings, and ultimately they are more likely to be enduring in their therapeutic benefits (Mathews et al., 1993).

The distinction may be quite subtle, for example, between "Close your eyes and relax" and "As you become more relaxed you will find that your eyes begin to close." Erickson was just as masterful at speaking as he was at listening (Erickson, 1994), and he used the subtleties of language to fine-tune the degree of openness of a directive and also the discrepancies between content and process to "trap" a client's unconscious into a collaborative relationship toward healing. Erickson's subtle use of content and process made it nearly impossible for a client to resist an indirect hypnotic suggestion. For example, "At first you will not notice any change" implies that the client will eventually experience a change. If the client resists, at any level of consciousness, then the change will occur immediately. More likely, when the change does not occur at first, as directed, the client automatically will be led to expect some future change. This is a simple example of a "bind" (also known as a double- or N-bind; Koopmans, 2001), whereby the clinician introduces a conflict between the content and process levels of a directive. This type of conflict, or bind, traps the client into a self-induced change in experience or behavior. Saudi (2005, p. 42) describes a few of the various of binds arising from the deliberate confluence of content and process that were documented in Erickson's therapy transcripts:

> Erickson had some 50 years of clinical experience and research in the use of indirect suggestion. He employed several terms of indirect suggestion in the same sentence or phrase in order to enhance their effectiveness. He considered them excellent tools for exploring the nonverbal potential related to the autonomic nervous system.... From the indirect forms: dissociation and cognitive overloading, apposition of opposites, metaphors, covering all possibilities of response, open ended suggestions, the implied directive, contingent suggestions and associated networks, compound suggestions, double bind,

implication, truisms, and associative focusing. It is interesting to note how much he learned from his environment; for example how he got interested in what he called later the double bind technique. He wrote that when he was a child he noticed his father asking him: "do you want to feed the chicken first or the hogs, and then do you want to fill the wood box or pump the water for the cows first." It was giving him the privilege to decide. Erickson continued: "in hypnosis the double bind could be direct, indirect, obvious, obscure or even unrecognizable."

Even if we were given 50 years of practice, it is not likely that any of us would become this adept at the use of binds within indirect suggestion. Nevertheless, many examples of simple indirect suggestion already have been described under "simple techniques." For example, all of the "sensory-transformation" techniques involve indirect suggestion, such as adding numbness, turning down pain, spreading pain out, or moving pain to a better location. What makes these techniques uniquely Ericksonian is the way you select and implement them, fine-tuning your selection of transformation to fit the personality, current needs, and specific pain experience and then fine-tuning the degree of openness and bind within your suggestion.

For example, you could suggest to one patient that she begin to notice a thickening of those "stabbing needles" in her back, an imperceptible thickening at first, about 1%, and then up to 2%, and so on, to the point where they become as thick as fingers—pressing on her back in a mildly annoying but tolerable manner. Here, you have a relatively specific shift in the metaphor (from needles to fingers), a subtle suggestion for initial change that is difficult to resist, and beyond that there is not much extra bind. With another patient, you may ask her to tell you when the pain changes in any manner and what is happening to the needles at that time. If she tells you that the pain is increasing, that the needles are becoming sharper, you may instruct her that this is good and to allow them to keep becoming sharper still. And as they do, she may notice that they either become thinner and thinner until they eventually either break or that they become thin enough to disappear altogether. In this case you are far more open-ended in terms of both content and process at the outset, with a higher degree of bind, using the client's own imaginary momentum (increasing pain) to drive the transformation of the needles to an innocuous form (to become so thin that they can no longer inflict pain).

In a similar vein, Erickson frequently used indirect suggestion to manipulate the temporal nature of a pain experience in addition to or instead of sensory transformations. This approach is particularly helpful in cases where pain is recurrent, as the contemplation of the return of pain between bouts can be quite destructive, defeating the purpose of the relief between bouts and at the same time adding to the discomfort that is experienced when the pain finally does return (Erickson & Rossi, 1980). For example, Erickson and Rossi (1980) describe a specific case involving time distortion, where a woman was experiencing bouts of pain approximately every 20 minutes that would last for between 5 and 10 minutes. Erickson worked with the woman first outside of the context of pain by helping her to play with her perception of time, either by distraction with an engaging task or by focusing on a less interesting topic. From this simple experience, he gradually worked with her to improve her ability to notice when the attack was coming and to engage herself in tasks that involved a degree of dissociation from pain combined with active engagement in other tasks. With practice, she became adept at making her attacks feel quite short in comparison with her time between bouts.

Using Momentum and Timing Erickson's sessions typically were much longer than the standard 50 minutes, and most writers attribute the length of session to his use of natural rhythms and momentums in consciousness (Mathews et al., 1993, Rossi, 1989; Saudi, 2005). Erickson and Rossi (1979, 1980) describe a number of examples of the use of timing to move along with a client's momentum in the detail they deserve. However, the general principle of using momentum is to always yield to and move along with client "resistance." Indeed, resistance would always be reconceptualized as belonging to the therapist in this respect rather than to the client. Resistance is a simple indication that you are fighting rather than using your client's momentum, which is self-defeating on your part. However, it is understood that some clients do have stronger or more difficult "momentums" that can seriously limit your available modes of helping. Again, Erickson stressed the fact that his approach involved no magic fixes and that strong client momentums running counter to interventions are to be accepted. In these cases, it behooves the clinician to respect reality and to expect smaller therapeutic gains and instead to enter an even deeper process of empathy in which these momentums can be better understood, engaged, and perhaps used to some benefit.

In the case with the sharpening and thinning needles, the suggestion for increasing pain and sharpness was an example of a suggestion that moved in the direction of the client's "resistance"; suggestions for needle blunting would have failed. If clients tend to dissociate from the areas in their bodies where the pain exists, consider helping them to enhance that dissociation. If a patient resists a particular metaphoric representation of a pain, such as seeing it as a radio (which may be turned down), it is likely that there is another competing image that may be harnessed. Finally, once an image is "harvested," such as a steel rod in the back, resistance to one transformation may lead to momentum toward an opposite transformation; for example, if melting won't work, try freezing it, or if neither of these work, try making it even stronger to see where that takes you. Or try changing the temperature gradually, using the client's inertia as momentum; begin with imperceptible heating or cooling and build slowly. Alternatively, increasing strength in the rod could make it feel heavier, allowing the patient to sleep on his or her back without rolling over, which could promote better sleep. One never knows where a client's own momentums will lead. But as a rule, Ericksonian therapists are always willing to join hands with these resistances and move along with them, which is far more practical than trying to swim upstream against the currents of another person's imagination.

Using Metaphors   According to Erickson's daughter, "Metaphorical and indirect interventions are probably the most widely recognized part of Ericksonian psychotherapy" (Erickson, 1994, p. 152). The essential function of metaphors is to package the problem or, better still, the solution to the problem in such a way that the client's outlook on the problem has shifted in some beneficial way. Particularly useful are those metaphors that shift the client's outlook in the direction of influence, control, or, more generally, some changeable nature of the problem situation.

Erickson typically developed metaphors with his clients in a story-like manner or by selecting anecdotes from his personal experience, from his formative years, from informal social situations, or from his prior clinical work. At other times he would deliberately query the client to find fitting metaphors that would be healing in the context of pain. For example, Erickson and Rossi (1980) describe a case of severe dental pain in an adult female. Erickson first asked this woman about the details of her current dental discomfort and then shifted to her earliest discomforts at the dentist as a child. This provided a first-level metaphor for her current pain—"child at dentist"—which was particularly salient and relevant to this client. He then asked her to describe in great detail her favorite childhood activity from that period of time, which yielded a second metaphor: "child at play." He had her rehearse the imagery of that favorite activity and then trained her to conjure up that imagery to shift the emotional context of her current experiences at the dentist. Beyond the harnessing of a well-fitting autobiographical metaphor of childhood play to overlay the adult dental experience, Erickson took a relatively simple technique, shifting the emotional context of pain through imagery, and made it deeper and more effective in this case. He created a powerful yet indirect associative link in his interviewing among pain at the dentist as an adult, pain at the dentist as a child, and the joys of childhood play. In this manner, Erickson brought to bear an unused unconscious linkage, or metaphor, for this woman's current pain. Undoubtedly, his approach was more effective when accomplished through this indirect, three-way associative link than it would have been had he simply directed her to imagine in an open-ended manner a joyful time in life without going through the connecting experience of going to the dentist as a child.

In another case, Erickson simply used the metaphoric experience of one's hand going to sleep for a terminal cancer patient in chronic pain to help her learn to put her entire body (except her head) to sleep when the pain flare-ups were at their worst. Again, the key consideration was taking a practical approach, listening to the woman's account in a deep manner, connecting with her unconscious momentums and resources around the pain and its natural fluctuations, and then using a well-fitting metaphor of a body part going to sleep, which was within this woman's accessible frame of reference. Neither of these examples involved deep, symbolic metaphors. The dental drill was not a dragon to be vanquished; the cancer pain was not a lion to be tamed. Yet in each case some small aspect of the client's experience, a well-tailored package of metaphoric relief, was grown into a larger experience that could assist with a current case of pain. It is in this creative application of experiential metaphors that Erickson's work may be considered to provide the foundations for each of the other deep techniques that follow in this section.

Inner Advisor

Making contact with an "inner advisor" can provide patients with a powerful source of relatively unfiltered information about the meaning of their pain. Such information may be helpful directly in transforming pain experiences, or it may assist the patient in making specific life changes to help alleviate pain. Such life changes may be clearly related to pain; for example, an inner advisor may give advice about better pain-coping strategies. Life changes also may be more existential in nature, for example, pertaining to the patient's life directions in career or relationships. Since pain signals an imbalance in the patient's biopsychosocial systems, healing insights from a patient's inner advisor may span the full range of these systems.

Looking inward for deeper knowledge about one's life, and indeed many of the deep techniques to follow, may seem strange or esoteric to some patients. It is important to listen to the concerns of these clients and to address them in a direct manner. In some cases, education about imagery may be helpful (see, e.g., the suggestions in Chapter 2). In other cases it may be helpful to simply point out that the inner advisor technique has been a common method of treatment in the best pain clinics for nearly 60 years (Baer et al., 2003; Jaffe, 1980).

Inner advisor techniques bear a close resemblance to Jungian active imagination techniques (Jaffe, 1980) as well as to the pan-spiritual traditions on which active imagination was based (see Baer et al., 2003, for a comprehensive review of the various examples of this technique). Regardless of the tradition from which the inner advisor is understood, this entity is viewed as a delegate from the patient's unconscious. Thus, the inner advisor can readily access and share pain-related information that has been cut off from the more conscious biopsychosocial systems of the patient.

Baer et al. (2003, p. 159) describe the rationale for communicating with the inner advisor:

> The presenting problem and corresponding symptoms are actually seen as a message from the unconscious that perceives itself to have been driven into opposition or conflict. Through the use of imagery, the patient takes a conscious attitude of listening to and cooperating with the unconscious, thus changing the nature of the presenting problem .... Thus, it can be stated that the goal of therapy using the inner advisor technique is increased communication with the unconscious.

Jaffe (1980) similarly regards the goal of the inner advisor technique as integrating the various systems of the self to renew balance, flexibility, and healing:

> How can you reconcile the different talents, potentialities, and selves lying within? As with health itself, the key seems to be balance. If you push yourself into too narrow a mold, or deny aspects of yourself that require expression, you will soon discover messages from those parts of you that have been denied. Very often, these messages surface in the form of a physical symptom or ailment. If you seek more than symptomatic relief, your unbalanced life-style needs exploration and change. (p. 230)

Who is the inner advisor? This point must be clarified with the patient before one begins the actual imagery procedure. The inner advisor is an omniscient inner healer, essentially the patient's inner physician. Jaffe (1980, p. 236) describes the inner advisor as:

> ... the part of us that actually does the healing, that mends the bones and coordinates the fight against stressors and external invaders.... The inner advisor has accumulated all the wisdom and knowledge of our body and psyche that usually escape our more limited, ordinary consciousness.

The procedure for meeting and communicating with an inner advisor is fairly simple and follows the general script of any tangible meeting (Baer et al., 2003). First, one finds a meeting place. This immersion in the meeting place is deepened by attending to its sensory features, such as objects in the room, sounds, temperature, and textures. An area within the larger space is identified for the actual meeting, perhaps on some chairs or on a hilltop. Once the meeting area is prepared, the patient is guided to look around and spontaneously report on the first living creature that emerges, whether it is heard, felt, viewed, or touched. Next, the patient is guided through a dialogue with the creature. This dialogue flows from the role of this creature as an advisor, and it may include identifying the name of the advisor and establishing terms of the consultation, such as the ideal communication method, the types of appropriate questions, and the frequency of any future meetings. It is advisable for the clinician to record the details of the communication in notes, as patients are likely to forget particular important aspects of the conversation once they return to a typical state of consciousness. The dialogue proceeds until a transition toward closure occurs spontaneously. The encounter typically closes with an expression of gratitude toward the advisor and arrangements for subsequent meetings.

In some instances, an inner advisor may appear more spontaneously. In the following case study, the patient, John, described his pain as a dog chewing on his spine. What begins as a dialogue with this dog, a symbolic representation of the pain, evolves into the dog assuming the role of inner advisor:

> [The] initial goal was to have the dog stop chewing on his spine. Over the next few sessions, the dog began to reveal critically important information. According to the dog (named Skippy), John never had wanted to be a physician—his own career choice was architecture—but he had been pressured into medical school by his mother. Consequently, he felt resentment not only toward his mother, but also toward his patients and colleagues. Skippy suggested that this hostility had in turn contributed to the development of his cancer and to the subsequent pain problem as well. During one session, Skippy told John, "You're a damn good doctor. It may not be the career you wanted, but it's time you recognized how good you are at what you do. When you stop being so resentful and start accepting yourself, I'll stop chewing on your spine." These insights were accompanied by an immediate alleviation of the pain, and in only a few weeks' time, John became a new person, and his pain progressively subsided. (Bresler, 1984, p. 227)

After the meeting with the advisor, it is important to process the experience. Topics to discuss include the meaning of any information given, emotional reactions to the encounter, specific information provided about the patient's body, and specific coping strategies that the patient now may wish. The imagery experience as well as the discussion of the experience should follow the patient's own natural pace. You cannot force issues without distorting the potential repairs that the patient may glean from the experience. Even if the advisor never arrives, one must respect the natural process as it unfolds. A nonarrival experience may be processed as any other; it may lead to some wisdom in its own right, to a modified renewed attempt to meet, or to the selection of better-fitting techniques.

When using the inner advisor technique, as well as each of the deep techniques to follow, one must be careful to avoid imposing an agenda on the patient or the patient's naturally unfolding imagery. The primary goal of these techniques is to reconnect patients with various aspects of themselves. Any intrusion by the clinician into the physical realm of the here and now will pull the patient toward a more conscious ego state and will "stir the pot" of any relevant unconscious material.

This is not to say that the clinician should be passive or disengaged with the process. In some situations, the clinician even may wish to communicate directly with the inner advisor or to engage actively in other ways. The clinician simply must take care not to impose his or her will on the patient's process because doing so would pull on the conscious aspects of the patient's identity—those aspects that have a relationship with the clinician. For example, it is perfectly fine for the clinician to ask clear and direct questions of the inner advisor, but it is not advisable to interfere with the form of the advisor, the role of the advisor, or the relationship between the advisor and the patient. The unconscious can be viewed as being easily spooked by involvement with conscious aspects of the patient's world. Therefore, interactions with the unconscious processes of patients can be readily spoiled through outside influence, particularly by the clinician who plays a powerful role within the conscious experience of the patient. This engaged but noninterfering stance of the therapist is common to all the deeper techniques to follow.

Dialogue with Pain

Dialogues with metaphoric images of pain are a corollary procedure to meetings with inner advisors (Rossman, 2000). The procedures are similar, and the underlying theoretical rationale is nearly identical. Each involves representing a bodily experience as an imaginary being with whom the patient may then establish an interactive relationship aimed at conflict resolution. One can use each technique, select one or the other in collaboration with the patient, or choose a blend of techniques. For example, in the case just described, an inner journey to a backache revealed a dog chewing on the patient's spine, a metaphoric pain creature that then assumed the role of an inner advisor.

Since pain serves a number of functions, including self-protection (Baer et al., 2003), within these techniques pain is considered to be a messenger rather than an adversary. The situation is analogous to an indicator light in a vehicle that signals some deeper engine problems. Within the engine of a human life, pain is an indicator light for biopsychosocial imbalance and conflicts, and if it is given a voice, it may speak to the deeper imbalance.

Jaffe (1980) makes an important point about the connection between a dialoguing process with pain and any underlying injury or illness: "This self-inquiry does not deny that there are physical reasons for the illness.... But his dialogue is another pathway, another source of information that might aid in the healing" (p. 233). The degree to which pain is directly related to a physical injury or illness is unimportant because the patient's relationship with pain will always reflect psychosocial conflicts.

Rachel Remen effectively describes the nature of this relationship:

> If you have a chronic illness, you already have a relationship with it. That relationship is often not the best it could be and may be characterized by mistrust, hostility, and fear. Dialoging with the symptom or with an image that represents it opens up lines of communication that may have been closed and may lead to an improvement in the relationship. This improvement is often experienced as a decrease in pain, anxiety, or depression, and in some cases, as improvement in the illness itself. (Quoted by Rossman, 2000, pp. 130–131; also see Remen, 1981)

Rossman (2000, p. 131) further emphasizes that the key is to maintain a "diplomatic" attitude. Both the pain and the patient must be given full opportunity to express feelings and opinions in an open manner. Thus, it is this "relationship" with pain that is the primary focus in a dialogue process.

The procedure for a dialogue with pain begins with a relaxation induction. Next, the patient is guided to focus on the pain. This focus should be phenomenological, allowing the patient to experience the pain in an open and subjective manner, free from any clinical or diagnostic language. It is also important to assist patients in maintaining focus on pain sensations rather than on any particular body part or injury site. If the patient is drawn instead to the site of pain, an inner body journey may be a more effective technique (see previous section for a variety of inner-body journeys). Once patients are sufficiently immersed in the subjective experience of pain, they are guided to allow the pain to have a voice and to become a metaphoric being. This goal is achieved through a variety of prompts, such as, "Allow the pain to have a voice and to become a creature of some sort." Finally, the patient may be guided to engage in a dialogue with the pain, exploring questions such as the following:

- "Why are you here?"
- "What do you need?"
- "What should I do to allow for healing to occur?"

Any negative feelings between the patient and the pain may be explored and resolved in a frank and assertive manner (Baer et al., 2003; Jaffe, 1980).

As an alternative to a verbal dialogue in the imagination, patients can be guided through a process of writing a *letter to pain*. This modification could be preferable for a number of reasons. Some patients resist immersion in imagery in general. Some patients struggle with conjuring up a voice or corpus for their pain in the imagination. Others simply prefer writing letters to a more direct and spontaneous dialogue. Letters allow patients to select their words more carefully and to avoid any direct or emotionally charged conflicts. Whatever the reason, the basic underlying principles of a dialogue through letters or a face-to-face interaction within the imagination are equivalent. The clinician simply provides some guidance through the process of a correspondence; patients begin by asking questions of their pain, and then they respond to those questions as they assume the role of their pain.

Regardless of the medium, be it verbal or in writing, communicating with pain often will feel somewhat foreign to patients; it will seem as if the pains have minds of their own. This makes sense when one considers illness as a loss of integrity in the biopsychosocial systems of the individual, a loss of connection with various sources of information within these systems. Jaffe (1980, p. 233) describes this situation:

> Very often, a sickness contains significant information about the nature of a personal crisis and what must be done to resolve it. Illness is an important signpost or message about something taking place in the inner self. It expresses a basic split, and a lack of integration and development in a person.

A dialogue with pain provides a means of reconnecting. One also should be prepared for the degrees of conflict or disconnection that are often revealed through this procedure. Inner dialogues are typically not easy or positive at the outset (Jaffe, 1980). Pain, for example, may request from patients that they make major life changes to renew balance, such as quitting their jobs or leaving their spouses. Such information will require serious problem solving in the nonimaginary here and now. Obtaining the information from the dialogue with pain is only a starting point in such situations.

Jaffe (1980) describes such a case: a successful businessman whose stomach cramps ironically were triggered by success on the job. These cramps had started in junior high, when he made the decision to become serious about academics and to neglect aspects of his emerging identity that were carefree and expressed themselves in his interest in basketball and playing guitar. Through a dialogue with his pain, this patient came to understand that his cramps were reminding him of these lost aspects of his identity.

Rather than quit his job, the patient softened his relationship with work. He resumed his former interest in guitar and other recreational activities. In subsequent dialogues with pain, he came to understand that he needed to find other ways to meet his emotional needs. As he reduced his complaints about cramps to family members, he began to open up and make himself more vulnerable to emotional support. This led him to learn an even broader array of new coping behaviors. Through his dialogue with the cramps, he was able to unravel his relationship with those cramps, to replace the cramps with healthier and more appropriate strategies, and to reclaim lost parts of his identity. In broader terms, he resolved a conflict with pain, he became more flexible, and he regained a sense of personal integrity.

The following vignette (Rossman, 2000, pp. 133–135) is a good example of the exact language that can be used to guide a patient through a dialogue with pain. It is noteworthy that within the vignette the patient is guided to merge the self with the pain image, to actually "stand in the shoes" of the pain. Such deep changes of perspective clearly are possible only within the realm of the imagination, and clinicians are encouraged to take full advantage of the metaphysical opportunities for conflict resolution that are uniquely possible within this arena. The vignette begins after the standard induction procedures: Patients are relaxed, travel in the mind to a suitable meeting location, and then become immersed in the experiences with pain:

> When you are ready, direct your attention to the … pain … as you focus on the sensations involved, allow an image to appear that represents this symptom …. Simply allow the image to appear spontaneously, and welcome whatever image comes—it may or may not make immediate sense to you …. Just accept whatever comes for now….
>
> Take some time just to observe whatever image appears as carefully as you can …. If you would like it to be clearer, imagine you have a set of controls like you do for your TV set, and you can dial the image brighter or more vivid …. Notice details about the image…. What is its shape? … Color? … Texture? … Density? … How big is it? … How big is it in relation to you? … Just observe it carefully without trying to change it in any way…. How close or far away does it seem? … What is it doing?
>
> Just give it your undivided attention …. As you do this notice any feelings that come up, and allow them to be there…. Look deeper…. Are there any other feelings present as you observe this image? … When you are sure of your feelings, tell the image how you feel about it—speak directly and honestly to it (you may choose to talk out loud or express yourself silently) …. Then, in your imagination, give the

image a voice, and allow it to answer you…. Listen carefully to what it says….

Ask the image what it wants from you, and listen to its answer…. Ask it why it wants that—what does it really need? … And let it respond …. Ask it also what it has to offer you, if you should meet its needs…. Again allow the image to respond….

Observe the image carefully again…. Is there anything about it you hadn't noticed before? … Does it look the same or is it different in any way? …

Now, in your imagination, allow yourself to become the image…. What is it like to be the image? … Notice how you feel…. Notice what thoughts you have as the image…. What would your life be like if you were this image? … Just sense what it's like to be this image….

Through the "eyes" of the image, look back at yourself…. What do you see? … Take a few minutes to really look at yourself from this new perspective…. As the image, how do you feel about this person you are looking at…. What do you think of this person? … What do you need from this person? … Speaking as the image, ask yourself for what you need….

Now slowly become yourself again…. The image has just told you what it needs from you…. What, if anything, keeps you from meeting that need? … What issues or concerns seem to get in the way? … What might you do to change the situation and take a step toward meeting the image's needs? …

Allow an image to appear for your inner advisor, a wise, kind figure who knows you well…. When you feel ready, ask your advisor about your symptom and its needs, and any thoughts, feelings, or circumstances that may make it hard for you to meet these needs…. Ask your advisor any questions you might have, and listen carefully to your advisor's responses…. Feel free to ask your advisor for help if you need it….

Now mentally review the conversation you have had with your symptom and your advisor from the beginning…. If it feels right for you, choose one way that you can begin to meet your symptom's needs—some small but tangible way you can fill some part of its unmet needs…. If you can't think of any way at all, ask your advisor for a suggestion….

When you have thought of a way to begin meeting its needs, recall again the image that represents your symptom…. Ask it if it would be willing and able to give you tangible relief of symptoms if you take the steps you have thought of…. If so, let the exchange begin…. If not, ask it to tell you what you could do in exchange for perceptible relief.... Continue to dialogue until you have made a bargain or need to take a break from negotiating....

Consider the image once more.... Is there anything you have learned from it or about it? ... Is there anything that you appreciate about it? ... If there is, take the time to express your appreciation to it.... Express anything else that seems important ... and slowly come back to your waking state and take some time to write about your experience....

After the dialogue with pain, patients should be encouraged to explore and process any additional insights and tangible changes that have occurred as a result of the dialogue with pain. Deeper processing of the experience may range from returning to imagery for ongoing dialogues with the pain, to examination of the experience through expressive forms of psychotherapy such as drawings of the encounter, or simply to discussing the encounter in depth with the clinician.

Focusing

"Focusing" is a comprehensive approach to psychotherapy and thus is broader than an imagery technique for pain management. Nevertheless, its overlap with guided imagery is clear, and it is well suited to the practice of pain management.

For those with a broader interest in psychotherapy, it is useful to note that focusing therapy has close ties to the humanistic traditions in psychotherapy and also relies heavily on experiential and body-focused therapeutic traditions (Tynion, 2002). The approach was developed by Eugene Gendlin (see Gendlin, 1981) and his colleagues at the University of Chicago, in collaboration with Carl Rogers (e.g., 1951), who extensively investigated the processes underlying successful psychotherapy (Tynion, 2002). One key predictor of positive outcomes was a process experienced by the patient during sessions that they termed *felt sense*. They found that early in the therapy process, typically by sessions 1 or 2, patients bound for positive therapeutic outcomes would tend to become less verbal, analytical, or cathartic and instead would become more focused on their emotions and other body-centered experiences, a marker for the process of felt sense. Gendlin (1981) describes felt sense as being distinct from more typical gut reactions; it is "the broader, at first *unclear*, unrecognizable discomfort, which *the whole* problem (*all that*) makes in your body" (p. 69, italics in original).

Theoretical Framework

Focusing as an approach to therapy is centered on activating felt sense within a patient and then facilitating information exchange between that felt sense and the more explicit and conscious identity of the patient. Cornell (1996, p. 3) describes focusing as:

> a body-oriented process of self-awareness and emotional healing. It's as simple as noticing how you feel—and then having a conversation with your feelings in which *you* do most of the listening. Focusing starts with the familiar experience of feeling something in your body that is about what is going on in your life. When you feel jittery in your stomach as you stand up to speak, or when you feel tightness in your chest as you anticipate making a crucial phone call, you are experiencing what we call a "felt sense"—a body sensation that is meaningful.

In its emphasis on forming an anthropomorphic representation of an important bodily sensation and then facilitating a "conversation" with that representation, focusing and the dialogue with pain techniques previously described are similar.

However, focusing is unique in a number of respects. Above all, the approach is far more detailed and specific in its procedures than any of the imagery interaction approaches discussed thus far. This specificity and detail in procedure is aimed at conjuring up a fuller and more integrated physical experience to gain access to the deepest sources of information prior to any attempts to engage in that experience through dialogue. To accomplish this goal, the technique specifically aims to leave the conscious ego out of the process until the felt sense is fully "there" and thus ready to be engaged by the patient.

The approach is also far more specific about the role of the clinician or guide, who attempts to remain completely detached from the experiential processes that are occurring within the patient. With the inner-advisor and dialogue-with-pain techniques already described, the clinician strives not to take over the interactions between patient and imagery, but the focusing approach (and the metaphor techniques to follow) calls for a radically nondirective stance from the clinician.

Basic Procedure

Because focusing is rather complex and sophisticated, we present only a basic and procedurally oriented description here. This description is intended to provide the steps a clinician would follow in the use of focusing as an imagery procedure with patients who are in pain (for a more complete account of focusing and related concepts, see Gendlin, 1981, 1996; Tynion, 2002; for an empirical review see Hendricks, 2002). Iberg (2001, p. 267) provides a strong overview of the approach and the underlying theory:

The initial symbols that fit the felt sense may be primitive, in the sense that they are "childish"? Or immature when compared with the normal thought processes of the person.... The emergent material must be able to form its own symbolization (utilizing the wealth of extant symbols and experiences that anyone has, drawing analogies, making metaphors).... Only after the emergence begins with its own just-right symbolization can the material change and become "adult" and consistent with the rest of the patient's explicit conscious contents.

The detailed procedures used in focusing are intended to produce a body-focused metaphor. The clinician then assists the patient toward engaging this metaphoric symbol in a loose and receptive interaction, until the metaphor becomes whole or complete. At this point the metaphor will provide a perfect fit between the conscious understanding of the patient, who is within an adult ego state, and the pain experience, which is considered to have been isolated and thus stuck in an immature state. Once this fit is achieved, the process is complete. Integrity is restored, and balance will automatically follow.

The specific procedure of focusing therapy involves six steps called "movements" (Gendlin, 1996). The first is labeled *clearing a space*. If the patient is calm and alert, one can dispense with the process of guided relaxation and proceed directly. In clearing a space, patients are guided to ask themselves, "How am I feeling right now? Why don't I feel great? What is getting in the way? What is bothering me right now?" (Tynion, 2002, p. 195). Patients should be assisted as needed to remain in a state of mindfulness throughout this initial process. Mindfulness in therapy comes originally from the Buddhist traditions of meditation and "involves intentionally bringing one's attention to the internal and external experiences occurring in the present moment" (Baer, 2003, p. 125). Along the same lines, patients are assisted in letting go of anything other than this state of mindful reflection, such as a connection to a particular thought or feeling and most generally to imposing their wills on any internal experience. The patient does not search for answers to the questions posed; rather, they are simply listed and then put aside as the patient opens to awareness of any experiences that follow. This openness is what is meant by the term *clearing a space*.

The second movement is referred to as *the felt sense of the problem*. This stage involves the patient's first opportunity to connect to a felt sense. After the patient has completed the first movement successfully and is relaxed, alert, and open, the next question is, "Which one [of the things that are bothering the patient] feels the worst to you right now?" The patient is directed to focus on the body after this question is posed while still remaining within a general state of mindful reflection. Further clarifying questions may include, What is "[t]he most painful, or the biggest, or the heaviest, or the prickliest, or the most 'stuck'" (Tynion, 2002, p. 195). If no body sensation emerges as the strongest, the patient may simply pick one from the list of different problems they generated while clearing a space.

For some pain patients, the problem will be clear: It will be pain. And the felt-sense stage will begin by allowing the strongest of their pains to emerge. For others, one may wish to cast a broader net, allowing the patient to highlight any problem that comes up, be it physiological, psychological, or social. Regardless, patients are not to enter into a connection with their problems at this stage. Rather, they are directed to stand back from the problem and the bodily sensation that follows it and to focus on a holistic sense of the sensation within their bodies.

The instructions call for the patient to wait at least 30 seconds for it to take shape as a somatic experience (Tynion, 2002). The goal is to allow the body to catch up to the head in a sense, because the bodily sensation is critical to the process. This waiting and focusing on bodily sensations can be very difficult for some patients. For even the mildest of clinical situations, many automatic thoughts will attempt to engage the patient's will as the waiting for the body experience continues. Patients should be coached as needed to just let such nonbodily experiences come and go. It may be helpful to inform patients who are having difficulty detecting the initial felt sense that it most typically arises from the midsections, such as the stomach, chest, or throat. Another approach that can be helpful is to guide patients in focusing their awareness on their big toes, moving to the knees, and then up to the centers of their bodies where they are most likely to find the felt sense. Once the felt sense is found, it typically will seem fuzzy at first, defying logic, words, or other labels. Gendlin (1981) calls this locating the "edge" of the problem. This marks the end of the second movement.

The third movement is called *finding a handle* and involves identifying a word or phrase to describe the felt sense. *Handle* refers to a nickname of sorts, which captures the essence of the felt sense in symbolic fashion, like the handle one uses as an identity on C.B. radio. *Handle* also carries the connotation derived from door handle, which allows the door to be opened. Tynion (2002) suggests that during this stage, "usually, a word or phrase (e.g., 'Jumpy,' 'heavy,' 'an empty feeling,' etc.) will present itself, although the description might also be in the form of a sound or an image" (p. 196). Patients try to identify a single label that captures the entirety of the experience. Intuition rather than logic is used to determine the level of fit between the handle and the experience, and when the handle does fit, the original experience of the problem typically changes automatically. One important difficulty for patients is maintaining awareness of the bodily feeling while searching for the handle. If patients begin to get too much "in their heads," they can simply be guided to refocus on the felt sense within their bodies.

The fourth movement is referred to as *resonating the handle and the felt sense* (Tynion, 2002). This movement focuses on titration of the handle until one achieves a perfect fit with the felt sense. This perfect fit is what is meant by "resonating." One of three things may happen at this stage: (1) One may find a perfect fit on the first try; (2) one may find a partial fit, which can be made perfect by modifying the handle with additional information; or (3) one may find a partial fit and then waiting brings a different handle that provides the perfect fit. Gendlin (1981, p. 57) describes this process of resonation:

> The sense of rightness is not only a check of the handle. It is your body just now changing.... Give it the minute or two it needs to get all the release and change it wants to have at this point. Don't rush on. You just got here.

The fifth movement, *asking*, begins at the point of a felt shift, a very positive physical sensation resembling release that occurs at the end of the fourth movement when the perfect fit between handle and felt sense is made. This release should spread into the patient's entire outlook. In the context of pain management, this means that pain should be less distressing in a direct sense and that one's relationship with the pain should shift in a positive direction as well.

If this shift has not yet occurred through significant time and resonating in movement four, then movement five focuses instead on beginning a receptive dialogue with the felt sense, essentially asking this sense what its handle is and waiting for a response. Typically the response takes a minute or two, which can feel long and awkward. So clinicians must be prepared to guide their clients to remain patient during this stage. Acts of will toward obtaining an answer sully the process and disrupt a truly receptive and mindful state. During this process, patients will remain within the felt sense or return to it repeatedly as distractions come and go. One continually refers to the felt sense by the latest iteration of its handle, for example:

> If the handle for your felt sense was "heavy," repeat that word to yourself until the felt sense is saliently there. Then ask the felt sense "What is it about the whole problem that feels so heavy?" Often, you may feel flooded with answers in your head. If so, just let them go by. These answers are "old tapes" that come from your mind. Wait, and repeat the question if necessary. (Tynion, 2002, p. 197)

The felt sense will be the source of the answer, not the mind or the emotions. If no felt shift occurs, Tynion (2002, p. 197) suggests that the clinician should guide the patient in asking the following three questions:

1. "What is the worst of this?" (Or using the handle "sticky," e.g., "What is the 'stickiest' thing about this?").
2. "What does the felt sense need?" (Or, "What is needed to make this okay?").
3. "How would my body feel if this whole thing was okay?"

If there is still no perfectly fitting handle at this point and no felt shift occurs, then the procedure stops here. The end result, like the rest of the process, cannot be forced. Significant progress may still occur following patients' experiences in the prior steps, and one may repeat the procedure either immediately or within another session. Felt senses and shifts even may occur during patients' day-to-day lives following the session, as they improve in their ability to enter into mindfulness and to become more receptive to the bodily sensations that are associated with their problems.

If a felt shift does occur during the fourth or fifth movements, however, then the sixth and final movement, *receiving,* involves greeting the handle and the shift in a friendly manner, such that the patient "will be likely to continue to experience other felt shifts" (Tynion, 2002, p. 198). One may stop the session here or may repeat the process through another round. Felt shifts are sequential according to Tynion (2002), so patients may "bookmark" their place and pick up later. If the patient chooses to continue, the next questions to ask are, "Does that take care of the whole problem? Is it solved?" or "What is the whole sense of *that*?" (Tynion, 2002, p. 198, italics in original). Then one simply repeats steps 2 through 6 again.

Case Example

The following is a hypothetical case example of a patient with a chronic-pain condition, followed by a vignette demonstrating dialogue during a focusing session. Susan is a 33-year-old Latino American woman presenting for psychotherapy following her separation from her husband, Marcus, of 10 years. The marriage ended after Susan, a successful attorney, discovered that her husband was planning to leave her for a younger woman. Her husband also disclosed numerous other past infidelities. Moreover, Marcus had taken large sums of money from Susan and her loved ones over the years purportedly for failed business ventures, which Susan now suspected he had hidden away in preparation for the day he would eventually abandon her. Susan's situation was made more complex due to her sense of shame at having been deceived. Susan was not reporting the degree of negative emotions (e.g., grief, anger) that one would expect in her situation. However, she was experiencing a dull intermittent pain in her chest. Her physician was able to rule out any medical condition that would explain these symptoms. After several weeks of traditional talk-oriented psychotherapy, focusing was used to address this pain. The following is an edited facsimile of a portion of this work:

Clinician: [Movement 1: Clearing a Space] Now that you are seated in a comfortable and relaxed position, let's begin. I'd like you to ask yourself: "How am I feeling right now?" Ask yourself what is bothering you most right now? What is in the way? Don't try to answer these questions. Just let the answers come on their own.

Patient: Okay. Well, I'm disappointed that Marcus did what he did. I feel kind of sad about it. Okay…. I guess I'm lonely … and I feel bad for my parents, like I feel bad that I'm putting them through this….

Clinician: [Movement 2: The Felt Sense of the Problem] Okay, now ask yourself which one of those problems feels worst to you right now? Which one is the biggest? Again, don't try to answer these questions. Just ask them. Then focus upon your body to see what feelings or sensations emerge.

Patient: Okay…It's kind of hard not to answer. I can tell that it's the part with my parents that is the worst of it. And that's strange to me, because I should be more upset about Marcus leaving me.

Clinician: That's fine. Good. Just let these answers come and go, and focus the spotlight of your attention onto your body instead. Be patient and wait to see what you sense in your body as you focus upon the biggest of your problems.

Patient: Okay…. [30-second pause] okay I'm not feeling anything, am I supposed to be feeling anything?

Clinician: Don't try to feel anything. Just focus on the problem, the biggest one, and wait. Be very patient. Sometimes it may take several minutes, which may seem like a long time. Just wait and see.

Patient: [after about a minute] Okay yes, I feel the pain in my chest. Yes, it is there now, it is connected to the problem with my parents. It is not that bad, but it is there, I can feel it right across here [gestures with her left hand].

Clinician: [Finding a Handle] Okay, very good. Now simply allow yourself to continue to focus upon that feeling in your chest. Do not try to do anything. Let any thoughts or emotions float by. Now see if any word can be used that would capture your sense of that feeling in your chest. Again, don't try. Don't think. Just open your mind to allow a nick-name or handle to come to you that would describe that feeling.

Patient: It's heavy. Like a weight. Just heavy, that's all….

Clinician: [Resonating the Handle and Felt Sense] Okay, now does "heavy" capture the whole thing? The whole feeling in your chest? Or is "heavy" just part of the feeling? How good is the fit?

Patient: It fits pretty well, but not entirely. Most of it, almost all.

Clinician: How much would you say it fits? Give me a percentage?

Patient: About a 90% fit I'd say. It is heavy, but that's not quite it.

Clinician: Okay, keep your mind and body open. Focus on the feeling across your chest and let the missing parts come to you. Take your time. It could take several minutes again. Don't try to come up with anything. If nothing ends up coming that's fine.

Patient: [after a minute] It's hot; heavy and hot. Oh [a look of discomfort comes across her face] it's a brand. Brand fits perfectly, 100%. It feels like a hot metal brand pushing down across my chest, that's the heavy part. It's like a brand they use to mark cattle.... [She starts to cry] ... For the first time I know it wasn't my fault....

Susan went on to process the meaning of the feeling of being branded across the chest. Metaphorically she had been branded with a scarlet letter, indicating her lack of worth and shame. These feelings were triggered by the abandonment and betrayal by her husband. However, the most significant negative aspect of this experience was the shame and lack of self-worth that was activated within her relationship with her parents. A number of early developmental memories were explored subsequently, including the feeling that she did not measure up within her family compared with a sibling and also shame related to being sexually abused by a neighbor. She also recalled a number of typical teenage "betrayals" of her parents' trust (e.g., sneaking out of the house, lying to parents), for which she had developed intense unconscious reactions of guilt and shame. The betrayal by her husband had left Susan in an interpersonal situation similar to each of these early memories, where she needed to turn to her parents for support but could not due to the conflict created by intense shame and a core sense of herself as being unworthy within her family. Once she identified the felt sense of being branded across the chest in a more complete manner, the discomfort lifted immediately and she was able to more fully explore and process these early experiences.

Eidetic Imagery

According to Ahsen (1973), an eidetic is a specific type of image that represents an episodic memory relating to a key developmental situation. These images hold the unresolved, conflicted information that lies at the heart of psychodynamic explanations for hysterical symptoms. However, rather than seeking to resolve these conflicts through verbal, talk-based techniques, eidetic psychotherapy aims to identify these key experiences and to transform them more directly through imagery. Ahsen's triple-code model suggests that these eidetics ideally should contain images, somatic events, and meaning. In the cases of developmental trauma, one or more of these components becomes unyoked, such as the repression of affect around the image. Thus, these images are degraded and stereotypic, like a painting without the color or a story that goes round and round with no ending. Theoretically, the goal is to reconnect the dislodged elements of the image so that it can be transformed from its degraded and problematic state and reabsorbed into the healthy flow of consciousness.

The following is a summary of the basic steps, procedures, and goals of eidetic psychotherapy (for a more complete description of these procedures and their rationales, see Ahsen, 1973; Ahsen & Lazarus, 1972; Sheikh, 1986). Eidetic psychotherapy begins with an unstructured interview that allows patients to freely discuss various aspects of their pain phenomenon, such as their current life situation, symptoms, and past experiences associated with the pain. Once patients have had a chance to tell their stories, the imagery phase of treatment begins. The basic sequence in eidetic imagery is to summon the pain symptoms, to identify conflicted developmental images associated with the first emergence of the symptom (eidetics), and then to transform these images in a healing direction.

The first phase of treatment is called the *age projection test* and is designed to find unconscious themes that are trapped in the symptom (Ahsen, 1973). In the first step of this test, *composing the symptom*, the therapist gathers the information necessary to bring the symptom out within the session, like a conductor who engages various parts of an orchestra to conduct a symphony. The patient is asked to talk about the symptom in terms of physiological sensations, psychological manifestations, and worries/concerns. As is the case in other approaches, it is important to direct patients to use their own language and to avoid technical jargon and diagnoses that may serve to detach them from the phenomenological aspects of their pain. The therapist keeps notes in three columns for the three areas previously listed, recording the exact words to describe these aspects of the pain experience. Ahsen (1973) suggests going through a detailed checklist (e.g., "How does the pain affect your head, nose, eyes, mouth, neck, shoulders, movement, talking, feelings, sleep, eating") for less introspective patients who have difficulty describing their pain. Finally, patients are asked to list nicknames, in addition to their first and last names, that people have used for them at various phases of their life. These nicknames are used to gain access to the various parts of the self-concept, particularly to those detached, forgotten selves that may have better access to possible eidetics than the current self.

Once this information is recorded, the therapist instructs patients on what they should expect from the procedure—that they will be relaxed, with their eyes open or closed, "attending to the therapist's words which will be spoken to him during this relaxed state of attention" (Ahsen, 1973, p. 255).

Furthermore, patients are told that as the therapist repeats certain words, they will gradually see an image of themselves somewhere in the past. They are instructed to just relax and attend to the therapist, allowing this image to develop on its own with no volition of their own. Finally, the therapist conducts the symptom by slowly and rhythmically repeating the descriptive words from the three columns previously generated, together with the nicknames in sequence. The goal is to repeat these highly specific descriptions and personal nicknames in such a way as to bring the symptom and related personal memories to the forefront of consciousness. Ideally, the words are repeated until the symptoms and related discomfort are brought to a high pitch. Therapists must use their intuition and sensitivity to determine the point at which this level is achieved, and then they must suddenly switch to a guided description of the opposite of being in pain. Ahsen (1973) suggests, "At this stage the therapist talks about the times when the patient was healthy and happy, and he did not have these symptoms" (p. 255).

Once patients reach this step, they are guided toward self-images during their healthy year, before the onset of their pain disorders. It is often necessary to encourage them to repeatedly see these self-images, perhaps 10 to 15 times, until they become sufficiently clear and absorbing. A useful test of vividness and immersion at this stage is to repeat the image until personal objects, such as clothing, become vivid. Next, patients are guided through an exploration of the year following this new image to find a key eidetic experience that "discloses meaning, the origin, and the character of the symptom" (Ahsen, 1973, p. 256). If this exploration uncovers useful eidetics, the task turns to their transformation within the imaginal realm. Again, this may be done through a variety of techniques depending on the specifics of the eidetic, the patient, and the therapist. However, these transformations usually will involve a reexperiencing of the traumatic memory with a more functional emotive, cognitive, and behavioral response by the patient. For example, if a patient uncovers a traumatic memory involving anger at an abusive parent, the patient can be guided to express this anger within the safe and versatile confines of the imagination. Furthermore, patients may be guided to attend to any difference in symptoms that emerges as they shift back and forth between the original image and the new image. Finally, the new, healing images that are uncovered during this procedure may be rehearsed between sessions to encourage their immersion into day-to-day consciousness.

While the aforementioned procedures may be sufficient with some patients, others require an additional step. Ahsen (1973, p. 256) describes a final phase: "In the last phase of the test this image is used in association with parental images to evolve a ritualistic movement of the image. This movement finally throws light on the meaning of the symptom. This phase is useful especially in case the initial projection of the image failed to elucidate the cause of the hysterical symptom." In this final phase, patients face their parents in their parental home around the time of the emergence of the symptom. First, they stand before their parents, crying in an attempt to evoke pity from them. Next, they remove an item of clothing, which should be made vivid through repetition prior to its removal. They throw this item on the floor in front of their parents and say, "Take it away! I don't want to wear it!" (Ahsen, 1973, p. 256). They follow the parent to see where the item has been taken, and they identify any object that stands out in the vicinity. Finally, any direct memories associated with this object are explored for ways that it may be tied to the symptoms and their possible meanings. For example, if the clothing is placed on a dresser in the patient's sister's room and her yearbook is vivid near the dresser, memories associated with the patient's sister's yearbook could be explored.

Though this procedure may seem somewhat arbitrary, the rationale is rather simple. The parental images are thought to be central to a person's self-image because of their proximity to the development of the self from conception through childhood. Furthermore, these images and the home that contains them are the most stable context within the psyche because they are perceived repeatedly early in the patient's development. Thus, when the parent image is used to tie the symbolic representation of the symptoms (e.g., the unwanted article of clothing) to an object within this stable schematic context, one is likely to arrive at a reliable symbolic connection for the pain disorder from the correct developmental period. Furthermore, this connection is made in a manner that is sufficiently symbolic to bypass a patient's customary defenses.

Clean Language and Metaphor: The Work of David Grove

David Grove's metaphor techniques are aimed at deep transformation and integration of patients' self-systems. Metaphor transformations involve the reprocessing of deep symbolic content, whose true meaning may actually remain unknown to the patient and the guide during the imagery session, and these approaches aim for deeper transformation of emotional processing and world meaning rather than for the more circumscribed goal of pain relief.

Grove's metaphor techniques have been revised a number of times over the years, under the rubric of *metaphor therapy, clean language* (Grove & Panzer, 1989; Tompkins & Lawley, 2000), and most recently *emergent knowledge* (for a description of Grove's latest work see Wilson, 2008). On a practical level, metaphor therapy, clean language, and emergent knowledge principles share the underlying assumption that individuals interpret their worlds through metaphors, dream-like images that filter experience. These systems also rely on the spatial dimensions of the imagery experience, such as location, size, or shape. In this manner, metaphors that contain important information about a person's autobiographical experiences may become detached from one another. This detachment may lead to disintegration among the biopsychosocial systems of the individual, whereby important metaphors are trapped within discrete areas of the body and, in an isomorphic manner, within discrete areas of the consciousness as well. Clean language refers to the approach used by the therapist to bring these systems back into contact with one another so that they can heal, and emergent knowledge refers to the systems-based philosophy on which the approach most recently has been grounded.

Grove and the proponents of the clean-language philosophy draw on concepts from contemporary systems science (i.e., emergence theory) to explain how metaphors may be used therapeutically. Indeed, emergent knowledge uses the term *emergence* to draw attention to the belief that consciousness arises from lower-level bioenergetic processes (e.g., neurophysiology) and then feeds back on these lower-level processes in the form of boundaries or constraints. Similar to other deep approaches previously described, metaphor therapy has the goal of restoring integrity within flows of information both within the individuals and between individuals and their environments. Although Grove and his colleagues do not mention self-organization explicitly, emergence is a facet of the broader theory of self-organizing systems (Guastello, Koopmans, & Pincus, 2008), making the rationale similar to the one developed in Chapter 3 and by Rossi (1997).

Basic Procedures

Within Grove's metaphoric therapy approach, metaphors are defined as containers of information. In particular, certain emotion-laden metaphors pertaining to the body are considered to be foreign objects. The information pertaining to these metaphors is stored in the body, outside of episodic or other mental memory systems. Their foreignness to the rest of the body–mind is what is believed to create their negative emotional power. Finally, these metaphors are referred to as *epistemological metaphors*; they are involved in a person's meaning-making systems (Grove, 1989; Linn, 2008).

The first step in the process is to ask questions that will elicit such a foreign, body-related, emotion-laden, and epistemological metaphor. As a container, the metaphor, containing emotional or mental information, can then be moved outside of the patient's body where it belongs. For example, butterflies in the stomach or a knot in the shoulder is not "you," nor is it your body. Instead, these are thoughts and feelings pertaining to some situation. They are foreign sensations. When situations overwhelm the mental and emotional processing capabilities of the individual—for example, in cases of trauma and particularly childhood trauma—such information may be mistakenly stored in an unprocessed manner within the individual's body.

These experiences come in, but they usually do not leave. Putting this information into a metaphor during treatment allows one to trap the butterflies or to isolate the knot. Then the metaphor can be removed from the body and placed back into the content of the traumatic memory or, if necessary, with another metaphor that can do something with them. For example, butterflies will do well in a field, and a knot can be unwound with hands.

To elicit the first metaphor, one asks questions that allow the somatic experience of the patient to take on the form of a metaphoric container, something that can be drawn. In response to the patient's description of the pain, the clinician asks the following questions (Grove, 1989):

1. First the clinician asks: "And what would you like to have happen?" A patient may respond: "I want it to stop." This simple question deepens the immersion of the patient into the experience and begins to activate the sense of foreignness of the experience.

2. Next the clinician asks: "And when you have [body sensation or feeling], how do you know you have...?" This question establishes the epistemological and phenomenological basis of the experience. For example, the question "And when you have pain, how do you know you have pain?" will bring a response such as: "I can feel my shoulder *tightening*." *Tightening* is a key word here; it is subjective and meaningful to the patient.

3. Next the clinician establishes the location in the body with: "Where do you have the pain?" and "Whereabouts is pain?" Grove generally asks these types of "where" questions three times or so to be sure that the exact location is determined. A patient may be even more specific than *shoulder* in identifying tightening and may specify that the pain originates in the shoulder blade and then reaches up over the top of the shoulder.

4. Next, the clinician asks: "And does *it* have a size or a shape?" The word *it* is carefully selected as an aspect of clean language that establishes the metaphor as a separate entity from the patient. Separating the metaphor in this manner allows it to be engaged without also engaging the ego state of the patient. A patient could respond, for example: "It is a big square knot, like the kind one uses to tie down a tent." Even if the metaphor seems clear from the patient's natural language, there always are details that can make the container more robust. This robustness may be maximized by engaging the image directly through the use of clean language.

These are the four basic questions that are repeated in eliciting metaphors. A number of follow-up questions are advised as well, such as: "And is it on the inside or the outside?" "And what's it like?" "And what kind...?" "And is there anything else about..?"(Grove, 1989). These questions serve to elicit a clearer metaphoric container. Other questions may be asked as well, and the clinician's style of interviewing is slow, nonreactive, yet attuned. The aim of all questions, scripted or improvised, is to objectify the bodily experience within a metaphoric container, to separate the metaphor from the patient through the clean use of pronouns like *it*, and to give the metaphor a specific location in the body.

This initial eliciting process is focused on locating an appropriate metaphor in the space of the body–mind, which, in the case of pain, will almost always be at a location somewhere within the body. In the second phase, one considers the location of the metaphor in time. Grove's rationale assumes that the relevant metaphor will exist within the patient's memory just before some trauma. His cases typically involved trauma such as child sexual abuse. However, the approach could be applied to trauma with higher physiological loadings as well, such as bodily injuries. In the case of pain, the first metaphor for that pain will exist at a time just before some traumatic event, at $t - 1$, with t representing the exact point of the trauma. Grove (1989) suggests that the replay of symptoms contained within the metaphor has the function of blocking the patient from reexperiencing the trauma at t. Consequently, symptoms tend to be reexperienced in a rigid and recurring manner over time. If cues from within or without the patient are moving the memory systems toward some aspect of the trauma, the pain will reemerge and detour that memory process to protect the patient. The end result is avoidance, which increases the traumatic impact and leads to more avoidance over time (see Chapter 2 for the role of avoidance in the maintenance of pain syndromes).

The result in the patient's body–mind is a fractured set of metaphors, typically more than one, which needs to be put back together, reintegrated, and then moved forward in time and also outside of the body. Moving the metaphor to t allows the experience to mature along with the rest of the patient to resolve the trauma. Essentially one is identifying the metaphor, which is usually fragmented, and creating a process through which it can be reassembled within the neighboring ego systems of the patient.

Grove suggests that one can tell when the metaphor is moving forward in time toward t because things seem to go from bad to worse within the patient's account. Similarly, the patient's language will become more active and intense; for instance, a knot may be "tightening," "pulling," or "burning."

Once the metaphor is created, it is located within the body, and it is found to be at $t - 1$, the guide begins to engage the metaphor in a clean dialogue. The approach is not patient centered, like most forms of therapy. Rather, the approach is metaphor centered (Grove, 1989). By interacting directly with the metaphor, using rules of clean language to avoid activating other aspects of the experience or the ego of the patient, the metaphor may be assisted in becoming unraveled, in unpacking some of its information, and in moving toward t. Using the knot as an example, one can ask: "And what would a knot like to have happen?" "And what would a knot like to do?" "And as that happens, what happens next?" Follow-up questions to move the metaphor toward t include: "And how long will that take?" "And what happens after that happens?" (Grove, 1989).

The clinician's goal is to locate the experience of the patient and to never contaminate it. Contamination can occur not only through the clinician's specific agenda or by expressing a reaction but is also thought to occur through any language that elicits the perspective of either clinician or patient. The objective is to engage the experience and the metaphor, not the patient. Once you locate the experience within the body, you attempt to establish that experience as separate from the body. You begin to relate with it as separate. Then you draw out a metaphor by asking about size, shape, location, and so on. Finally, you begin to unravel the metaphor, to relate to it by asking, for example, what its purpose is, or what it would like to do. These questions help to create a more coherent and goal-oriented state within the metaphor. Finally, questions are asked to facilitate movement in time toward t.

Because all of the information within us (e.g., thoughts and feelings) has the potential to be contained within metaphor, one must be extremely careful not to enact these other metaphors when a patient's primary epistemological metaphor is engaged during treatment. As with all images, metaphors naturally mix and merge when they come into contact with one another. Therefore, clean language allows for a pure treatment of the patient's own epistemology. The situation is akin to the surgical removal of a foreign object, which demands a perfectly sterile environment to avoid contamination of the patient's body. The approach digs rather deep, so one needs to be sure to remove the true metaphoric information package, not to tug at another metaphor that comes from the patient or from the clinician.

The following are some clean language rules of thumb. Do not use the word I. I brings the patient into the here and now, away from t or $t - 1$. I also injects you, the clinician, into the situation. Similarly, do not use the pronoun *you*, even in response to the patient using the word I, once you have the metaphor. *You* goes to the adult part of the patient. Since metaphors exist at $t - 1$, the metaphor may not exist within the adult patient in your office. You want to communicate with the metaphor, not the patient or the patient's current ego state. You are trying to establish a relationship with the metaphor, not the here-and-now patient. Finally, you should use the subjective and passive tone in all questions asked. You are nondirective and open in this manner because neither you nor the patient knows what information is wrapped up in the metaphor. Therefore, patients need to be able to say no or yes or nothing to any question posed. Resistance is the metaphor saying, "Don't ask that question; it is not relevant" (Grove,

1989). Any question that is not open-ended imposes on the metaphor from the clinician's metaphors; it forces the metaphor to lose its epistemological, meaning-making role within the patient's consciousness.

Finally, clean language involves identification of epistemological metaphors "owned' by earlier selves, and the process involves discovering the owner of the metaphor. Remember, the approach is information centered, not patient centered, so you talk to the knot, for example, not to the patient who has the knot. Then the knot will let you know what else is happening and who else is involved. You are encouraging the metaphor to grow toward the level of the adult, in mnemonic time, but you must engage it first. Because the metaphor typically belongs to earlier selves within the individual, Grove instructs clinicians to speak very slowly, gently, and simply when engaging metaphors. The younger you suspect the owner of the metaphor to be, the slower and cleaner your language should be (Grove, 1989).

One practical advantage of the use of clean language and of working with metaphors is that one can do deep symbolic work without activating the defenses in patients or even gaining access to a high degree of their detailed traumatic memories. Working with metaphors provides a sort of analgesic protection around the traumatic experiences, and the work is largely content free because one is working with implicit memory contained within the metaphors.

In his video, Grove (1989) shares another insight concerning work through metaphors: Somatic metaphors do not work in isolation. The metaphor exists within the memory of the adult; thus, the adult or observing ego of the patient is involved. On the other hand, the metaphor is treated like a separate entity, a container of information within the patient that resembles a foreign invader or a disease process. This distinction between the patient and the metaphor is what is maintained through the use of clean language. Finally, there is a context to the episodic memory at $t - 1$, the time in the patient's memory just before the traumatic experience when the metaphor and its symptoms become activated in meaning making. The context contains the various aspects of the memory, such as other people, location, and different features of the location.

To review, there are three aspects involved at $t - 1$: (1) the metaphor; (2) the patient; and (3) the memory context. One can infer which aspects patients are describing by the language they use. If you hear a somatic or feeling word, then you know you are hearing an experience within the patient and, thus, a metaphor. If patients use personal pronouns such as I, he, or she, then they are describing themselves. If they describe things outside of themselves with pronouns such as it or he (e.g., "He is chasing"), then you can infer that the focus is on context.

The response of the clinician depends on which aspect is in focus at the time. If a feeling word is used, then the clinician responds with the metaphor responses, such as establishing a location and growing the metaphor toward *t* by asking what it wants or what happens next. If patients describe themselves or their bodies, within the process, (e.g., "I want to hide"), then you respond to the body using clean language (e.g., "And you want to hide"). A variant on focus on the body of patients occurs if they describe just a body part (e.g., "A shoulder won't move"). Following the principles of clean language, the clinician then responds directly to that body part (e.g., "And when *a* shoulder won't move, what does *a* shoulder want to do?").

The pronouns are important. The clinician uses a personal pronoun like *you* only when patients describe their whole selves as being in the memory. The difference can be quite subtle. For example, "I'm feeling hot" is clearly a feeling inside the person, so the response that targets the feeling is, "And when you're feeling hot, whereabouts is hot?" If the patient says, "I'm hot," then the better response could be, "And when you are hot, what happens next?" If the patient describes the context, "It's getting hot outside," then the clinician's response goes to context: "And when it's hot outside, what happens next?" As a final rule, the clinician should respond to the last phrase of the patient, which takes priority over prior information. For example, if the patient describes the first episode of pain and says, "It starts to hurt, up in my shoulder, and I remember it is spring and the birds are chirping outside of my window," then the clinician responds to the birds: "And when birds are chirping outside of a window, what happens next?"

Sometimes patients will supply numerous experiences and metaphors but very little ego-related content or context. If this is the case, the clinician can explore integrations among various metaphors. The clinician can simply ask the patient if the various metaphors that have been collected thus far will go together in various combinations. Grove (1989) uses the example of a patient who feels a whirlpool of confusion in the head and a rock in the stomach. A clinician could ask, for example, "And can a whirlpool go to a rock? And what would a whirlpool do with a rock if a whirlpool goes to a rock?" In his example, the whirlpool cleaned the rock, leading to a decrease in the negative experience associated with the rock. Remember, metaphors and their associated symptoms are viewed as unsuccessful internal attempts at healing. Therefore, they can be used as medicine, all the while maintaining clean language not to impose purpose or meaning on them during the dialogue process. Whirlpools go to rocks and either do something or do not. The patient and the therapist need not become involved directly.

Ultimately, the clinician will need to shift the focus of questions to follow the patient's lead. Furthermore, if patients respond with "I don't know," then the clinician may simply query another source within the memory. For example, the clinician may ask in an open-ended manner, "And when you don't know, what happens next?" or "And when you don't know, how can you tell that you don't know?" If the patient responds, "I feel foggy," then the clinician can query the experience of being "foggy" with, "And whereabouts is foggy?" Likewise, the clinician could go outside of the patient to engage context with "And what keeps you from knowing?"

The clinician simply works within this mapping in time and internal space to collect the distinctive metaphors and to work toward allowing them to become more integrated. Integration occurs by moving the information within the metaphors around within time and information space—among the domains of patient, somatic experience, and context. Metaphors in particular are grown forward in mnemonic time and are grown outward from within the body toward the surrounding context where they are assumed to originally belong. The clinician facilitates such movement by following the rules of questioning described thus far by using clean language.

Within the patient, pain is believed to be exacerbated by what Grove (1989) refers to as an *enmeshment*. An enmeshment is a fusion that may occur among information pertaining to the body, the metaphor, or the context of an experience. The term *enmeshment* can be considered to be equivalent to a conflict, to a rigid flow of biopsychosocial information, or to a tangle or knot within biopsychosocial space. Such a knot restricts the flows of information therein.

In technical terms (see Chapter 3), the topological surface describing such a constriction would be described as a fixed-point attractor surrounded by a repellor, a modified saddle attractor (Guastello, 2002). A common example in nature would be a whirlpool or tornado. At the center, where the metaphor is located, one would find a deep hole that sucks information in. Thus, the metaphor and the pain associated with it are reexperienced repeatedly in a rigid manner, moving around quickly toward a center. Once triggered sufficiently, it is nearly impossible to break free of pain on one's own. Around the hole one would find strong repelling forces composed of the patient's ego state and the surrounding context in memory. These areas would serve to deflect information, which would tend to be blown away or to disintegrate. The process is both rigid and chaotic at the same time, as information is fused near the center of the metaphor and fragmented in the surrounding biopsychosocial areas.

As the imagery procedure unravels the information within the metaphor, the various aspects of memory may become whole again, distinct, and healed. The various aspects of the pain-related memory are stretched out from one another spatially and also in mnemonic time; the trauma is reintegrated within the here and now. The outermost chaotic areas of the "memory tornado" are brought into contact with the rigid inner areas at t, returning the system to a state of balance.

In summary, the three phases of Grove's metaphor therapy are the following. First, the *separation* phase involves separation of the metaphor from the person. At this time, the clinician asks questions aimed at identifying, locating, and engaging metaphors within the person. The first question of the patient is: "What do you want to have happen?" with regard to pain. Subsequent questions aim at identifying features of the metaphor, such as location, size, color, shape, what it wants, and what happens next.

Next, the *individuation* phase involves questions that extend the significance of words or phrases of the patient downward, to greater depth, and toward greater distinction among metaphor/feeling, person/body, and context (information outside of body). Each aspect is queried separately depending on the nature of the patient's unfolding description. Just like metaphor questions, questions that can develop or deepen the body can pertain to age, clothing, what the person wants, or what happens next. Similar questions may be asked to develop contextual factors.

In the final phase, *maturation*, the aim is to work through, unpack, and defuse metaphoric information to promote reintegration and healing. There are two ways in which this may occur. The primary method is to move the three gathered and deepened sources of information forward in time, toward t. The primary question here is, "And what happens next?" More generally, each of the deepening questions may serve to move the metaphor, body, or context forward in time. Metaphors will tend to move from within the body to the outside context as healing occurs. Expect things to go from bad to worse and then for metaphors to migrate out of the body, back into context.

The alternative process involves a lack of context. In these situations, context dissolves as the metaphors move toward time $- t$. In these situations, one guides the process of combining various metaphors, without actually moving through t. For the sake of clarity, we refer to this alternate phase as the *combination* phase. The clinician asks, for example, if a "needle" will go to a "balloon" or if a "rock" will go to a "river." If the answer is yes, then the clinician asks what the needle or rock does and what comes next. Finally, the clinician may wish to query subsequent metaphors that have emerged after such transformations. For example, if a "rope" is woven into a "sweater," the clinician could ask if a sweater would go to the patient's body, and the patient could respond that when it goes there it brings warmth and comfort. One never knows which metaphors will go together, what they may become, and what they may do. The process is quite creative in this sense, but at the same time it is highly structured through the rules of clean language.

Case Example

The case example that follows involves a woman with recurring pain in her upper back, just under the left shoulder blade. The pain is associated with stiffness in the jaw on the opposite side, which runs down her neck. This pain emerges during times of stress and also at other times in an inexplicable manner. On occasion the pain has been intense enough to limit her physical activity. Modified excerpts from an imagery session with her are interspersed with explanatory text:

> Guide: And now I want you to focus on your body and allow the discomfort you typically feel to emerge. When you can begin to feel the pain, describe it to me in your own words without the use of any medical jargon. Then tell me what you want to have happen with your pain.

The session begins by asking the patient to describe her pain and what she wants to have happen with it over time. Medical jargon can distance a person from the experiential aspects of their pain, so it is avoided. This gathering of descriptive language can be done prior to the actual imagery session, during an eyes-open interview or at the start of the imagery process. In either case, it is usually best to use a notepad to record the actual language used by the patient, particularly adjectives and adverbs that pertain to any experiences. These descriptive terms will provide useful information about the metaphors that contain the pain-related experiences:

> Patient: It starts to feel tight, right here in my jaw, like there's something pulling down on it and then tightening it, so it gets stiff.

The patient is using the pronoun *it* to describe her experience. This conveys the start of a natural separation of the patient from the metaphor. If she had demonstrated greater fusion with the image, such as "*I'm* tightening up," then further use of clean language to address the "tightening" rather than the patient herself would be required. However, this patient uses a clean description of a feeling, so the guides choice of "it" is simple:

> Guide: And a jaw is *tight*, and something is pulling *down*, and *tightening*, and in *tightening*, and it gets *stiff*?
> Patient: Yes (starts to show facial expressions indicating mild stress and discomfort).

Deep metaphor approaches, particularly Grove's, emphasize the connections between physical and metaphysical space and time. Movement is facilitated within the process across the space of information (e.g., metaphors within the body) and mnemonic time (e.g., memory for events in time). Terms within the patient's verbiage are repeated and emphasized (shown in italics in the dialogue) to facilitate awareness and immersion within those aspects of the imagination. The guide uses the patient's own language and uses those descriptive terms to massage the consciousness, bringing the metaphoric content to the forefront of the patient's awareness:

Guide: And whereabouts in a jaw is tight and stiff and pulling down, when a jaw is tight and pulling down and stiff?
Patient: In the bottom of my jaw, all along the bottom right here (patient brushes along the bottom of her jaw with her index finger).

Here the guide is attempting to identify the location of the metaphor within the body of the patient. The patient has already said it is in "the jaw." However, the specific location within the jaw and any extensions (i.e., pulling down) into other areas will be identified through this process of deepening the immersion into or "separating" the image. The patient uses the pronoun *my* to describe her jaw. However, the focus will stay with the metaphor, not the patient, because she did not switch targets to her whole self, as would have been the case if she had instead said something like "I'm stuck" or "I don't know." These types of responses would have allowed the guide to respond with the pronoun *you* and to explore these experiences further, with "And when you don't know, how do you know that you don't know?" or "And when you are stuck, how do you know you are stuck?" Or the guide could query the patient rather than the experience with "And when you are stuck, what do you want to have happen?" The first two queries would have led to further epistemological experiences and metaphors within the patient. The third would have led the patient's memory of herself forward toward *t*. Instead, the next question will query the physical aspects of the metaphor in the jaw, beginning with size or shape:

Guide: And when the bottom of a *jaw* is *tight*, and *tightening*, and *pulling down*, and *stiff*, does *stiff* have a *size* or a *shape*?

Now the guide attempts to identify a metaphoric object that will be a container for information pertaining to tightness and pulling down within the patient's jaw. Several feelings are described (i.e., "pulling," "tight," and "stiff") spontaneously in sequence. Therefore, each is repeated in temporal order, and the next query follows the final experience in the sequence, "stiff." Sometimes the patient will provide the metaphor spontaneously, and then the guide will engage the metaphor and attempt to move it forward in time by asking what it wants or what happens next. Other times, the patient will require more time to respond, and the guide will need to repeat the request for a size or shape after a long pause. Again, if the patient does not know, one can either query the experience of not knowing, or, if the patient is referring to the self, then the self may be asked what it wants to do when it does not know. The dialogue continues with the patient's identification of a metaphor:

Patient: Yes, it's like a metal rod….
Guide: A metal rod.
Patient: Yes, a metal rod, and at the end is tied a string that goes down into my back, pulling under my shoulder and it hurts right there (pointing).

The patient has attached a string to the rod, which follows naturally in time with discomfort under the shoulder blade. Since the patient has spontaneously moved forward in time and the two metaphors are connected, the guide will proceed with these queries:

Guide: And a metal rod, and a string, and *tied*. And *pulling* under the shoulder…and hurts under a shoulder. And is a metal rod light or heavy? Hot or cold? Thick or thin?

At this point in time, the guide is attempting to obtain more information about the rod, for example, weight, temperature, and thickness:

Patient: It's thin but very hard and stiff. It runs along the bottom of my jaw, and it is very cold, freezing cold. It hurts, but the cold kind of makes it feel numb.
Guide: And *thin*, and it's *hard*, and … it's … *stiff*, running on the bottom of a jaw, and … it's … *cold, freezing cold*, and it hurts, and it is numb.
Patient: The string is thin but very strong, like fishing line. And under the shoulder it is all in a knot. When it pulls on that knot it hurts.
Guide: And a thin, hard, stiff rod runs along the bottom of a jaw … and freezing cold … and numb … and a thin … strong string … a fishing line … goes under a shoulder and pulls on a knot … and a knot hurts … and when a knot hurts … what … happens … next?

The guide is attempting to intensify the clarity and emergence within the spatial, temporal, and experiential aspects of the imagery. The question also engages the metaphor into a clean language interaction with the guide. Then the guide simply asks "What happens next?" This is the process of maturation toward *t*, when the biopsychosocial "injury" or trauma originally occurred. What will follow is either a shift to the patient's ego ("I want to scream"), a shift to the situation or context of the imagery scenario ("It won't let me scream"), another image will unfold, or the patient will stay with a final experience suggesting that *t* may have been reached. Within this patient, the rod simply continued to pull upon the knot, which became tighter and tighter, until eventually the rod softened up as it became warmer from the friction of pulling. Over time, the patient reported that it stopped pulling.

One could infer that the information contained in the jaw was attached to a traumatic experience from around the time that the pain symptoms first emerged in the patient's life. The trauma may have been primarily physical or psychological in nature. Regardless, simply moving the activity of the rod forward in time matured it and allowed it to soften, and its stiffness dissipated out of the patient.

Despite the rod's maturation, however, within this patient the knot remained, and further queries aimed at individuation and maturation of the knot led nowhere. Therefore, the guide used the alternative process of combination to assess where a knot may wish to go. In many cases, one may find numerous metaphors that can be gathered, each related to a subsequent experience in the pain process. One would then query which of these other images, each containing potential for healing, would go to a knot. However, in this case, the patient had no other images, just a knot that stayed a knot. The rod and string were gone. For this patient, then, the aim was simply to allow that knot to go wherever it wanted to go by asking, "And where would a knot like to go?" An alternate question could have been to ask the knot what it would like to do or what it would like to have happen. In the case of the patient above, the knot wanted to go into the ocean, along with the string dangling along behind it. Responses to "What happens next?" led the knot into the ocean, where it sank to the bottom, and came to rest in a bed of sand. The subsequent prompt of "What happens next?" resulted in the image of a fish that came along and ate the knot and string. After a final prompt, the fish defecated the digested knot, and these remains were dispersed through ocean currents. This transformation of the metaphoric knot under the shoulder blade led to immediate relief of the pain episode that was occurring at the outset of the session and to a shift in the experience of subsequent pain episodes, which became more diffuse across the upper back.

This patient continued to experience some discomfort associated with the tightening of the jaw, and the metal rod became cold again on occasion. However, this remaining discomfort was more manageable, and consequently the patient completed treatment after two sessions. It is possible that the metal rod was anchored by a more strongly emotionally charged set of episodic developmental memories (i.e., subjectively traumatic memories from childhood), which she was not yet ready to explore even in a metaphoric format. Nevertheless, a follow-up assessment at 6 months and 1 year indicated that this patient did not have any significant recurrence of the shoulder pain, and she was able to manage her neck aches and headaches with occasional massage therapy.

It is worthwhile to note that there are many other methods that may be useful in the transformation of metaphoric images associated with pain. Indeed, Grove's own techniques have continued to evolve over the years. As long as one uses clean language to separate and engage with metaphors and one allows these metaphors to mature and transform in imaginary time and space, one may use these approaches creatively. This may be of comfort to clinicians who understandably could find the previously described procedures to be quite complex. For example, when patients identify several distinct metaphors associated with the pain process, the guide can simply ask if each of the metaphors will "go to" any of the others. In this case, one is exploring the more nonlinear process of combination from the outset (Grove, 1989). For example, if the patient had identified a fish swimming in the stomach and a hailstorm moving down the shoulders in response to the prompt "What happens next?" the guide simply could have asked, "And does a hail storm go to a metal rod? And does a fish go to a knot?" Typically, it is good to query each combination. For example, a rod going to a fish may involve a different process than a fish going to a rod.

It is noteworthy that patients almost always will be able to answer yes and no in response to queries about what goes to what. Typically the guide does not even need to understand what the metaphors may be representing or what the outcomes will be if one item does go to another. If a particular metaphor does go to another, one has the opportunity for transformation. The guide simply needs to ask, for example, "And when a fish goes to a knot, what happens when a fish ... goes ... to a ... knot?" In the case just presented, the patient probably would have said that the fish eats the knot followed by the prompt, "What happens next?"

In summary, although the techniques are quite detailed and sophisticated, the overall process and goals of these deep metaphoric approaches to treatment are rather simple. First, patients describe their pain experiences in common language and identify what they want to happen. Next, the separation phase involves identifying the location within the body and the physical aspects of the metaphor. As the metaphor emerges, it is engaged by the guide and moved forward in time in the processes of individuation and maturation respectively. These phases are repeated with different metaphors, as movement in space and time continues, by asking what the metaphor (or the ego or context) wants to do next or what happens next. Finally, the patient explores possible transformation through combination by asking which ones can go together and then what happens next.

Comparative Analysis

As a practical matter, it is useful to compare and contrast Grove's metaphor therapy and the numerous other metaphor-based transformational approaches to managing pain. First, approaches based on Carl Jung's active imagination are similar to Grove's work in that each relies on the notion that consciousness is active and that the heart of its activity rests within the ongoing flows of metaphors within the imagination. However, the two approaches differ in the origins of healing symbols. Jung believed that the source of renewal and healing in the imagination came primarily from the collective unconscious, in the univeral archetypes existing beyond the individual. Grove's metaphor therapy relies on metaphors generated from the autobiographical, meaning-making experiences of the patient.

Grove's approach is also far more specific and circumscribed in its procedures compared with most approaches based on Jungian theory. This specificity centers on the use of clean language and is intended to allow clinicians to better engage the deepest aspects of a patient's metaphoric imagery without any interference through engagement of the patient's or the clinician's dominant ego state. The use of clean language to draw out metaphors, purely from within the patient and with no influence from the therapist, is a primary distinction between Grove's work with metaphors and numerous others, particularly Ahsen's eidetic imagery, Erickson's hypnotherapy, and, to a lesser extent, Gendlin's focusing approach.

Gendlin (in Rossi, 1997) clearly highlights some of the similarities and contrasts between Ericksonian hypnotherapy and focusing in his formal role as a discussant for Rossi's presentation on nonlinear dynamics in hypnotherapy. First, he broadens the context of nonlinerity beyond the Ericksonian methods of cultivating and using the client's past experiences in therapy; he states, "It is not just hypnosis that is nonlinear; all experiencing is nonlinear. Any moment is a mesh of thousands of aspects that have never been separate" (p. 158). Gendlin then discusses the fact that focusing is grounded in the notion that within experience, the part is in the whole, and whole is in the part. This would be expected if memory, levels of experience, and, most broadly, body–mind self-regulation processes are self-organizing. Self-organizing systems tend to emerge into fractal structures, which are self-similar across scales. Clinically, this means that when a clinician is able to help a client to work through some vague felt sense, the working through of that experience will propagate across the whole of the body–mind systems of which that felt sense is a part.

The differences in approach that Gendlin identifies between focusing and Ericksonian hypnotherapy may be extended to eidetic imagery and Grove's metaphor therapy. First, in focusing there is no trance: The client is fully conscious and awake. There typically will be some degree of trance in eidetic imagery, depending on the client's conscious access to the time in life when the original eidetic memory was created. In contrast, Ericksonian hypnotherapy almost always involves a degree of trance, and Grove's metaphor therapy should always involve trance. However, whereas Ericksonian hypnotherapy relies on trance to gain access to the unconscious, in Grove's metaphor therapy the trance is somewhat incidental to the process. In metaphor therapy, trance likely emerges naturally as the conscious ego of the client becomes separate from the metaphor through the individuation process.

Gendlin (in Rossi 1997) proposes an interesting theoretical rational for his disdain for the use of trance. He suggests that there is an inverse relationship between access to therapeutic material and ability to work that material through in a beneficial manner: "When in a hypnotic state, you may access a lot, but you can not make enduring changes to the more wakeful conscious processes of the individual. If you work with the conscious individual, you can't get at as much, but what you do get you can work with. In focusing, this is why you have the conscious person and also the body engaged at the same time in communication with one another. Each needs the other" (quoted in Rossi, 1997, p. 160). If this proposition is true, it appears that Gendlin gets around this impediment by facilitating a process between one small but potent part of the subconscious (felt sense, which contains the whole of the problem) and the client in a fully conscious state: the best of both worlds. Ahsen approaches this problem by gaining access to key areas of the unconscious, key developmental memories tied to the "injury" and then by enhancing the patient's ability to act therein through the power of imagery. Erickson appears to have used the strategies of efficiency and working with momentum, along with his own superior clinical acumen to circumvent this limiting depth-to-will ratio. Grove, by contrast, seems to have bypassed the limitation altogether. His approach dispenses with the need for either the conscious individual or the unconscious to be involved in therapy, facilitating change instead by directly activating the intrinsic dynamics within the metaphors themselves.

Gendlin (in Rossi 1997) makes a second distinction in the approaches: It lies in the use of suggestion. No suggestion is used in either focusing or in Grove's metaphor therapy, whereas Ericksonian hypnotherapy is centered around suggestive techniques (primarily indirect) and Ahsen's eidetic approach is open to their collaborative use within the imagination. In focusing, the body most typically says no to any particular handle that the client may come up with. This provides useful information that allows for the further resonating of the handle until a felt shift occurs. Gendlin makes the point that indirect suggestion brings Ericksonian hypnotherapy closer to focusing in this respect, yet the essential difference remains. Gendlin writes:

> I relate to the client's body only through the client. I don't elicit things directly from the client's body without consulting the client. I am like a lawyer, not like a doctor.... A lawyer would not go to court and sue someone in my name without my approval or my knowledge. (Rossi, 1997, p. 160)

This point about the difference in roles and relationships of the guide provides a final key distinction among the approaches. Within eidetic imagery, the therapist relates to the client within the imagination, a traditional imagery guide role with enhanced precision and depth, due to the use of preparatory procedures such as age projection and composing the symptom. In Ericksonian hypnotherapy, the therapist typically is engaged with the client's unconscious, attempting to elicit some healing imagery from the client's experiential learnings. The innovation and artistry of Erickson's work lay in his ability to leave his own agenda aside and to find images that provided a deep and sensitive fit for the client. One could argue that this moved Erickson's work far into the direction of being "clean" compared with other hypnotic work at that time. However, it is this aspect of the work that is most challenging for Erickson's students to replicate or to teach.

In Grove's metaphor work, it may appear that the guide is creating a metaphor and engaging it without actually "relating" with it. The only things that actually relate are the metaphors among themselves, and even this is not always necessary. Because the guide uses clean language, the ego states of neither the client nor the guide are involved in a relational process. The guide is only receptive, there is no "I" that relates to the metaphor. There is no agenda either in process or in content; there are only heuristics that serve to create metaphors and then move them wherever it is that they want to go. Essentially, Grove's approach provides a basis for the guide to become a therapeutic agent of change without actually forming a relationship at all, not with the client, not with the unconscious of the client, and technically not even with the metaphor itself. In this respect, Grove's approach is most unique.

In its general goals and rationale, however, metaphor therapy is similar to the other techniques previously outlined, particularly to focusing. The differences lie primarily in approach. Each aims to elicit deep body-nested metaphoric images and to create a context in which they can heal. For example, the felt shifts that occur during the fourth movement of focussing may be considered to be equivalent to the phenomenology of healing within Grove's approach to transforming metaphors.

One could make the case, however, that Grove's approach is more complete or "teachable" than any of the other approaches inasmuch as clean language provides rule-governed heuristics for what to say in different clinical situations. The process is radically open-ended, whereas the therapist's job is quite structured. Clean language also provides a means to maintain the depth of the process while not contaminating it, whereas the others require the therapist to stay balanced within a process of mindful detachment. Focusing relies on the therapist to stay out of the way of the process by not imposing any theory, interpretations, or sympathy, as does Ericksonian therapy in being technique and theory free. Eidetic psychotherapy relies on the proper identification of an eidetic memory upon which to focus. Alternatively, the clean language used in metaphor therapy makes any imposition by the therapist impossible. Though clean language procedures may be difficult to acquire at first once one is comfortable with the approach, reintegration within the patient is more or less inevitable and automatic.

Grove's approach is similar to other symbolic transformation approaches that exist in the literature. But the basic distinction lies in the depth of Grove's approach. For example, Weaver (1973) and Greenleaf (1978) each have used the transformation of symbolic content in imagery to treat a variety of issues. In the case of pain, the general principle they follow is to enter the imagination and to make the vague experience of pain clearer through encapsulation within a metaphoric image. Once the image for each of the aspects of the pain experience emerges, each of those aspects then can be manipulated within the imagination toward the goal of transformation, which in turn probably will bring about a transformation of the original experience of pain to which the information is attached. Specifically, one asks questions about the size, shapes, colors, smells, weight, and other sensory aspects of the metaphor to enhance the clarity of the information attached to those painful experiences. Once the metaphor is clear, it may be transformed in a number of different ways depending on what transpires during the therapeutic process.

Bellissimo and Tunks (1984) describe a nearly identical approach for treating pain through imagery, except that they recommend a more specific focus on the affective information within the pain experience and maintaining a state of detached awareness or mindfulness. For example, their approach begins with travel inside the body as a molecule that eventually arrives at the sites of pain. Once patients have arrived at these sites, they are asked to describe the imagery therein and the feelings they evoke, with no intention toward modifying those feelings. Alternatively, patients can be asked to attend to a vague and holistic sense of the pain. Next, patients are instructed to zoom in on the specific location of the pain and to allow the sensations there to take on a symbolic representation as a metaphoric image. Finally, patients are instructed to focus their attention on the crux of that image and the feelings that are attached to that aspect.

For example, a hypothetical patient with a terminal illness could describe pain vaguely as a throbbing; this throbbing could be located within the ribcage. The throbbing could emerge symbolically as a frog sitting within the ribcage and causing the throbbing pain with each expansion of its lower lip (as it fills with air in preparation for a croak). In focusing on the crux of this image, the patient identifies a crown sitting on the frog's head and identifies feelings of regret, tragedy, and lost opportunity, because this frog never had the chance to become a prince.

Indeed, this simple process of engaging metaphors attached to experience is similar to all of the imagery approaches, from Jung's active imagination to Grove's metaphor therapy. The key differences lie in the specific "road maps" that are used by clinicians to guide and understand the process of transformation. Jungians rely on notions such as renewed balance that arises from contact with metaphoric imagery from the collective unconscious. Ericksonians try to unlock efficient healing potentials within the unique unconscious experiences of each client, whereas Ahsen, Gendlin, and Grove each propose that the transformation of metaphors allows for trapped aspects of the patient's ego to be matured and brought back into harmony with the dominant adult ego.

Our theoretical explanations from Chapter 3 would suggest that the body–mind reacts to overwhelming trauma by creating unresolved conflicts including rigid and disintegrated flows of biopsychosocial information. The transformation of symbolic images allows the flows of information within the body–mind to become reopened and reconnected. This leads to healing by renewing flexibility and integrity of conflicting body–mind systems. Each of these explanations has a significant degree of overlap. None is mutually exclusive. Therefore, each approach may potentially be helpful in guiding imagery work with patients in pain.

CHAPTER 8

Imagery for Children in Pain

When the dog bites,
When the bee stings,
When I'm feeling sad,
I simply remember my favorite things,
And then I don't feel so bad.

Julie Andrews
(in The Sound of Music)

Until the last few decades, the prevailing view was that children's pain was less intense and less enduring than adults' pain due to the immaturity of children's central nervous systems (Alvarez & Marcos, 1997; LeBaron & Zeltzer, 1996). This belief led many medical practitioners and researchers to conclude that children were less vulnerable than adults to trauma from intense procedural pain or to the development of chronic-pain syndromes. These mistaken beliefs about children in pain delayed research and the development of effective treatments.

Children's pain parallels that of adults in a number of respects. For example, children have the same beneficial response to regular steady dosing with pain medications (as opposed to dosing as needed; for a complete review of the use of analgesics in children see Shechter, Berde, & Yaster, 2002). Also, acute pain due to injury and disease is the most common source of pain, as is the case with adults, and the risks of developing a chronic pain syndrome increases when the traumatic aspects of pain extend into the psychosocial domains (McGrath & Hillier, 2002). Pain plays an adaptive role in children's day-to-day lives, even more so than in the lives of adults: The typical bumps and bruises of childhood produce healthy, adaptive expectations about pain as well as safer and more adaptive habits. Finally, children's pain experience and distress are greatly impacted by contextual factors, including levels of perceived control, the visibility of wounds, subjective meaning, social responses, and affective states.

On the other hand, children's experiences with pain differ from those of adults in a number of respects, and treatment should be modified and tailored to fit a child's unique developmental, family, and biophysical processes. Treating children's pain in the same way as adults' pain may lead to numerous iatrogenic complications. For example, children respond differently to medications, relate differently to treatment providers, understand language differently, and use different methods of coping than adults.

One beneficial difference between children and adults is that children appear to respond more strongly than adults to imagery techniques in pain management (for a comprehensive review of the effectiveness of imagery techniques for children's pain see Alvarez & Marcos, 1997). Furthermore, the limitations, potential side effects, and other risk factors associated with using high and prolonged doses of pain medications in children make guided imagery an ideal intervention for children in pain (Kemper, Cassileth, & Ferris, 1999). This is not to say that medications should never be used in managing children's pain. Rather, children are even more likely than adults to require additional procedures above and beyond medications (Schechter et al., 2002).

Common conditions underlying children's pain include headaches, stomachaches, inflammatory conditions (e.g., arthritis), sickle cell anemia, and cancer treatments. Nevertheless, children also suffer from pain conditions in which clear-cut medical causes are absent (e.g., "central" or "neuropathic" pain conditions). Children in pain without clear-cut medical causes may be subject to even greater misunderstanding and stigma than adults in pain, as parents, medical personnel, and other caregivers are more likely to attribute lying, exaggeration, or attention seeking to children with these types of pain syndromes.

As we know, disbelief or contempt for the sufferer is likely to aggravate pain, and this is even more common with children. Indeed, children's neurological, psychological, and social sensitivities may leave them more vulnerable to the negative impacts of trauma, self-criticism, helplessness, and social isolation that can accompany chronic-pain conditions (LeBaron & Zeltzer, 1996). As a result, these factors are more likely to fuel the development of chronic pain conditions in children than in adults, counter to most stereotypes of childhood resilience to pain. For example, cognitive-developmental factors make it more likely that children will jump to the conclusion that pain is a form of punishment, inflicted for some misbehavior.

Similarly, the experience of pain may be seriously detrimental to a child's growing sense of confidence and independence.

Within these developmental risks, however, there also lie potential benefits. Children's sensitivity to psychosocial factors allows them to experience an even stronger benefit from treatments directed at the motivational-affective and cognitive-evaluative dimensions of the pain experience. As a result, pediatric clinicians have been strongly urged to apply the biopsychosocial model and to individually tailor treatments to fit the needs of their child patients: "Our treatment emphasis should shift from an exclusive disease-centered focus to a more child-centered focus ... [because] complex and dynamic interactions occur among cognitive, behavioral, and emotional factors" (McGrath & Hillier, 2002, pp. 534–535). For example, in a typical child's case, biological factors impacting pain are likely to include the degree of tissue damage and the invasiveness of the medical procedure. Psychological factors include the child's emotional regulation abilities, beliefs about pain, and expectations for the procedure, and each of these will vary greatly among children. Social factors include family expectations, family relationship structures, staff behaviors, descriptions of procedures, and emotional states of care providers. The complexity created by the unique constellation of relationships among these factors creates the necessity for tailored assessment and treatment planning.

Developmental Factors

When using imagery with children, the therapist first must consider children's developmental levels, along with their medical and psychosocial needs, to determine which techniques, if any, would be most beneficial (Wall, 1991). Understanding a child's developmental levels and processes will also help the clinician to recognize the unique aspects of the child's pain experience, to track the child's response to any interventions, to shift the interventions accordingly, and to assist parents in "tuning in" to their child's pain and treatment experiences. An understanding of developmental factors, particularly cognitive and socioemotional development, will provide a window into the child's world, a window through which adults may understand the child's pain experience and provide the greatest degree of support, comfort, and relief.

Detailed descriptions of the broad areas of cognitive and socioemotional development (i.e., attachment theory) are found in the foundational works of Piaget (1952) and Bowlby (1982), respectively. Entire courses could be taught on various domains of child development, but our focus is on integrating these distinct domains in a manner that is most useful to clinicians in working with children in pain. Toward this goal of integration and practicality, three general propositions are useful in understanding how children develop.

First, in each of the domains of child development, development generally moves from simplicity to complexity. For example, compared with an older child or adolescent, a younger child in pain will have simpler mental representations of that pain (e.g., the pain is a big scary monster rather than a big scary monster with big teeth that lives in a cave and eats bones for lunch), less diversity in the various emotional reactions to the pain (e.g., fear rather than fear mixed with shame and anger), and fewer options for coping (e.g., seeking comfort exclusively from the primary attachment figure). As children develop, they branch out developmentally, and increasing complexity brings increased flexibility. New habits lead to new habits, which lead to refinements of those new habits across the various domains in an exponential progression of growth, just as trees and other natural systems grow from fragile simple structures to more complex, flexible, and robust structures.

A second general principle of child development is that with increasing complexity in the various domains comes increasing integrity among them. More specifically, when a child experiences some negative affect within a social situation, increased complexity in emotional expression will bring about more flexible problem solving and selection from among a wider range of options for solving the problem and relieving the negative affect. For example, a more mature child who is about to undergo a painful medical procedure may experience a combination of fear and anger, which may lead the child to conclude that the procedure has not been handled in an ideal manner, and to request more detailed clarification about the procedure and advanced warning of when the next procedure will occur. A younger child may simply throw a tantrum, pulling the parents into a difficult situation. Flexible affect leads to flexible cognition, which leads to flexible behavior and to flexible social relations. Developmental complexity spreads among the various domains, leading to greater exchange of information among these domains over time. Therefore, within the context of healthy developmental processes, complexity and integrity go hand in hand.

In regard to imagery techniques, younger children will require techniques that are more domain specific than older children or adults. For example, imagery directed at helping children understand the meaning of their pain (e.g., that it is not their fault) may be less likely to spread to the affective or behavioral arena. As a result, younger children may require a greater variety of relatively simple techniques, each addressing relaxation, beliefs, or coping in a more specific and isolated manner.

The end result of increasing levels of developmental complexity and integrity is improved self-regulation within the child, a third general aspect of child development. As children develop flexibility and connectivity within and across their developmental domains, they will tend to be better at responding to a variety of challenges. This process may be best exemplified by the proclivities of children in the "terrible 2s" or the "stresses and storms" of adolescence. These developmental periods are characterized by discontinuous shifts in children's ability to self-regulate. In 2-year-olds, this shift is driven by qualitative changes in the motoric, cognitive, and language domains, for example, which for the first time allow a child to reach levels of beginning competence in locomotion, concrete thought, and telegraphic speech, respectively. These abilities allow for a qualitative jump in the ability to respond to and adapt to the environment—to self-regulate.

In the adolescent, pushes and pulls for independence are largely driven by the emergence of formal abstract thought, along with the relatively flexible and abstract sense of personal identity that accompanies such thought processes. For the first time, teens are capable of abstract self-examination of values, for example, an advanced cognitive-emotional mode of self-regulation. This is not to say that 2-year-olds or teens no longer need parents and peers. Rather, jumps in self-regulation allow children to better choose and acquire the manner, type, and degree of assistance they require from important others. The simplest implication of increasing self-regulation abilities for the use of imagery techniques with children is that younger children will need higher levels of external support within the imagery process, particularly from their parents. At the same time, all children will have a strong need for participation and control within the treatment process.

With these three general principles in mind—complexity, integrity, and self-regulation—let us look more specifically at the application of imagery techniques at the various stages of development. Wall (1991) describes techniques that are appropriate depending on a child's level of cognitive development (Piaget, 1972). Inasmuch as cognitive development interacts with the affective, behavioral, and social domains, Piaget's four stages of cognitive development provide useful benchmarks with which to discuss imagery procedures for children.

During the *sensorimotor period* (birth to 2 years approximately), children's mental processes are extremely simple and rudimentary. Essentially, sensorimotor children's mental imagery is limited to information that is currently available to their senses. One could say that children in this age range are living "completely in the moment." Cognitive capacity during this period is limited to the ability to hold a few simple vague images in mind based largely on recent experience. They are not able to *operate* on those images, to animate them, or to cause them to interact at will. Because they are unable to focus their attention on internal images or to develop these images into a fantasy, techniques that require such activities are too difficult (LeBaron & Zeltzer, 1996). Furthermore, the various domains of development are not well integrated at this age, nor are children in this stage good at self-soothing. As a result, parents are the first option for delivering interventions for children under the age of 2, and intervention strategies are simple and domain specific. For example, parents may be instructed in the use of strategies that direct children's attention away from themselves rather than in encouraging them to have internal control of an event. Because their thinking is still very dependent on sensory information, the delivery of actual sensory input to offset the experience of pain is ideal. Distraction may be the most effective strategy if the child's imagery is overwhelmed by a focus on the pain-inducing stimulus (e.g., a needle), for example, by engaging the child in play with a favorite toy or stuffed animal. If the child is becoming overwhelmed by negative affect, gentle shushing or singing in the ear along with the comfort of rocking and patting might be best. If they require more predictability or control, it may be useful to count along with them during medical procedures of set duration (Wall, 1991). In any case, repetition and consistency in soothing methods are critical for younger children (LeBaron & Zeltzer), as the simple internal representations of children in this stage are built on the repetition of experience.

Children in the *preoperational period* (2 to 7 years) are able to willfully conjure images, but they are not yet able to hold and manipulate them well. Krueger (1987, p. 38) illustrates the progression of understanding that occurs during the period from ages 2 to 7:

> The younger child at a preoperational level of cognitive development would attempt to comprehend his or her illness essentially in terms of external cues, such as operating-room lights, surgery gowns, or medical instruments. An older child at a higher level of cognitive growth would think and imagine more about the internal parts of his or her body to understand the illness and pain.

Along with simple mental representations, the language comprehension of preoperational children is also quite limited, so parents and health-care professional must be cautious in their choice of words to describe pain or medical procedures. Krueger (1987) describes an apt example in which a 5-year-old girl thought that her knee was literally on fire when she heard a doctor use the word *inflamed*.

Along with the simplicity of thought at this stage, preoperational children are not able to effectively transform their images. For example, they may be able to imagine some good healing medicine and to imagine some illness within their bodies, yet they may be unable to put the two together within the imagination. Nevertheless, children at this stage are drawn toward using their imaginations, engaging in fantasy, making up stories, and taking on different roles. However, they typically require objects to fully engage in fantasy, such as dolls, costumes, or picture books. Such objects may be conceptualized as prosthetics, providing necessary assistance to the developing imagination: The child may wish to dress up as a superhero, to become immersed within a favorite story, or to interact with a figurine.

Along with this pull to fantasy, children in this age range also demonstrate qualitative increases in their ability to be self-determining compared with children in the sensorimotor stage. As a result, preoperational children benefit from simple but accurate information about medical procedures and the causes of pain, from rehearsal and from the provision of choices whenever possible. Along with a strong desire to practice self-regulation, children in this stage become increasingly integrated and thus may benefit from interventions that are more holistic and less domain specific. For children who are in the 2-year to 5-year age range, such techniques may include talking to the child through puppets, telling stories, using toys, engaging in a favorite activity, or projecting favorable images on a TV screen (Wall, 1991). Such stories and activities may be delivered prior to procedural pain as a form of practice or rehearsal, during the pain as a form of direct transformation of the experience, or after the procedure as a means of working through or processing the experience to mitigate levels of traumatic residue.

Regardless of the specific technique, parents ideally will continue to be the primary facilitators of imagery, along with the practitioner, and children should be encouraged to interact with the external sources of positive stimulation. In particular, children should be encouraged to become engaged with the affects, coping behaviors, and meaning of any pain-related narratives that are acted out with the puppets, picture books, or videos.

Around the age of 5 years, children transition from dependence on external objects for imagination to the development of the ability to fantasize without external props (LeBaron & Zeltzer, 1996). They begin to develop the ability to form internal representation of objects, allowing imagery techniques that are closer to the adult variety to be used effectively (Wall, 1991). The same general principles will apply with respect to parental involvement, self-determination, and immersion, yet prosthetics, such as puppets, may become unnecessary.

Children who have reached the concrete operations stage of development (ages 7 to 12 approximately) are better equipped to use techniques that employ visual imagery, because their ability to hold images in their minds increases dramatically during this time (LeBaron & Zeltzer, 1996; Wall, 1991). However, abstract themes continue to be difficult for children at this age and should be avoided in most cases. Though not quite abstract in thought, children in this age range begin to display increasing levels of flexibility within and integrity among their developmental domains. As a result, they should be encouraged to provide more input regarding who is present with them during times of pain and how much support they will receive from those people (LeBaron & Zeltzer, 1996). A child who already has been through several painful cancer treatments, for example, may unexpectedly choose to do the treatment without a parent in the room but may want to have the parent available on request. Furthermore, children in this age range are better able to explore the range of emotions associated with their pain, better able to examine their misattributions regarding pain (i.e., they will almost always think initially that the pain is their fault due to oversimplified conceptualizations of cause and effect (Alvarez & Marcos, 1997), and better able to seek out information if they are encouraged to ask questions about the pain and any medical procedures. With this increased level of cognitive, affective, behavioral, and social competence, children in this age range may become more collaborative in the treatment process.

Imagery techniques that have been suggested for this age group include sensory transformation techniques (e.g., "Imagine your arm is a branch of an oak tree"), travel to favorite places, listening to music, and engaging in favorite physical activities within imagery (Wall, 1991). Essentially, any of the "simple techniques" described in Chapter 5 may be applied to children in this age range, given modifications to the language levels and desired content of the child.

Individuals who reach the *formal operations stage* (adolescence into adulthood) often develop the capacity for abstract reasoning, which allows them to imagine and transform such abstract concepts as identity, love, and the abstract relational aspects of self with pain, such as conflict and control. It is important to bear in mind that not all adults reach this level of cognitive development, and such adults may prefer the simpler techniques in Chapter 5.

Because abstract thought is the highest level of cognitive development, imagery techniques traditionally used with adults can be used with adolescents who have reached this developmental phase, with a couple of caveats in mind. First, adults and teens will differ in their levels of abstract reasoning abilities, even if the same formal operations stage has been reached. Teens who have abstract thought are not necessarily well equipped to handle such thought. Thus, therapists should adjust any techniques to fit their clients' individual levels of cognitive development. Furthermore, even those with strong abstract-reasoning abilities tend to find it easier to manipulate concrete rather than abstract images. Thus, therapists should attempt to help clients identify concrete metaphors that may represent both painful and healing images. Finally, developmental regression is likely to be observed in patients who are in pain (LeBaron & Zeltzer, 1996). As such, individuals who generally have reached formal operations may fall back to a more concrete level of cognitive development when they are in pain, requiring simpler techniques.

The view of pain presented in Chapter 2 conceptualizes pain as a rigid biopsychosocial process that reduces the complexity, integrity, and self-regulatory mechanisms of the individual. In other words, pain by definition will lead to developmental regression, and this regression will involve more developmental domains in more chronic cases. This is hypothetically the reason chronic pain within individuals leads to greater levels of dependence, lower personal efficacy, simpler coping behaviors, rigid beliefs, and so on. As such, children and adults alike who generally may appear flexible, integrated, and autonomous will likely shift in the direction of rigidity, disintegration, and dependency when they are in pain. Therefore, the rule of thumb always should be to err on the side of using simpler rather than deeper techniques, particularly with children and adolescents.

The Family System

Because children are immature across the developmental domains, their experience of pain and responses to treatment are highly dependent on social rather than internal processes. In other words, children's reactions to pain will depend on reactions within the family system (McGrath & Hillier, 2002). On the broadest level, different families will have different understandings of and reactions to both pain and image therapies. As a result, imagery practitioners must assess not only the child's beliefs about pain and imagery but also the beliefs of important family members. For example, practitioners should ask the child's caregivers about other family members who have experienced pain, particularly chronic pain, as pain syndromes tend to run in families. Specifically, parents who are surviving with chronic pain tend to have children who respond to pain with "higher impairment and disability … increased pain complaints, reduced effective coping, and increased disability and impairment" (McGrath & Hillier, pp. 537–538). Treating the child as an individual without addressing the family's culture of pain to some extent probably will not be beneficial. Furthermore, simply involving the family in the treatment process may not be sufficient. Some families may require intervention that will modify the family's relationships to allow for the benefits of imagery with the child to be more fully realized.

One may wonder how family relationships can impact an individual child's pain and response to imagery. First, it is important once again to consider the child's development within the context of the family, which serves as a contextual niche in which the child's developmental processes are nested. Let us examine these processes in greater detail. Generally speaking, older children tend to experience pain in a more acute manner than younger children, while at the same time they are better able to man-age their pain (McGrath & Hillier, 2002). As such, the degree of final dis-comfort is equivalent in children across the age ranges. The younger the child, the less coherence there is in the child's affects and cognitive pro-cesses, two of the three processes underlying pain perception according to the gate-control theory (Melzack & Wall, 1965, 1996). The amorphous nature of their pain perceptions renders those perceptions more malleable. This malleability of experience helps to explain the relative effectiveness of imagery in treating children's pain. On the other hand, it is this same amorphous state that makes children less able to self-regulate compared with adults. Therefore, it is important to consider the ratio between chil-dren's malleability of experience and their coping abilities in determin-ing the likely reactions to pain and image therapies. Furthermore, because children rely on parents and other family members to provide them with ways of interpreting their experiences and coping, the child's experience of and responses to pain will depend on the family. It will make little sense to work toward transforming a child's pain experience through imagery if the family culture washes such transformations away. Nor will it make sense to shore up the child's coping processes if the parents' style of sup-porting the child is in conflict with such processes.

More specifically, a wide variety of caregiver reactions to pain and pain treatments will lead inadvertently to lower efficacy expectations in the child, increasing dependence, and to more negative interpretations of the pain. Thus, it is beneficial to provide information about children's pain and image therapy in an open-discussion format at the outset of treatment with as many family members present as possible. Through this process of information exchange, the clinician may gain a better understanding of the beliefs, expectations, and meanings surrounding the child's pain. These family reactions serve to inform the cognitive-evaluative dimension of the child's pain experience. Clinicians should attend to the affective reac-tions and other impacts on the family as a whole, which serve to inform the child's motivational-affective dimension of pain. At the same time, any family relational processes that serve to self-regulate these dimensions and assist the child in coping should be assessed.

Now that we have explored in detail the ways the family system feeds into a child's experience of and reactions to pain, let us examine what occurs at the broader level of the family as they react to a child in pain. The term *family systems* is commonly used in various treatment settings involving children; however, the term is rarely defined in any clear or empirically oriented manner. Consequently, there are a great number of purportedly unique approaches to working with a family system, each having its own set of techniques, rationales, and supporters within the therapeutic communities. At the same time, few of these approaches are empirically testable at a level deeper than simple clinical outcomes, and for the most part the various approaches appear to be equivalent in this respect (Sprenkle & Blow, 2004).

For the sake of the current discussion, we apply a more integrative and empirically oriented framework known as the *Five-R model* (see Pincus, 2001; Pincus & Guastello, 2005; Pincus, Fox, Perez, Turner, & McGee, 2008, for a complete description and empirical support of the model). The Five-R model defines the family system as a self-organizing information processing system. Consider the information flows within a family discussion. From such discussions, information exchanges lead to the emergence of more global aspects of family relationships (i.e., shared affects, expectations, meaning). In this manner, family systems are expected to display self-similar dynamics to a child's self-organizing biopsychological information processing systems (see Chapter 3). In many respects, one would expect the information processing dynamics within the child to be a reflection of the family dynamics. As pointed out in Chapter 3, such dynamics involve the process of self-organization, by which global order emerges from the interaction of component parts within the system (i.e., mind emerges from information flows among neurons), which then serves to feed back down to constrain these component parts (i.e., mental processes serving to regulate subsequent neuronal interaction patterns).

When conceptualized as self-organizing and thus self-regulating information processors, family conversation patterns, patterns of family relationships, and broader culture within each family take on a deeper and more specific meaning. At the same time, one can make direct predictions about the ways the family system will impact the child; for example, levels of flexibility and integrity in the flows of information about the child's pain within the family system is associated with levels of flexibility and integrity within the flows of information in the imagery of the child.

The Five-R model suggests that one can intervene at five different levels of information flow within the family:

1. *Rules* directly govern the flows of information (e.g., who may speak to whom, when, and about what).
2. *Roles* are the collection of rules carried by any particular individual (e.g., child versus parent roles).
3. *Relationships* are the various constellations of role configurations (e.g., parent–child relationship, spousal relationship).
4. *Realities* are the broad coherent patterns of information flow within the family system that manifest as family narratives or cultures.
5. The family's *response patterns* are the observable sequences of information exchange among members during discussions.

Although one can intervene within any of these nested and overlapping aspects of the family system, clinicians may wish to watch for particular relational dynamics that may signal more pressing relational concerns. Such relationship dynamics would warrant a referral to more formal family intervention beyond the issue of pain management for the child. These relational processes focus around control, closeness, and conflict (Pincus & Guastello, 2005; Pincus et al., 2008). Control, closeness, and conflict processes within healthy family systems tend to involve reasonable levels of balance. For example, dysfunction in the self-regulation of information exchange occurs in families engaged in the following:

1. Levels of interpersonal control are either too high (e.g., authoritarian parents) or too low (e.g., permissive parents; see Baumrind, 1983).
2. Levels of closeness are either too high (e.g., enmeshment) or too low (e.g., disengagement; see Pincus, 2001).
3. Levels of conflict are either too high (volatility) or too low (i.e., avoidance; see Pincus & Guastello, 2005).

Generally speaking, the healthiest families are those balanced with respect to flexibility and structural integrity. These families balance control to allow for democratic interactions. They balance intimacy and distance. And they exhibit moderate levels of conflict through which they can adapt and grow. Finally, the relational processes surrounding the child generally should move in the direction of increasing flexibility in control strategies, closeness or support of the child, and conflict-management strategies as the child matures. This increasing flexibility in family–child relations allows for the increasing psychosocial regulation abilities growing within the child. Families that are highly controlling or highly enmeshed in relation to the child's developmental needs are more likely to have high levels of conflict and rigidity in their interaction patterns and children from such families would be less able to self-regulate. Such family dynamics would signal the need for a full course of family therapy beyond any imagery interventions for pain. Such family interventions would ideally focus on assisting the family in resolving conflicts, allowing for the emergence of more flexible exchanges of information and more flexible control and closeness within the family relations.

However, we must not forget the influence of the child on the family. Self-organization works in both directions, from the top down and also from the bottom up across scales. Therefore, one would expect in some cases that pain dynamics *within* the child could lead to the emergence of rigid interaction processes *among* family members. For example, a child in pain may lead parents to provide higher levels of closeness with that child in the form of worry, concern, nurturance, and support. Similarly, parents may respond to this child with stricter control methods or rules that are designed to keep this child safe as well as to relieve the parent's concerns about the child's health and comfort. Unfortunately, if these accommodations are taken too far or for too long a period of time, they may serve to increase the intensity and chronicity of the child's pain. For example, such rigid relational shifts may interfere with the child's growing sense of autonomy and confidence with respect to pain.

In milder situations, involving the parents in the treatment process as co-therapists may provide them with a more effective channel through which to convey their support of the child and gain a feeling of control. Most parents who are given knowledge of pain and the processes by which imagery works are able to assist the child in the use of imagery when appropriate, to prompt the child toward its use, or to feel more comfortable with the child engaging in self-regulation independently. Involvement in the use of imagery for pain may allow the parent to dispense with oversupport or overcontrol in response to the child's pain and to resolve pain-related family conflicts.

Effective Approaches to Treatment

It is important to examine some imagery treatment outcome studies in detail because such analysis leads to greater clarity concerning what techniques will tend to work for which children, how well they will work, and how they work. Furthermore, gold standard treatments from such studies represent good models for clinicians to follow in treating various types of pain.

Abdominal Pain

Functional abdominal pain is defined as abdominal discomfort lacking in clear-cut physiological causal mechanisms. It is the most common chronic pain condition in children, impacting between 10% and 20% of school-aged children at some point in time (Oster, 1972) and four of every five pediatric patients seen in outpatient visits for complaints of pain (Anbar, 2001).

Anbar (2001) describes both positive and negative outcomes from a general imagery treatment protocol used in several adolescent patients seen in an outpatient setting for abdominal pain. The approach involves a single session of self-hypnosis instruction involving five distinct steps. Step 1 involves an induction and engagement of the teen in favorite-place imagery, using language to enhance each of the five dominant senses. Step 2 is training in progressive muscle relaxation carried out within the imagination of the adolescent's favorite place. Step 3 involves the selection by the patient of a key word that may be used in the future during times of abdominal pain to trigger the reemergence of both the favorite place and the muscle relaxation practiced therein. Step 4 involves conjuring up some degree of abdominal pain through suggestive imagery (e.g., a focus on the abdomen and the specific sensations felt by the teen patient), followed by practice in using the key word for relaxation. The session concludes with Step 5, clinician's praise and instructions for daily practice over the next several weeks.

Anbar (2001) describes the cases of two 14-year-old patients in detail: One involves a near complete resolution of the abdominal pains within a 3-week period, and in another the imagery had no apparent impact, possibly due to a lack of follow-through in post session practice. Though it is difficult to draw firm and general conclusions from case studies, these results suggests that even a brief and simple imagery procedure aimed at cued relaxation potentially can be effective for chronic and recurrent pain in adolescents. Furthermore, the lack of response in the adolescent who did not follow through highlights the need to fully engage adolescents in the treatment process.

A more recent and comprehensive study of abdominal pain in children examined the response to imagery treatment of 10 children ranging in age from 5 to 18 years (Ball, Shapiro, Monheim, & Weydert, 2003). All of the children were referred due to recurrent and chronic treatment-resistant abdominal pain. The imagery intervention consisted of four weekly sessions, each lasting approximately 50 minutes. The imagery procedure involved symbolic transformation: The creative content was child selected, but the process was similar across all of the children. Following a relaxation induction, the children were guided to imagine their pain as some object. Engagement in imagery was enhanced by querying each of the five dominant senses in relation to this pain object. Next, the children were guided to imagine a pain destroyer, specifically tailored to work against their particular pain object, and this destroyer was clarified and engaged using activation of the five senses. Finally, the pain destroyer was allowed to do its job, engaging the pain object in a process of total annihilation.

The most positive benefit observed was an average decrease of 67% in pain frequency 1 month after treatment was completed, from an average of 20 episodes to 6.5 per month. The intensity of those remaining flare-ups was unchanged. In regard to trajectories for improvement, 7 of the 10 children had clinically significant improvements immediately after the 4 weeks of treatment, and 2 additional children reached levels of significance at the 1-month follow-up. This posttreatment boost was part of a general *sleeper effect* found within the study: The positive responders continued to improve during the month following active treatment. In considering this rather robust and enduring treatment effect, one should also consider the fact that the average levels of response were dampened by a single nonresponding child who accounted for most of the posttreatment flare-ups.

It may be particularly interesting for clinicians to consider more closely the observed sleeper effect in this study. This effect suggests that some aspect of this rather brief, simple, and child-focused imagery intervention was *swallowed up* by the child and family systems, setting their self-regulating dynamics on a new trajectory that continued to shift beyond the active phase of treatment. In addition, the results of this study suggest that clinicians may expect rather dramatic and positive results from symbolic transformation imagery in children, even with severe and treatment resistant cases of abdominal pain.

Headaches

Another common source of childhood pain is headaches, which affect children in a similar manner and with similar frequency as adults. Tourigny-Dewhurst (1993) furnished a detailed case study describing the use of imagery in an 8-year-old African American girl who began suffering frequent and intense headaches shortly after being placed in a gifted and talented education (GATE) program at her school. The case conceptualization included a formal *Diagnostic and Statistical Manual of Mental Disorders,* 4th ed. (*DSM-IV*) diagnosis of generalized anxiety disorder (APA, 1994); the worries largely focused on school performance were believed to be driving the headaches. At the outset of treatment, the child was experiencing high intensity headaches an average of 4 to 5 hours per day.

The treatment entailed five weekly sessions and one posttreatment follow-up session. The imagery techniques used were of the behavioral variety. They involved the child's mother as a cofacilitator, and the general procedure was practiced via tape recording twice daily between sessions. In the first week, progressive muscle relaxation was taught along with some body-focused imagery designed to identify the muscle tension triggers of headaches. This was intended to provide the child with increased body awareness and the ability to foresee the onset of a headache so that she could employ her imagery as a preventative measure.

Next, sequences of imaginary control strategies were taught: (1) thought stopping; (2) relaxation imagery; and (3) covert self-reinforcement. Thought stopping was taught through graduated guidance. First the therapist modeled for the child by yelling "stop!" at the child, while she was engaged in purposeful worry out loud. Next, the child shouted a loud "stop!" at herself while engaged in worry. Finally, the "stop!" was made covert, carried out within the child's imagination. In the third week of treatment, a new tape was made in session. This tape contained the same thought-stopping procedure followed by a simple relaxation imagery procedure. In the fourth week, the covert self-reinforcement was added. The child engaged in the same cued awareness of muscle tension signaling anxiety, thought stopping, relaxation, and finally an imaginary scene in which she was involved in a favorite activity without headache pain.

Prior to this final self-reinforcement session, the headaches had already decreased from the baseline of 4 to 5 hours per day of high-intensity headaches to 2 times per week for 1 to 2 hours of low-intensity headaches. At the final termination session, the mother and daughter reported no headaches during the past week. Once again, this study illustrates the strong effects that simple and brief imagery procedures can have in children, even those with rather severe levels of pain. A critical component of this treatment probably was the engagement of the mother in the treatment process, particularly since this child was only 8 years old. Also it was helpful that this child was allowed to teach her class at school some of the relaxation techniques she had learned. This role probably enhanced her feeling of comfort and competence with her peers, a key developmental concern for school-aged children. Finally, this case illustrates the importance of helping headache sufferers who also have significant levels of anxiety and tension to identify their tension headache triggers and to employ imagery as a preventative strategy. Knowing the anxiety-tension triggers of headaches allows the sufferer to experience headaches as more predictable and controllable and allows imagery to be engaged as a self-corrective measure.

Migraine headaches are another common cause of pain in children, occurring in approximately 7% of the child and adolescent population (Olness, Hall, Rozniecki, Schmidt, & Theoharides, 1999). For children with migraine headaches, *self-regulation* treatments, including imagery, have been found to be both more effective and also safer than the use of pharmacological agents (Duckro & Cantwell-Simmonds, 1989). The physiological mechanism through which imagery and other self-regulation treatments are assumed to work in migraines is the activity of mast cells, which regulate vasoconstriction and dilation, specifically blood flows in response to stress. Because mast cells had been implicated in adult migraines and in the effectiveness of imagery in adult treatment, Olness et al. (1999) set out to examine their potential role in mediating the effectiveness of imagery in children with migraine headaches.

Olness et al. (1999) randomly assigned 27 children between the ages of 5 and 12 (average age 10) with chronic and persistent migraine headaches (controlling for sex across groups) to either a 3-week active phase relaxation-imagery treatment condition (followed by 9 weeks of self-guided practice) or to a 12-week treatment-as-usual control condition. The first sessions focused on teaching the children progressive muscle relaxation, followed by engagement in a pleasant imagery scenario chosen by the child. Examples of such scenarios included a skiing trip and playing with animals such as koala bears and unicorns. A key word was selected from these enjoyable scenarios for the purpose of cued recall. These sessions were taped, and parents were engaged to facilitate twice daily, 10-minute practice sessions between office visits. In session 2, the relaxation-imagery skills were reviewed, and biofeedback was added to provide evidence to the children and parents that the imagery skills they had been practicing were indeed leading to significant decreases in bodily stress. Next, the children were guided through a sensory-transformation technique that they selected from a menu of different options (e.g., dissociation from the pain, the use of a "magic" analgesic glove, switching the pain off). Again, the procedure was taped, and twice daily practice was assigned. Session 3 involved review of the skills in the first two sessions and preparation for daily practice over the next 9 weeks. Children were asked to keep a daily log to track improvements and compliance.

The treatment group included 10 children who responded very well and 4 children who did not respond at all. At the 12- and 24-week follow-ups, the most significant benefit was observed in headache frequency for the responders, which had dropped from approximately five times per week to less than once per month at the end of the 12 weeks, and these gains continued through the 24-week follow-up. Furthermore, 8 of these 10 responders showed reduction in urine tryptase levels, a metabolite associated with mast cell activity. The 4 nonresponders and 13 children in the control condition showed no change in their migraine frequency or intensities and no differences in tryptase levels. Overall, these results suggest that brief, self-guided imagery techniques may be used with remarkable success for a majority of children with migraine headaches and that imagery typically serves to change the regulation of blood flow through the activity of mast cells.

Procedural Pain

A number of studies have examined the effectiveness of imagery to manage children's responses to painful medical procedures. For example, Kuttner, Bowman, and Teasdale (1988) compared ego-affirming fantasy imagery, concrete distraction, and a control condition in the pain responses of children (ages 3 to 10) undergoing bone marrow treatments for leukemia. The fantasy imagery involved storytelling, in which the child was engaged in creating an *ego-affirming* fantasy, for example, having superpowers like flying or carrying out acts of heroism. The distraction technique involved simple training in maintaining a focus on an external (i.e., a point in the room) or internal object (i.e., an imagined object) unrelated to the pain.

Overall, each simple imagery condition led to significant improvements over the treatment-as-usual control condition in reducing both pain and anxiety in response to treatment. There was, however, an interesting differentiation in the responses of older children compared with younger ones. The younger children (3- to 7-year-olds) as a group responded in a very strong and positive manner to absorption within the ego-affirming fantasy stories but not to distraction, whereas the older children (7 to 10) had the opposite response. The distress ratings for the younger group on a standardized measure (with 20 to 30 being the severe range) dropped from a mean of 15 to a mean of 7 after a single intervention. For the older children, the average decrease was from 10 to 7.5 on the same scale. Similar improvements were observed over time in both pain intensity ratings and procedure-related anxiety. These results suggest that younger children more easily than older ones engage in playful fantasy-related imagery and that older children may require more reality-bound procedures.

Lambert (1996) carried out a controlled study of hypnotic imagery on the postoperative pain, anxiety, and length of hospital stay in 7- to 19-year-olds (average age was 13) admitted for various routine surgeries (e.g., tonsillectomy). The treatment condition involved a single imagery session (under 30 minutes in length) carried out 1 week prior to surgery. The imagery sessions were standardized for process but not for specific content; the session began with immersion of the child within a relaxing activity or place, then the operative and postoperative procedure was rehearsed, and then suggestions for a positive postoperative course involving only low levels of pain were given. The children were instructed to rehearse their imagery prior to surgery, and all but one did so at least once. Children assigned to the control condition were given equal time to discuss the upcoming surgery in an open and nondirective manner.

The most clinically significant results were observed in lengths of hospital stay: 5 days versus 5.8 days on average for the imagery and control groups, respectively, and in postoperative anxiety levels, which increased for the control group and decreased for the imagery group. Though the same amount of medication was used across the groups, the reported levels of pain showed a small (but statistically significant) improvement for the imagery group compared with the control group (3.9 vs. 4.4 out of 10, respectively). Similar to findings in research with adults, the differences across groups may have been attenuated to a degree by the spontaneous use of imagery by each of the children in the control condition. The most frequent use of spontaneous imagery was to manage pain at night for sleep, which was used by 20 of the 26 children in the study, regardless of their group assignment. It seems that imagery is a natural and spontaneous response to pain in children just as it is in adults.

Huth, Broome, and Good (2004) found similar results in a subsequent controlled study on a similar population of 7- to 12-year-old children undergoing tonsillectomies surgeries. The imagery procedure was simple and standardized, consisting of a 30-minute audiotape containing a relaxation induction followed by a trip to a park or other favorite place. The audiotape was used 1 week prior to surgery, just after surgery, and 1 day after hospital discharge. Huth et al. (2004) used more sophisticated statistical techniques than prior studies to control for extemporaneous factors (e.g., levels of medication use) in testing the impacts of imagery on standardized measures of pain intensity, pain-related negative affect, and anxiety. All three of these measures showed a significantly larger decrease in the imagery group compared with a clinical attention placebo condition. The relative benefits of imagery were attenuated somewhat by the fact that all of the children were taking pain medications postsurgery and by the fact that pain levels were low and temporary in the control group. Still, the imagery group displayed 28.3% less pain, 10.5% less anxiety, and 8.5% less negative affect postsurgery compared with the clinical attention control condition.

Techniques

A few examples of specific guided imagery techniques for children's pain may serve as prototypes for clinicians to borrow from across different treatment contexts. The following examples are modified examples of scripts provided by Klein (2001). Each approach may be modified in any number of ways, depending on factors including the age of the child, the type of pain, the treatment context, and levels of family involvement.

The Paintbrush

Most children have had numerous positive experiences with painting by the time they are entering middle childhood. These positive and relaxing common experiences make using a paintbrush to "paint away" pain sensations an ideal technique. Following a standard progressive muscle relaxation induction, the following is a portion of a script involving the paintbrush:

> In your imagination, you can see all of your favorite colors, like a rainbow or the colors in a set of paints. Pick your favorite color from all of these good colors. Tell me, which color is it? Now picture a room filled with buckets of all of these different colors of paint. Walk up to the bucket that holds your favorite color. And look over on the other side of the room. You will see there a table with a nice paint brush. Just the right size, and with long soft bristles for brushing on your paint.
>
> Dip your brush into bucket of paint. Tap the extra paint off into the bucket. We are going to do some magical painting with this paint. First pick a little patch of your skin where you have no pain; maybe on your arm or on your leg. Now take the brush and paint a little spot on that part of you. Spread the paint slowly and smoothly; back and forth, back and forth. And as you paint that spot, feel the goodness of that magic paint. It brings comfort and nice feelings to that spot.

That spot that is painted is the most relaxed it can be [an alternate procedure here is to brush numbness into the site]. How does it feel to you? The paint feels good on your skin [an optional approach here is to give the child an actual paintbrush or bit of fabric to brush against the skin]. This magic paint not only feels good on your skin. This magic paint can brush away pain.

Dip your paint into the bucket again, and tap away the extra paint. And now, touch the brush against the part of you that hurts. Feel the paint sink into your skin, making your feel calm and relieved. Wherever the brush touches will start to feel better, little by little. Breathe in and out along with your brushing, back and forth, in and out, slowly, calmly. And with each brush feel the magic paint doing its work.

Imagine that you are painting this magic colorful medicine over any part of your body that hurts. As those parts become covered with that beautiful color, they become calmer and feel better. Tell me what it feels like when the paint sinks in? Is it warm or cold? Is it slow, or fast? How is it working? Where else do you want to paint?

Now feel the paint sink deeper, filling your body with that beautiful color. With each breath in, the paint spreads. See it fill your whole body. It fills you up. Every tiny part. And as it does, the comfort and relaxation spreads too.

You can use your magic paint and brush any time you want. Just close your eyes and paint any part of you that hurts. Give the paint time to sink in, and let it spread all over. They are always there in your imagination. They will always be there for you when you need them.

The Dolphin

Children are more preoccupied with animals than adults in their day-to-day lives and also in their dreams and imaginations (Van de Castle, 1983, 1994). This makes the use of positive and relaxing images of animal friends within the imagination an ideal scenario for children's pain relief. The following is a modified script used by Klein (2001) based on an encounter with a dolphin:

In your mind, imagine yourself standing on a beautiful beach. Hear the gentle waves washing up on the shore. Hear the birds flying over your head, and the gentle breeze, and the waves as they break and splash. Smell the salt, and the sand, and feel the warm air on your skin. The sky is thick with big, white, puffy clouds, gently floating by. This is the most beautiful beach you have ever seen.

Look out over the ocean. Look deep into the water, stretching out forever. Notice all of the colors of the sea—the dark blues, light blues, the greens, and even some black and some yellow, as the sun shimmers on the far off waves. And as you look deeper and deeper into the water, the ocean stops. The waves slow and become still. Everything is calm and still.

You walk out into the still ocean water, wading in to your ankles. Feel the perfect temperature of the water. Not too cold, not too warm, just right for you. Wade out deeper until your legs are in the still water, now your belly button, up to your chest and then dive under. And as you swim under this beautiful magic ocean, you find that you can breathe under water. It is like you are a mermaid or merman. It is like the ocean is your home. And you are able to glide along under and on top of the water like never before, as if you were a dolphin, at home in the sea. Your swimming further and further into the water calms you. Enjoy this feeling of peace and calm.

And as you do, look to your side. It is a dolphin that has come to swim with you. You look into the dolphin's eye and he calms you. It is like he knows you, and at once you are like best friends. Notice how easily he swims along with you, his smooth grey skin, and strong dolphin's tail. Feel his friendship, his calm, and his strength as you swim together in the beautiful sea.

The dolphin invites you to his home, beneath the waves. And you are surprised that you can understand what the dolphin is saying. And the dolphin can understand you too. The dolphin asks you if anything hurts. You feel comfortable, that this is your friend, and that the dolphin cares for you. You tell the dolphin that you wish you could feel even more comfortable.

Then the dolphin swims closer to you and touches you with a flipper. The dolphin is pointing down, down to a place on the sea floor where there is no pain. You follow the dolphin down, deeper and deeper. The light from the sky above grows dim, as you see the sea floor. There is a spot on the sand on the bottom of the sea. The dolphin brings you to this place to rest. You feel the water all around you and breath in deep. And as you breathe, you feel the weight of the ocean fill your body. With each breath, your body grows heavier and heavier; you are like heavy anchor resting on the ocean bottom. And with each breath, your body feels comfortable, more and more calm and comfortable.

The dolphin tells you that this is your place to rest. Stay there and rest a while. Feel the warmth of the sea, the dull sounds of the deep ocean, and look around you to see gentle fish swimming by .... Enjoy this calm and magic place....

And when you are ready, the dolphin comes to lead you home. Hold the dolphins fin, as it pulls you along up, up toward the surface of the water. You are too calm and relaxed to swim back to the beach, so the dolphin will give you a ride. Feel the dolphin's strength underneath you, as it swims in toward the beach, where you started. See the ripples of the water next to you, as the dolphin speeds along. And feel how good your body feels, how heavy and relaxed, as you glide along through the warm ocean waves.

When you arrive at the beach, the dolphin leaves you on the sand. It looks back to say goodbye. It tells you that it will come for you, whenever you need to return to your place beneath the sea. Your magic underwater place of calm and of comfort.

Candles

Birthdays are well known to almost all children, and blowing out the candles is central to birthday party scripts, holding particular significance and joy. Therefore, blowing out candles is an ideal metaphor for pain relief in children of all ages as in the following script adapted from Klein (2001):

In your mind, see a big beautiful cake. This cake has been made just for you. It is sitting in front of you on a big table. It is your perfect cake. Picture its shape. Is it round or is it a rectangle? Is it a single sheet or is it two layers? What flavor is the cake? What color is the frosting? Describe this perfect cake to me.

It is your cake. So you may do what you want. The first thing you want to do is taste it. Reach out with your finger. You can't wait. And dip your finger into the frosting. Tell me, how does it taste? It is sweet, yes? It is the most delicious frosting you have ever imagined.

Now you notice that there are candles on top of the cake. It is not your birthday, but the candles have been lit for you. Just like your birthday, you are going to blow these candles out. But in this story, these are magic candles. And you will need to blow them out one at a time. This will take more than just one big blow, more than one big breath. You will blow these candles out each with one strong short puff of air. Show me how you can do this once, for practice. Good, that's it, just one big puff, all at once, right at a single candle.

Each of these candles is magic. When you blow them out, you blow away your pain. Try just one to see. How many candles are on the cake? Okay, now pick just one candle to blow out. As you watch it go out you will feel your pain go out too one candle at a time. Once all of the candles go out, you will feel as comfortable and relieved as you can possibly be. Ready? Aim your lips right at this one candle and: Blow! Good. Feel your pain go out a little bit as the flame of this one candle is gone. Now go to the next candle and: Blow! Remember, short strong puffs of air. As each candle goes out, any discomfort or scary feelings go out with them. Now let's blow out the rest, one by one .... As each candle goes out, see the tiny bit of smoke go up from the candle. As it floats up, each bad feeling that you have floats away with it. With each blow you feel more calm, relaxed and comfortable. And as the last candle goes out, all you have is this beautiful cake. Your body is relaxed from your head down to your toes. You are calm and as happy as can be.

General Guidelines

Beyond providing justification for the use of imagery in treating children's pain, clinical effectiveness studies such as those just reviewed can be of use to individual clinicians in routine practice settings. In the most general sense, these results suggest that we may use imagery techniques with great confidence with children in pain. Rather than viewing the use of a child's imagination in pain treatment as an alternative treatment, the available evidence supports the use of imagery as a standard first-line intervention for children. In addition to the direct effectiveness of imagery on pain frequency and intensity, imagery appears to work on the associated features of pain as well, such as negative affect and anxiety. Similarly, the results are positive with respect to physiological changes, such as reduced mast cell activity, lowered levels of physiological arousal, and reduced postoperative recovery times. The strong and broad effectiveness of imagery in treating children's pain warrants great confidence from imagery practitioners in children's medical settings.

With respect to age groups, the results suggest that imagery works as well for toddlers as for older children and perhaps even better in certain instances. Imagery is effective for a range of pain types and severity. Finally, despite the specific factors involved effective procedures tend to be simple and easy to deliver—in some cases even through the use of standardized audiotapes.

Nevertheless, the results provided herein should inform realistic expectations as with any medical treatment. Imagery does not always work, and it typically does not work in a perfect or complete manner. Generally, 10% to 30% of children are nonresponders to imagery for pain. Until research addresses the specific reasons for nonresponse, the responsibility will remain with clinicians to monitor responses to treatment and to take corrective action toward better outcomes in these cases.

In conclusion, we offer three suggestions to tie together the information presented within this chapter.

Suggestion 1: Keep It Simple.

Imagery for children typically looks more like storytelling than anything else. Indeed, the best procedures, particularly for younger children, may typically involve watching cartoons, reading books, or using dolls in a concrete manner providing for simpler engagement of the child's creative imagination (Syrjala & Abrams, 2002). The line between fantasy and reality is more blurred in younger children, so they may become immersed in healing fantasy more readily. By keeping it simple, the clinician can follow along with the child's own inherent imagination abilities and reduce the chances of interfering with them.

Suggestion 2: Provide Options.

Children have a developmental drive to become mature and become autonomous. In fact, when this drive is healthy and engaged, children often will seek to overreach their actual abilities (e.g., the terrible 2s). Feeling helpless, small, and powerless makes pain worse for everyone, particularly for children, inasmuch as these feelings work against this natural developmental drive. Therefore, consider the child to be an active member of the treatment team (McGrath & Hillier, 2002), along with parents or other important caregivers. In this manner, the child will experience a level of control and respect. In addition, this interpersonal process conveyed by the clinician will serve to counteract dysfunctional supports that may have evolved within the family system, modeling for parents the ability to provide support that is balanced and in tune with the child's own abilities at self-regulation, sense of competence, and strength.

Suggestion 3: Don't Just Talk, Play!

Adults respond well to words, creating imagery, and working through biopsychosocial conflicts in the context of conversations or conventional guidance through imagery. Children, on the other hand, respond far better within the context of play. Again, children have a far looser grip on the "real" world compared with adults. As a result, they require little induction to become engaged in creative imagination. They are already there, in their imaginations, waiting for you to catch up (LeBaron & Zeltzer, 1996).

For those clinicians who are more mature and have forgotten how play works, it may be helpful to point out the parallels between play and adult conversation. Both play and adult conversation involves listening, leading, and following. If the child suggests some fantasy in your presence, go along with this fantasy, just as you would if an adult patient introduced some idea to you. For example, if a child says, "This looks like a spaceship," consider this as an invitation to engage in imagery involving space travel. Just as you would not deny the assertion of an adult in polite company, do not deny any imaginary suggestions made within the context of play with a child. Instead, elaborate on such suggestions, saying, "It could be a spaceship if you like. Would you like to take a trip somewhere?" Even more so than with adults, it is important to follow the child's lead during imagination and not to ruin the spirit of free play toward which children are so naturally inclined.

But good play needs to be consistent in a number of respects. For example, children who have enjoyed an imaginary game or imagery scenario at a prior session probably will want to repeat it at a subsequent session. Because their memories are more rudimentary than those of adults, children require more repetition to learn. This is why they require so much routine and consistency in their daily lives and why, for example, they can tolerate watching the same movie over and over again while an adult is driven mad. Treatment settings should be as consistent as possible in terms of procedures, appointment time, and personnel (McGrath & Hillier, 2002). Just as you would not carry on an intimate conversation with a stranger, a child may not feel comfortable resuming an imaginative play scenario with an unfamiliar clinician, with a different caregiver, or within a different setting.

CHAPTER 9

The Gift of Pain and Suffering

Your pain is the breaking of the shell that encloses your
  understanding.
Even as the stone of the fruit must break, that its heart
may stand in the sun, so must you know pain.
And could you keep your heart in wonder at the daily
miracles of your life, your pain would not seem less wondrous
than your joy;
And you would accept the seasons of your heart, even
 as you have always accepted the seasons that pass over your
  fields....
Much of your pain is self-chosen.
It is the bitter potion by which the physician within you heals
  your sick self.
Therefore trust the physician, and drink his remedy in silence
  and tranquility:
For his hand, though heavy and hard, is guided by the tender
  hand of the Unseen,
And the cup he brings, though it burn your lips, has been
  fashioned of the clay
which the Potter has moistened with His own sacred tears.

Gibran
(1966, pp. 52–53)

Furst (2003) compares the act of living to "licking honey off a thorn." In the
process a few pricks from the thorns of life are unavoidable. Pleasure and

pain, joy and suffering are both an integral part of being human. Gibran's (1966, p. 29) metaphor sums up our condition: "The selfsame well from which your laughter rises was oftentimes filled with your tears." Yet we regard pain as the darkest side of life and invest considerable energy in its avoidance. Alleviating pain is at the heart of the healing professions, and the preceding chapters have discussed a plethora of techniques that have been successfully employed to this end.

In this closing chapter, we propose to turn away from scientific viewpoints and technical approaches and to look instead at pain and suffering from more philosophical and spiritual perspectives. We focus especially on unrelenting physical pain and suffering that flow from significant losses, injuries that gradually invade all aspects of life: mind, body, and spirit. We focus on injuries that threaten to shatter our very sense of identity as human beings and to forever change our path through life.

Each of the world's spiritual traditions views such experiences as blessings in disguise. These painful challenges threaten our survival but also offer unusual opportunities for growth and transformation. As Brazier (1995, p. 13) puts it, "By working with our grit, we become a 'true pearl.'" Similarly, the English poet William Wordsworth commented on the delicate connection between loss and rejuvenation: "So once it would have been-'tis so no more; I have submitted to a new control: A power is gone, which nothing can restore; A deep distress hath humanized my soul" (Palgrave, 1975, p. 332). It is interesting to note that in the Chinese language, the symbol used for disease and suffering also represents opportunity. From the Eastern perspective, pain is an integral part of life and the catalyst for growth (Sheikh & Sheikh, 2007).

Perhaps it is productive to reconsider the prevailing view of pain; maybe pain is not an enemy to be held at bay, to be removed or avoided at all costs, but rather an inevitable and natural force that prompts growth. This perspective finds support in science as well: Complex systems adapt in response to stresses over time. Such open systems break down and reemerge in response to challenge. And new growth brings renewed flexibility, integrity, and strength to withstand the next challenge. A metaphor for human growth through pain can be found in the plant world: The pruning of branches, particularly before the winter thaw, enhances the strength and complexity of the new growth. Ironically, organisms that are too perfectly adapted to their niche exist in a fragile state, as any small change can prompt their extinction. The ongoing pruning and regrowth within each of our lives may be a necessary process for our continuing growth and adaptation throughout our lives.

The Encounter

Fisher (2002) discusses three major elements that characterize our endurance of sustained pain and suffering and our experience of regrowth through pain and suffering. First, the pain intrudes upon and disrupts our carefully constructed, normal lives. The familiar boundaries of our identity that help us feel secure and provide meaning to our lives begin to disintegrate, and we lose the threads of our life narratives, the stories of who we are and why we live. Also we begin to lose our feelings for and connections to others. We find it difficult to communicate with those familiar to us, and consequently we feel isolated (Scarry, 1985; Soelle, 1975).

Next, Fisher (2002) observes that pain and suffering tend to promote self-scrutiny. Within one's hub of isolation, one begins to question life meanings and identity. Such questions may elicit feelings of injustice, outrage, and bewilderment to which the therapist can offer a compassionate ear but need not supply answers.

Finally, Fisher (2002) observes the emergence of new paths that may lead the sufferer into radically different directions. At this stage, the questions often change from "why?" to "how?" because the individual has apparently accepted the change and is open to new ways of coping. This process is described by many others: Harris (2007, p. 78) suggests that in all of us there is an inherent inclination to discover "new meanings, new selves, new ways of being in the world," and Merleau-Ponty (1992, p. 344) notes, "There is an inexhaustible reservoir from which meanings can be drawn."

The Clinician

A patient's discovery of a new path in life, new values, and a renewed sense of identity will depend significantly on the nature of the patient–clinician relationship as well as on the clinician's faith, maturity, and wisdom. It is easy to understand the clinician's aversion to a patient's pain and suffering. Even the best of us who are deeply committed to compassionate care are likely to experience the tendency toward self-protection. Such self-protection may manifest in withdrawal from our patients or in trying to do too much for them. Yet giving in to this impulse to self-protect creates distance between therapist and patient, either directly as the therapist withdraws from the patient's pain or, more subtly, as the therapist provides overcare and thereby moves the patient into a helpless and dependent position within the relationship. Any of these pain-avoidant responses by the therapist will limit the depth of any new meanings that they may decipher together (Harris, 2007).

Healing is essentially an intersubjective activity; it does not take place in isolation (Harris, 2007; Scarry, 1985; Soelle, 1975). When one joins patients in their subjective experiences of pain, one provides the opportunity for a pure expression, one that comes from the isolated worlds of those that Wright (2005) refers to as the "wounded storytellers." Healing involves the process of coming to understand one's suffering (Harris, 2007). Finally, any new life journeys the patient discovers will depend on "the sort of story one tells of one's suffering—and is told about oneself" (Harris, 2007, p. 70).

Like many others (e.g., Scarry, 1985), Harris (2007) stresses the importance of the imagination in developing empathy, compassion, and caring with patients. The joint imagination of the clinician and patient are the arena in which patients may express their pain, and where clinicians may assist them in finding new meanings to weave into the plotlines of their life stories. If skillfully employed, imagination can provide answers to questions of "why?" and "how" and suggest worthwhile alternative life paths.

Like the Buddhists, Harris (2007) emphasizes that the ability to achieve detachment from what has been plays a central role in the cessation of suffering. Letting go or "self-emptying," as Johnston (2003) puts it, opens new doors and permits change to occur. It permits living in the present without dwelling on the wrongs of the past or fearing the future. The process of detachment also involves the ability to forgive, which, according to many, is also central to healing. Harris (2007, p. 82) describes the role of forgiveness within the therapeutic process: "Forgiveness is an important practice for both healer and sufferer. Forgiveness from others heals the sufferer of her alienation and guilt; forgiveness of others heals the sufferer of his attachment, freeing him from corrosive emotions and toxic imaginings." As clinicians, it is worth the effort to familiarize ourselves with the power of forgiveness, to remain open to its potential to heal our patients, and to cultivate it within our own lives.

The Gift

The mechanistic and materialist approaches to health assign no meaning or value to pain and suffering. Suffering is seen as something to be eliminated rather than as a catalyst for a richer life (Madison, 2005). Without meaning or value in suffering, human life may exist only in tragic terms, where everything eventually comes to nothing and "the whole cosmic drama is, in the final analysis, futile and devoid of meaning" (Madison, p. 2). On the other hand, the existential/spiritual approaches, particularly of the Buddhist tradition, claim that pain and suffering can provide an extraordinary opportunity for growth. As Moulyn (1982, p. 31) puts it, "The intrinsic value of suffering lies in its propensity to clear a path toward mature inalienable happiness." However, this does not mean that pain and suffering are essential for growth. One would not encourage further suffering in the lives of our patients, and one should not consider those who have gone through these experiences to be more evolved than those who have not (Fisher, 2002). Rather, pain should be viewed from a balanced perspective. Pain is indeed quite uncomfortable, yet it is inescapable, and necessary. Pain is but a single, sorrowful path to joy.

Paul Brand (Brand & Yancy, 1993), who devoted his career to working with leprosy patients in India, discusses the value of bodily pain. He discovered that the loss of appendages due to leprosy was actually due to numbness rather than to any intrinsic process of the disease itself. In the absence of pain nothing warned patients of tissue damage. Brand offers numerous accounts of the horrible consequences of living without the sensation of pain. Many patients reported, "Of course, I can see my hands and feet, but somehow they don't feel like part of *me*. It feels as if they are just tools." It seems obvious that in addition to warning and protecting us, pain unifies us. Just as the "physical pain unifies our sense of having a body, we can conceive of the general experience of suffering acting as a unifying force that connects us with others....unifies us with all living creatures" (Dalai Lama & Cutler, 1998, p. 211) .

The Dalai Lama and many others (e.g., Gibran, 1966; May, 1958; Pascal, 1963; Wilde, 1946; Yalom, 1980) agree that pain and suffering play an important role in promoting growth, transcendence, and compassion. Indeed, virtually all world religions and secular philosophies converge on this perspective. Many salutary effects of suffering have been noted (Dalai Lama & Cutler, 1998; Harris, 2007; Wilde, 1946):

- It makes us sensitive, gentle, empathic, and compassionate, and thereby it helps us understand the suffering of others.
- It invites us to show our moral greatness.
- It builds character, breeds dignity, and can bring out the best in us.
- It shows us new and expanded ways of being in the world that lead to deeper meanings.
- It deepens our experience of life and brings us to a broader understanding of our identity.
- It can reduce our arrogance and conceit and enhance humility.

Of all the potential gifts of pain and suffering, compassion has been the primary focus of the Tibetan Buddhists. Compassion is not only a consequence of pain and suffering, but along with forgiveness, it perhaps also is the most powerful antidote to them. Consequently, it is not surprising that the Tibetan Buddhists have developed a broad range of meditation exercises to cultivate compassion.

In a classic Buddhist meditation for compassion enhancement, participants are instructed to view each individual, in fact each sentient being, as their mother. This arouses a "sense of fondness, cherishing, gentleness, affection, and gratitude" (Goleman, 2003, p. 283). In another Buddhist exercise called Tong-Len, we "mentally visualize taking on another's pain and suffering, and in turn giving them all of our resources, good health, fortune, and so on" (Dalai Lama & Cutler, 1998, p. 203).

It is a common misconception that our cultivation of compassion and loving kindness is done mainly for the sake of others. The Dalai Lama is quick to point out that we are the bigger beneficiaries of this practice. As soon as we experience a sense of caring in our heart, we feel greater inner strength and happiness (Goleman, 2003; Ricards, 2003). The experience of pain and suffering can soften us and make us more sensitive and empathic. This enhanced compassion in turn contributes to our true happiness. Recent research has supported the connection between a kind heart and happiness (Davidson & Harrington, 2002; Goleman, 2003; Ricards, 2003). As Ricards (2003, p. 210) remarks, "Joy and satisfaction are closely tied to love and affection. As for misery, it goes hand in hand with selfishness and hostility."

It is a hidden blessing that our pain and suffering almost certainly bring us face to face with the concept of mortality, prompting thoughts such as, "It hurts so bad; it feels like I am dying." Yet all major spiritual traditions teach that a meaningful life is possible only after we are able to accept the inevitability of death. Death is a basic condition of life. To this end, the Buddhists have developed many meditation techniques. They claim that contemplating our impermanence and letting go of our attachments to our egos liberate us from suffering and help us attain lasting happiness and contentment. Herman Feifel (1968, p. 68) says, "Life is not genuinely our own until we renounce it." Rollo May (1958, p. 47) maintained, "With the confronting of nonbeing, existence takes on vitality and immediacy, and the individual experiences a heightened consciousness of himself and his world, and others around him." Irvin Yalom (1980, p. 16) felt that "by keeping death in mind one passes into a state of gratitude for the countless givens of existence." George Santayana remarked, "The dark background which death supplies, brings out the tender colors of life in all their purity" (quoted in Yalom, 1980, p. 163). And Nietzsche (1974, p. 37) stated, "Out of such abysses, from such severe sicknesses, one returns newborn ... with a more delicate taste for joy, with a more tender tongue for all good things, with merrier senses, with a second dangerous innocence in joy."

As you work with individuals in pain, you will have the opportunity to experience each of the spiritual and philosophical lessons outlined herein: the ephemeral nature of suffering and transcendence, pain and joy; the power of detachment and reconnection; the power of forgiveness and the compassion that suffering may bring. Your patients will arrive at your office with opportunities for growth, forgiveness, and the creation of new paths through life and new life stories. If you are present and open to these possibilities, if you can maintain compassion and faith, and if you seek wisdom, then your work with your patients in pain will fill your life with meaning as well. You will acquire deeper ways of connecting with others and also with yourself. Such lessons will be as strong as the pain is deep. It appears that this truth is universal.

In conclusion we offer a meditation (Central Conference of American Rabbis, 1999, pp. 283–284):

> Birth is a beginning
> And death a destination.
> And life is a journey:
> From childhood to maturity
> And youth to age;
> From innocence to awareness
> And ignorance to knowing;
> From foolishness to discretion
> And then, perhaps, to wisdom;
> From weakness to strength
> Or strength to weakness-
> And, often, back again;
> From health to sickness
> And back, we pray, to health again;
> From offense to forgiveness,
> From loneliness to love,
> From joy to gratitude,
> From pain to compassion,
> And grief to understanding-
> From fear to faith;
> From defeat to defeat to defeat-
> Until, looking backward or ahead,
> We see that victory lies
> Not at some high place along the way,
> But in having made the journey, stage by stage,
> A sacred pilgrimage.

References

Achterberg, J. (1985). *Imagery in healing: Shanamism and modern medicine.* Boston: Shambhala.

Achterberg, J., Dossey, B., & Kolkmeier, L. (1994). *Rituals of healing: Using imagery for health and wellness.* New York: Bantam Books.

Achterberg, J., Kenner, C., & Lawlis, G. F. (1988). Severe burn injury: A comparison of relaxation, imagery and biofeedback for pain management. *Journal of Mental Imagery, 12*(1), 71–88.

Ahles, T. A., Blanchard, E. B., & Leventhal, H. (1983). Cognitive control of pain: Attention to the sensory aspects of the cold pressor stimulus. *Cognitive Therapy and Research, 7,* 159–178.

Ahsen, A. (1972). *Eidetic parents test and analysis.* New York: Brandon House.

Ahsen, A. (1973). *Basic concepts in eidetic psychotherapy.* New York: Brandon House.

Ahsen, A. (1984). ISM: The triple code model for imagery and psychophysiology. *Journal of Mental Imagery, 8*(4), 15–42.

Ahsen, A. (2000). Image and maze: Learning through imagery functions. *Journal of Mental Imagery, 24*(1–2), 1–60.

Ahsen, A., & Lazarus, A. A. (1972). Eidetics: An internal behavior approach. In A. A. Lazarus (Ed.), *Clinical behavior therapy* (pp. 87–99). New York: Brunzer/Mazel.

Albright, G. L., & Fischer, A. A. (1990). Effects of warming imagery aimed at trigger-point sites on tissue compliance, skin temperature, and pain sensitivity in biofeedback-trained patients with chronic pain: A preliminary study. *Perceptual and Motor Skills, 71,* 1163–1170.

Alcoholics Anonymous World Services. (1953). *Twelve steps, twelve traditions.* New York: Author.

Alexander, E. D. (1971). In-the-body travel: a growth experience with fantasy. *Psychotherapy: Theory, Research, and Practice, 8,* 319–324.

Allport, G. W. (1968). *The person in psychology.* Boston: Beacon Press.

Alvarez, C. B., & Marcos, A. F. (1997). Psychological treatment of evoked pain and anxiety by invasive medical procedures in paediatric oncology. *Psychology in Spain, 1,* 17–36.

American Psychiatric Association. (APA). (1994). *Diagnostic and statistical manual of mental disorders* (4th ed.). Washington, DC: Author.

Anbar, R. D. (2001). Self-hypnosis for the treatment of functional abdominal pain in childhood. *Clinical Pediatrics, 40,* 447–451.

Assagioli, R. (1973). *The act of will.* New York: Viking Press.

Avia, M. D., & Kanfer, J. H. (1980). Coping with aversive stimulation: The effects of training in self-management context. *Cognitive Therapy and Research, 4,* 73–78.

Baer, R. A. (2003). Mindfulness training as a clinical intervention: A conceptual and empirical review. *Clinical Psychology: Science and Practice, 10,* 125–143.

Baer, S. M., Hoffman, A. C., & Sheikh, A. A. (2003). Healing images: Connecting with inner wisdom. In A. A. Sheikh (Ed.), *Healing images: The role of imagination in health* (pp. 141–176). Amityville, NY: Baywood.

Bain, A. (1872). *The senses and the intellect.* New York: D. Appleton and Co.

Bak, P. (1996). *How nature works: The science of self-organized criticality.* New York: Springer-Verlag.

Bakan, P. (1980). Imagery, raw and cooked: A hemispheric recipe. In J. E. Shorr, P. Sobel, P. Robin, & J.A. Connella (Eds.), *Imagery: Its many dimensions and applications* (pp. 35–53). New York: Plenum.

Baldwin, M. W. (1995). Relational schemas and cognition in close relationships. *Journal of Social and Personal Relationships, 12,* 547–552.

Ball, T. M., Shapiro, D. E., Monheim, C. J., & Weydert, J. A. (2003). A pilot study of the use of guided imagery for the treatment of recurrent abdominal pain in children. *Clinical Pediatrics, 42,* 527–532.

Bandura, A. (1977). Self-efficacy: Toward a unifying theory of behavioral change. *Psychological Review, 84,* 191–215.

Bandura, A. (1986). *Social foundations of thought and action.* New York: Prentice-Hall.

Barber, J. (1996). Hypnotic analgesia: Clinical considerations. In J. Barber (Ed.), *Hypnosis and suggestion in the treatment of pain* (pp. 85–120). New York: W.W. Norton & Company.

Barsky, A. J., Goodson, D. J., & Lane, R. S. (1998). The amplification of somatic symptoms. *Psychosomatic Medicine, 50,* 510–519.

Bartlett, F. C. (1932). *Remembering: A study in experimental and social psychology.* Cambridge, England: Cambridge University Press.

Baumeister, R. F. (1998). The self. In D. T. Gilbert, S. T. Fiske, & G. Lindzey (Eds.), *The handbook of social psychology* (vol. 1, pp. 680–740). New York: McGraw-Hill.

Baumrind, D. (1983). Familial antecedents of social competence in young children. *Psychological Bulletin, 94,* 132–142.

Beck, A. T. (1991). *Cognitive therapy and the emotional disorders.* New York: Penguin Books.

Beers, T. M., & Karoly, P. (1979). Cognitive strategies, Expectancy, and coping style in the control of pain. *Journal of Consulting and Clinical Psychology, 47,* 179–180.

Bejenke, C. J. (1996). Painful medical procedures. In J. Barber (Ed.), *Hypnosis and suggestion in the treatment of pain: A clinical guide* (pp. 209–266). New York: W.W. Norton.

Bellissimo, A., & Tunks, E. (1984). *Chronic pain: The psychotherapeutic spectrum.* New York: Praeger.

Benson, H., & Friedman, R. (1996). Harnessing the power of the placebo effect and renaming it "remembered wellness." *Annual Review of Medicine, 47,* 193–199.

Benson, H. B., & Stark, M. (1996). *Timeless healing: The power and biology of belief.* New York: Scribner.

Berkowitz, L. (1989). The frustration-aggression hypothesis: An examination and reformulation. *Psychological Bulletin, 106,* 59–73.

Berkowitz, L. (1993). Pain and aggression: Some findings and implications. *Motivation and Emotion, 17,* 277–293.

Berkowitz, L., Cochran, S. T., & Embree, M. (1981). Physical pain and the goal of aversively stimulated aggression. *Journal of Personality and Social Psychology, 40,* 687–200.

Berkowitz, L., & Heimer, K. (1989). On the construction of the anger experience: Aversive events and negative priming in the formulation of feelings. In L. Berkowitz (Ed.), *Advances in experimental social psychology* (Vol. 22, pp. 1–37). New York: Academic Press.

Boothby, J. L., Thorn, B. E., Stroud, M. W., & Jensen, M. P. (1999). Coping with pain. In R. J. Gatchel & D. C. Turk (Eds.), *Psychosocial factors in pain: Critical perspectives* (pp. 343–359). New York: Guilford.

Borckardt, J. J., Younger, J., Winkel, J., Nash, M. R., & Shaw, D. (2004). The computer-assisted cognitive/imagery system for the use in the management of pain. *Pain Research and Management, 9*(3), 157–162.

Bowlby, J. (1982). *Attachment and loss: Vol. 1. Attachment* (2nd ed.). New York: Basic Books. (Original work published 1969)

Bradley, G. W. (1978). Self-serving biases in the attribution process: A re-examination of the fact or fiction question. *Journal of Personality and Social Psychology, 35,* 56–71.

Brand, P., & Yancy, P. (1993). *Pain: The gift nobody wants.* Grand Rapids, MI: Zondervan

Brazier, D. (1995). *Zen therapy: Transcending the sorrows of the human mind.* New York: Wiley.

Bresler, D. (1984). Mind-controlled analgesia: The inner way to pain control. In A. A. Sheikh (Ed.), *Imagination and healing* (pp. 211–230). Farmingdale, NY: Baywood Publishing Company, Inc.

Burger, J. M. (1991). Control. In V. J. Derlega, B. A. Winstead, & W. H. Jones (Eds.), *Personality: Contemporary theory and research* (pp. 287–312). Belmont, CA: Wadsworth Publishing.

Central Conference of American Rabbis. (1999). *Gates of repentance: The new union prayerbook for the days of Awe* (revised ed.). New York: Author.

Chapman, C. R., Nakamura, Y., & Flores, L. Y. (1999). Chronic pain and consciousness: A constructivist perspective. In R. J. Gatchel & D. C. Turk (Eds.), *Psychosocial factors in pain: Critical perspectives* (pp. 35–55). New York: Guilford.

Chodorow, J. (2006). Active imagination. In R. K. Papadopoulos (Ed.), *The handbook of Jungian psychology* (pp. 215–243). New York: Routledge.

Colman, W. (2006). Imagination and the imaginary. *Journal of Analytical Psychology, 51,* 21–41.

Cooke, R. (2001). *Dr. Folkman's war.* New York: Random House.

Corbin, H. (1970). *Creative imagination in the Sufism of Ibn 'Arabi* (R. Manheim, Trans.). London: Routledge & Kegan Paul.

Cornell, A. W. (1996). *The power of focusing*. Oakland, CA: New Harbinger Publications.

Cousins, N. (1980). *Anatomy of an illness*. New York: W. W. Norton.

Cupal, D. D., & Brewer, B. W. (2001). Effects of relaxation and guided imagery on knee strength, reinjury, anxiety, and pain following anterior cruciate ligament reconstruction. *Rehabilitation Psychology, 46,* 28–43.

Davidson, R., & Harrington, A. (2002). *Visions of compassion*. New York: Oxford University Press.

Deadwyler, S. A., & Hampson, R. E. (1995). Ensemble activity and behavior: What's the code? *Science, 270,* 1316–1318.

DeAngelis, D. L., Post, W. M., & Travis, C. C. (1986). Introduction. In S. A. Levin (Managing Ed.), M. Arbib, H. J. Bremermann, J. Cowan, W. M. Hirsch, S. Karlin, J. Keller, et al. (Editorial Board), *Biomathematics: Vol. 15. Positive feedback in natural systems* (pp. 1–25). New York: Springer-Verlag.

Dalai Lama & Cutler, H. C. (1998). *The art of happiness: A handbook for living*. New York: Riverhead Books.

Descartes, R. (1958). Discours de la methode (1637). In N. K. Smith (Ed., Trans.), *Descartes' philosophical writings*. New York: Random House. (Original work published 1637).

Descartes, R. (1958). Meditations de prima philosophia (1641). In N. K. Smith (Ed., Trans.), *Descartes' philosophical writings*. New York: Random House. (Original work published 1641).

Dolan, A. T. (1997). *Imagery treatment of phobias, anxiety states, and other symptom complexes*. New York: Brandon House.

Donahoe, J. W., & Vegas, R. (2004). Pavlovian conditioning: The CS-UCR relation. *Journal of Experimental Psychology: Animal Behavior Processes, 30*(1), 17–33.

Dossey, B. M., Keegan, L., Kolkmeier, L. G., & Guzzetta, C. E. (1989). *Holistic health promotion: A guide for practice*. Rockville, MD: Aspen Publishers, Inc.

Duckro, P. N., & Cantwell-Simmonds, E. (1989). A review of studies evaluating biofeedback and relaxation training in the management of pediatric headache. *Headache, 29,* 428–433.

Dworkin, S. F., Von Korff, M. R., & LeResche, L. (1992). Epidemiologic studies of chronic pain: A dynamic-ecologic perspective. *Annals of Behavioral Medicine, 14,* 3–11.

Eisendrath, P. (1977). Active imagination: A separate reality. *Art Psychotherapy, 4,* 63–71.

Ellis, A. (1977). Rejoinder: Elegant and inelegant RET. *Counseling Psychologist, 7,* 73–82.

Ellis, A. (1958). Rational psychotherapy. *Journal of General Psychology, 59,* 35–49.

Engel, G. L. (1977). The need for a new medical model: A challenge for biomedicine. *Science, 196*(4286), 129–136.

Epstein, G. (1986). The image in medicine. *Advances, 3,* 22–31.

Epstein, G. (1989). *Creative visualizations: Creating health through imagery*. New York: Bantam Books.

Erickson, B. A. (1994). Ericksonian therapy demystified: A straightforward approach. In J. K. Zeig (Ed.), *Ericksonian methods: The essence of the story* (pp. 1–45). London: Routledge.

Erickson, P., & Rogers, L. (1973). New procedures for analyzing relational communication. *Family Process, 12,* 245–267.

Erickson, M. H., & Rossi, E. L. (1979). Altering sensory-perceptual functioning: The problem of pain and comfort. In M. H. Erickson & E. L. Rossi (Eds.), Hypnotherapy: An exploratory casebook (pp. 94–138). New York: Irvington.

Erickson, M. H., & Rossi, E. L. (Eds.). (1980). *The collected papers of Milton H. Erickson on hypnosis, Vol. IV. Innovative hypnotherapy.* New York: Irvington.

Fanurik, D., Zeltzer, L. K., Roberts, M. C., & Blount, R. L. (1993). The relationship between children's coping styles and psychological interventions for cold presser pain. *Pain, 53,* 213–222.

Farthing, G. W., Venturino, M., Brown, S. W., & Lazar, J. D. (1997). *International Journal of Clinical and Experimental Hypnosis, 45,* 433–446.

Feifel, H. (1968). Death: Relevant variable in psychology. In R. May (Ed.), *Existential psychology* (pp. 58–71). New York: Random House.

Fernandez, E. (1986). A classification system of cognitive coping strategies for pain. *Pain, 26,* 141–151.

Fernandez, E., & Turk, D. C. (1989). The utility of cognitive coping strategies for altering pain perception: A meta-analysis. *Pain, 38,* 123–135.

Ferrucci, P. (1982). *What we may be.* New York: Tarcher.

Ferster, D., & Spruston, N. (1995). Cracking the neuronal code. *Science, 270,* 756–757.

Fisher, R. N. (2002). Introduction. In R. N. Fischer, D. T. Primozic, P. A. Day, & J. A. Thompson (Eds.), *Suffering, death, and identity* (pp. 1–3). Amsterdam: Rodopi.

Fletcher, G. J. O., & Ward, C. (1988). Attribution theory and processes: A cross-cultural perspective. In M. H. Bond (Ed.), *The cross-cultural challenge to social psychology* (pp. 230–244). Newbury Park, CA: Sage.

Flor, H., Birbaumer, N., Schugens, M. M., & Lutzenberger, W. (1992). Symptom-specific psychophysiological responses in chronic pain patients. *Psychophysiology, 29,* 452–460.

Fors, E. A., Sexton, H., & Gotestam, K. G. (2002). The effect of guided imagery and amitriptyline on daily fibromyalgia pain: A prospective, randomized, controlled trial. *Journal of Psychiatric Research, 36,* 179–187.

Frank, J. D., & Frank, J. B. (1991). *Persuasion and healing: A comparative study of psychotherapy* (3rd ed.). Baltimore, MD: Johns Hopkins University Press.

Freeman, W. J. (1995). *Societies of brains.* Mahwah, NJ: Lawrence Erlbaum.

Furst, A. (2003). *Kingdom of shadows* (cassette recording). Prince Fredrick, MD: Recorded Books.

Gatchel, R. J., & Dersh, J. (2002). Psychological disorders and chronic pain: Are there cause-and-effect relationships? In D. C. Turk and R. J. Gatchel (Eds), *Psychological approaches to pain management: A practitioner's handbook* (2nd ed., pp 30–51). Guilford: New York.

Gatchel, R. J., & Epker, J. (1999). Psychosocial predictors of chronic pain and response to treatment. In R. J. Gatchel and D. C. Turk (Eds.), *Psychosocial factors in pain: Critical perspectives* (pp. 412–434). Guilford: New York.

Gauron, E. F., & Bowers, W. A. (1986). Pain control techniques in college-age athletes. *Psychological Reports, 59,* 1163–1169.

Gay, M., Philippot, P., & Luminet, O. (2001). Differential effectiveness of psychological interventions for reducing osteoarthritis pain: A comparison of Erickson hypnosis and Jacobson relaxation. *European Journal of Pain, 6,* 1–16.

Geisser, M. E., Gaskin, M. E., Robinson, M. E., & Greene, A. F. (1993). The relationship of depression and somatic focus to experimental and clinical pain in chronic pain patients. *Psychology and Health, 8,* 405–415.

Gendlin, E. T. (1981). *Focusing* (2nd ed.). New York: Bantam.

Gendlin, E. T. (1996). *Focusing-oriented psychotherapy: A manual of the experiential method.* New York: Guilford Press.

Gibran, K. (1966). *The prophet.* New York: Alfred A. Knopf.

Gilligan, S. G. (1994). The fight against fundamentalism: Searching for soul in Erickson's legacy. In J. Zeig (Ed.), *The Evolution of Psychotherapy* (pp. 79–98). New York: Bruner/Mazel.

Goleman, D. (2003). *Destructive emotions: How we can overcome them? A scientific dialogue with the Dalai Lama.* New York: Bantam Books.

Gramling, S. E., Clawson, E. P., & McDonald, M. K. (1996). Perceptual and cognitive abnormality model of hypochondriasis: Amplification and physiological reactivity in women. *Psychosomatic Medicine, 58,* 423–431.

Green, D. M., & Swets, J. A. (1966). *Signal detection, theory and psychophysics.* New York: Wiley.

Greenleaf, M. (1978). Relaxation training in the control of high blood pressure: A report on techniques. *Transnational Mental Health Research Newsletter, 20*(1), 12–16.

Grove, D. (1989). Metaphors to heal by: A study course in epistemological metaphors, Tape 1. Edwardsville, IL: David Grove Seminars.

Grove, D. J., & Panzer, B. I. (1989). *Resolving traumatic memories: Metaphor and symbols in psychotherapy.* New York: Irvington Publishers

Guastello, S. J. (1997). Science evolves: An introduction to nonlinear dynamics, psychology, and life sciences. *Nonlinear Dynamics, Psychology, and Life Sciences, 1,* 1–6.

Guastello, S. J. (2002). *Managing emergent phenomena: Nonlinear dynamics in work organizations.* Mahwah, NJ: Lawrence Erlbaum.

Guastello, S. J. (2004). Progress in applied nonlinear dynamics: Welcome to NDPLS Vol. 8. *Nonlinear Dynamics, Psychology, and Life Sciences, 8,* 1–16.

Guastello, S. J., Hyde, T., & Odak, M. (1998). Symbolic dynamic patterns of verbal exchange in a creative problem solving group. *Nonlinear Dynamics, Psychology, and Life Sciences, 2,* 35–58.

Guastello, S. J., Koopmans, M., & Pincus, D. (Eds.) (2008). *Chaos and complexity in psychology: The theory of nonlinear dynamical systems.* Cambridge, England: Cambridge University Press.

Haber, R. N. (1979). Twenty years of haunting eidetic imagery: Where's the ghost? *Behavioral and Brain Sciences, 2,* 583–629.

Hackett, G., & Horan, J. J. (1980). Stress inoculation for pain: What's really going on? *Journal of Counseling Psychology, 27,* 107–116.

Haines, J., Williams, C. L., Brain, K. L., & Wilson, G. V. (1995). The psychophysiology of self-mutilation. *Journal of Abnormal Psychology, 104,* 471–489.

Haken, H. (1984). *The science of structure: Synergetics.* New York: Van Nostrand Reinhold.

Haley, J. (1994). Typically Erickson. In J. K. Zeig (Ed.), *Ericksonian methods: The essence of the story* (pp. 1–45). Levittown, PA: Brunner/Mazel.

Hardin, K. N. (1997). Chronic pain management. In P. M. Camic & S. J. Knight (Eds.), *Clinical handbook of health psychology: A practical guide to effective Interventions* (pp. 75–99). Seattle, WA: Hogrefe & Huber.

Hargadon, R., Bowers, K. S., & Woody, E. Z. (1995). Does counterpain imagery mediate hypnotic analgesia? *Journal of Abnormal Psychology, 104,* 508–516.

Harris, I. (2007). The gift of suffering. In N. E. Johnston & A. Scholler Jaquish (Eds.), *Meaning in suffering* (pp. 60–97). Madison, WI: University of Wisconsin Press.

Hayes, S. C. (2004). Acceptance and commitment therapy, relational frame theory, and the third wave of behavioral and cognitive therapies. *Behavior Therapy, 35,* 639–665.

Hayes, S. C., & Duckworth, M. P. (2006). Acceptance and commitment therapy and traditional cognitive behavior therapy approaches to pain. *Cognitive and Behavioral Practice, 1,* 185–187.

Hayes, S. C., Strosahl, K. D., & Wilson, K. G. (1999). *Acceptance and commitment therapy: An experiential approach to behavior change.* New York: Guilford.

Hendricks, M. N. (2002). Focusing-oriented/experiential psychotherapy. In D. J. Cain (Ed.) and J. Seeman (Assoc. Ed.), *Humanistic psychotherapies: Handbook of research and practice* (pp. 221–251). Washington, DC: American Psychological Assocation.

Hilgard, E. R., & Hilgard, J. R. (1994). *Hypnosis in the relief of pain.* New York: Brunner/Mazel, Inc.

Hill, H. F., Chapman, C. R., Kornell, J. A., Sullivan, K. M., Saeger, L. C., & Benedetti, C. (1990). Self-administration of morphine in bone marrow transplant patient reduces drug requirement. *Pain, 40,* 121–129.

Hochman, J. (2002). Ahsen's triple code model of dynamic imagery and mindbody connection in contemporary psychology. *Journal of Mental Imagery, 26* (1–2), 111–138.

Holroyd, K. A., & Penzien, D. B. (1986). Client variables and the behavioral treatment of recurrent tension headache: A meta-analytic review. *Journal of Behavioral Medicine, 9,* 515–536.

Horan, J. J. (1973). "In vivo" emotive imagery: A technique for reducing childbirth anxiety and discomfort. *Psychological Reports, 32,* 1328.

Howland, E. W., Wakai, R. T., Mjaanes, B. A., Balog, J. P., & Cleeland, C. S. (1995). Whole head mapping of magnetic fields following painful electric finger shock. *Cognitive Brain Research, 2,* 165–172.

Hugdahl, K., Rosen, G., Ersland, L., Lundervold, A., Smievoll, A. I., Barndon, R., et al. (2001). Common pathways in mental imagery and pain perception: An fMRI study of a subject with an amputated arm. *Scandinavian Journal of Psychology, 42,* 269–275.

Huth, M. M., Broome, M. E., & Good, M. (2004). Imagery reduces children's post-operative pain. *Pain, 110,* 439–448.

Iberg, J. R. (2001). Focusing. In R. J. Corsini (Ed.), *Handbook of innovative therapy* (pp. 263–278). New York: Wiley.

Jacobson, E. (1931). Electrical measurement of neuromuscular states during mental activities V. Variation of specific muscles contracting during imagination. *American Journal of Physiology, 96*, 115–121.

Jaffe, D. T. (1980). *Healing from within.* New York: Bantam Books

Jensen, M. P. (2002). Enhancing motivation to change in pain treatment. In D. C. Turk & R. J. Gatchel (Eds.), *Psychological approaches to pain management* (2nd ed., pp. 71–93). New York: Guilford.

Johnson, M. I. (2001). Transcutaneous electrical nerve stimulation (TENS) and TENS-like devices: Do they provide pain relief? *Pain Reviews, 8,* 121–158.

Johnston, N. (2003). Finding meaning in adversity (Abstract). *Dissertation Abstract International,* 65(01). (UMINO.AAT N6.86530).

Jung, C. G. (1960). *Collected works (vol. III). The psychogenesis of mental disease.* Oxford, England: Pantheon.

Kahneman, D., & Tversky, A. (1996). On the reality of cognitive illusions. *Psychological Review, 103,* 582–591.

Kantorovich, A. (1993). *Scientific discovery: Logic and tinkering.* Albany, NY: State University New York Press.

Kauffman, S. A. (1993). *The origins of order: Self-organization and selection in evolution.* New York: Oxford University Press.

Kauffman, S. A. (1995). *At home in the universe.* New York: Oxford University Press.

Kelly, S. F., & Kelly, R. J. (1995). *Imagine yourself well: Better health through self-hypnosis.* New York: Plenum.

Kemper, K. J., Cassileth, B., & Ferris, T. (1999). Holistic pediatrics: A research agenda. *Pediatrics, 103,* 902–910.

Klein, N. (2001). *Healing images for children.* Watertown, WI: Inner Coaching.

Kleinman, A., Brodwin, P. E., Good, B. J., & DelVecchio-Good, M. (1992). Pain as human experience: An introduction. In M. DelVecchio-Good, P. E. Brodwin, B. J. Good, & A. Kleinman (Eds.), *Pain as human experience: An anthropological perspective* (pp. 1–28). Berkeley, CA: University of California Press.

Koopmans, M. (2001). From double bind to N-bind: Toward a new theory of schizophrenia and family interaction. *Nonlinear Dynamics, Psychology, and Life Sciences, 5,* 289–325.

Korn, E. R.. (1982). *Pain management with relaxation and mental imagery (audiocasette).* La Jolla, CA: Psychology and Consulting Associates Press.

Korn, E. R. (1983). The use of altered states of consciousness and imagery in physical and pain rehabilitation. *Journal of Mental Imagery, 7*(1), 25–34.

Korn, E. R., & Johnson, K. (1983). *Visualization: Uses of imagery in the health profession.* Homewood, IL: Dow Jones-Irwin.

Kosko, B. (1993). *Fuzzy thinking: The new science of fuzzy logic.* New York: Hyperion.

Kuttner, L., Bowman, M., & Teasdale, M. (1988). Psychological treatment of distress, pain, and anxiety for young children with cancer. *Developmental and Behavioral Pediatrics, 9,* 374–381.

Kroger, W. S., & Fezler, W. D. (1976). *Hypnosis and behavior modification: Imagery conditioning.* Philadelphia, PA: J.B. Lippincott.

Krueger, L. C. (1987). Pediatric pain and imagery. *Journal of Child and Adolescent Psychotherapy, 4,* 32–41.

Kwekkeboom, K., Huseby-Moore, K., & Ward, S. (1998). Imaging ability and effective use of guided imagery. *Research in Nursing & Health, 21,* 189–198.

Lambert, S. A. (1996). The effects of hypnosis/guided imagery on the postoperative course of children. *Developmental and Behavioral Pediatrics, 17,* 307–310.

Lazarus, A. (1977). *In the mind's eye.* New York: Rawson Associates.

LeBaron, S., & Zeltzer, L. K. (1996). Children in pain. In J. Barber (Ed.), *Hypnosis and suggestion in the treatment of pain: A clinical guide* (pp. 305–340). New York: W.W. Norton Company, Inc.

Lerner, M. J. (1980). *The belief in a just world: A fundamental delusion.* New York: Plenum.

Levendusky, P., & Pankratz, L. (1975). Self-control techniques as an alternative to pain medication. *Journal of Abnormal Psychology, 84,* 165–168.

Levine, S. (1982). *Who dies? An investigation of conscious living and conscious dying.* New York: Anchor Books.

Levis, D. J., & Brewer, K. E. (2001). The neurotic paradox: Attempts by two factor fear theory and alternative avoidance models to resolve the issues associated with sustained avoidance responding in extinction. In R. R. Mowrer & S. B. Klein (Eds.), *Handbook of contemporary learning theories* (pp. 561–597). Mahwah, NJ: Lawrence Erlbaum.

Lindberg, C., & Lawlis, G. F. (1988). The effectiveness of imagery as a childbirth preparatory technique. *Journal of Mental Imagery, 12*(1), 103–114.

Linn, C. D. (2008). *The inherent logic of epistemological metaphors.* London: Cei Davies Linn.

Locke, E. A. (1971). Is "behavior therapy" behavioristic? (An analyis of Wolbe's psychotherapeutic methods). *Psychological Bulletin, 76,* 318–327.

London, P. (1964). *The mode and morals of psychotherapy.* New York: Holt, Rinehart, & Winston.

Lueger, R .J. (1986). Imagery techniques in cognitive behavior therapy. In A. A. Sheikh (Ed.), *Anthology of imagery techniques* (pp. 61–84). Milwaukee, WI: American Imagery Institute.

Maddux, J. E. (1991). Personal efficacy. In V. J. Derlega, B. A. Winstead, & W. H. Jones (Eds.), *Personality: Contemporary theory and research* (pp. 231–262). Chicago, IL: Nelson-Hall.

Madison, G. B. (2005). *On suffering.* Unpublished manuscript.

Mannix, L. K., Chandurkar, R. S., Rybicki, L. A., Tusek, D. L, & Solomon, G. D. (1999). Effect of guided imagery on quality of life for patients with chronic tension-type headache. *Headache, 39,* 326–334.

Manyande, A., Berg, S., Gettins, D., Stanford, S. C., Mazhero, S., Marks, D. F., et al. (1995). Preoperative rehearsal of active coping imagery influences subjective and hormonal responses to abdominal surgery. *Psychosomatic Medicine, 57,* 177–182.

Marks-Tarlow, T. (1999). The self as a dynamical system. *Nonlinear Dynamics, Psychology, and Life Sciences, 3,* 311–346.

Markus, H. (1977). Self-schemata and processing information about the self. *Journal of Personality and Social Psychology, 35,* 63–78.

Markus, H., & Nurius, P. S. (1986). Possible selves. *American Psychologist, 41,* 954–969.

Marino, J., Gwynn, M. I., & Spanos, N. P. (1989). Cognitive mediators in the reduction of pain: The role of expectancy, strategy use, and self-presentation. *Journal of Abnormal Psychology, 98,* 256–262.

Mathews, W. J., Lankton, S., & Lankton, C. (1993). An Ericksonian model of hypnotherapy. In J. W. Rhue, S. J. Lynn, & I. Kirsch (Eds.), *Handbook of clinical hypnosis* (pp. 187–213). Washington, DC: American Psychological Association.

May, R. (1958). The origins and significance of the existential movement in
psychology. In R. May, E. Angel, & H. F. Ellenberger (Eds.), *Existence: A
new dimension in psychiatry and psychology* (pp. 3–36). New York: Simon
and Schuster.

McCaffery, M., & Beebe, A. (1989). *Pain: Clinical manual for nursing practice.*
Philadelphia, PA: Mosby.

McClelland, J. L., & Rumelhart, D. E. (1985). Distributed memory and the representation of general and specific information. *Journal of Experimental
Psychology: General, 114,* 159–188.

McGrath, P. A., & Hillier, L. M. (2002). A practical cognitive-behavioral approach
for treating children's pain. In D. C. Turk & R. J. Gatchel (Eds.), *Psychological
approaches to pain management* (2nd ed., pp. 534–552). New York: Guilford.

McKim, R. H. (1980). *Experiences in visual thinking.* Monterey, CA: Brooks & Cole.

McMahon, C. E., & Sheikh, A. A. (1986). Imagination in disease and healing processes: A historical perspective. In A. A. Sheikh (Ed.), *Anthology of imagery
techniques* (pp. 1–36). Milwaukee, WI: American Imagery Institute.

McMahon, C. E., & Sheikh, A. A. (1986). Psychosomatic illness: A new look: In A.
A. Sheikh and K. S. Sheikh (Eds), *Healing East and West: Ancient Wisdom and
Modern Psycholosy* (pp. 296–324). New York: Wiley.

McNeil, D. W., & Brunetti, E. G. (1992). Pain and fear: A bioinformational perspective on responsivity to imagery. *Behavioral Research and Therapy, 30,*
513–520.

McNicol, D. (2005). *A primer of signal detection theory.* Mahwah, NJ: Lawrence
Erlbaum.

Meichenbaum, D. (1977). *Cognitive behavior modification: An integrative approach.*
New York: Plenum.

Melzack, R. (1999). Pain and stress: A new perspective. In R. J. Gatchel & D. C.
Turk (Eds.), *Psychosocial factors in pain: Critical perspectives* (pp. 89–106).
Guilford: New York.

Melzack, R., & Casey, K. L. (1968). Sensory, motivational and central control deter-
minants of pain: A new conceptual model. In D. Kenshalo (Ed.), *The skin
senses* (pp. 443–523). Springfield, IL: Thomas.

Melzack, R., & Wall, P. D. (1965). Pain mechanisms: A new theory. *Science, 150,*
971–979.

Melzack, R., & Wall, P. D. (1996). *The challenge of pain* (2nd ed.). London:
Penguin Books.

Merskey, H., & Bogduk, N. (Eds.). (1994). *Classification of chronic pain: descriptions
of chronic pain syndromes and definitions of pain terms* (2nd ed.). Seattle, WA:
IASP Press.

Merleau-Ponty, M. (1992). *Phenomenology of perception.* London: Routledge.

Merriam-Webster online dictionary (2008). Retrieved November 26, 2008, from
http://www.merriam-webster.com/dictionary/pain

Meyer, R. G. (1992). *Practical clinical hypnosis.* New York: Lexington Books.

Miller, E. (1983). *Change the channel on pain* (audiocassette). Stanford, CA: Source.

Miller, E. (1997). *Deep healing: The essence of mind/body medicine.* Carlsbad, CA: Hay House.

Miller, W. R., Benefield, R. G., & Tongigan, J. S. (1993). Enhancing motivation for change in problem drinking: A controlled comparison of two therapist styles. *Journal of Consulting and Clinical Psychology, 61,* 455–461.

Miller, W. R., & Rollnick, S. (1991). *Motivational interviewing: Preparing people to change addictive behavior.* New York: Guilford Press.

Moulyn, A. C. (1982). *The meaning of suffering.* Westport, CT: Greenwood Press.

Naparstek, B. (1994). *Staying well with guided imagery.* New York: Warren Books.

Narduzzi, K. J., Nolan, R. P., Reesor, K., Jackson, T., Spanos, N. P., Hayward, A. A., et al. (1998). Preliminary investigation of associations of illness schemata and treatment-induced reduction in headaches. *Psychological Reports, 82,* 299–307.

Newshan, G., & Balamuth, R. (1990–1991). Use of imagery in a chronic pain outpatient group. *Imagination, Cognition and Personality, 10,* 25–38.

Nietzsche, F. (1974). *The gay silence.* New York: Random House.

Nispett, R. E., & Ross, L. (1980). *Human inference: Strategies and shortcomings of social judgment.* Englewood Cliffs, NJ: Prentice-Hall.

Nolan, R. P., Spanos, N. P., Hayward, A. A., & Scott, H. A. (1995). The efficacy of hypnotic and nonhypnotic response-based imagery for self-managing recurrent headache. *Imagination, Cognition and Personality, 14,* 183–201.

Norenzayan, A., & Nisbett, R. E. (2000). Culture and causal cognition. *Current Directions in Psychological Science, 9,* 132–135.

Okifuji, A., & Turk, D. C. (1999). Fibromyalgia: Search for mechanisms and effective treatments. In R. J. Gatchel & D. C. Turk (Eds.), *Psychosocial factors in pain: Critical perspectives* (pp. 227–246). New York: Guilford.

Olness, K., Hall, H., Rozniecki, J. J., Schmidt, W., & Theoharides, T. C. (1999). Mast cell activation in children with migraine before and after training in self-regulation. *Headache, 39,* 101–107.

Online Etymology Dictionary (2008). Retrieved November 26, 2008, from http://www.etymonline.com/index.php?term=pain

Orlinsky, D. E., & Howard, K. I. (1986). Process and outcome in psychotherapy. In A. E. Bergin & S. L. Garfield (Eds.), *Handbook of psychotherapy and behavior change* (3rd ed., pp. 311–381). New York: Wiley.

Ost, L. G. (1987). Applied relaxation: Description of a coping technique and review of controlled studies. *Behaviour Research and Therapy, 25,* 397–410.

Oster, J. (1972). Recurrent abdominal pain, headache and limb pains in children and adolescents. *Pediatrics, 50,* 429–436.

Oster, M. I. (1994). Psychological preparation for labor and delivery using hypnosis. *American Journal of Clinical Hypnosis, 37,* 12–21.

Osterweis, M., Kleinman, A., & Mechanic, D. (Eds.). (1987). *Pain and disability: Clinical, behavioral, and public policy perspectives.* Washington, DC: National Academy Press.

Ostrander, S., Schroeder, L., & Ostrander, N. (1979). *Super learning.* New York: Dell Publishing Co.

Palgrave, F. T. (Ed.). (1975). *The golden treasury.* London: Macmillan.

Pascal, B. (1963). *Oeuvres completes.* Paris: Aux Editions Du Seuil.

Patterson, D. R. (1996). Burn pain. In J. Barber (Ed.), *Hypnosis and suggestion in the treatment of pain: A clinical guide* (267–304). New York: W.W. Norton.

Perry, B. D. (2002). Childhood experience and the expression of genetic potential: What childhood neglect tells us about nature and nurture. *Brain & Mind, 3,* 79–100.

Pettit, J. W., & Joiner, T. E. (2006). Interpersonal conflict avoidance. In J. W. Pettit & T. E. Joiner (Eds.), *Chronic depression: Interpersonal sources, therapeutic solutions* (pp. 73–84). Washington, DC: American Psychological Association.

Philips, H. C., & Hunter, M. (1981). The treatment of tension headache: I. Muscular abnormality and biofeedback. *Behavior Research and Therapy, 19,* 485–498

Piaget, J. (1952). *The origins of intelligence in children.* New York: International Universities Press.

Piaget, J. (1972). *The child's conception of the world.* Towowa, NJ: Littlefield, Adams.

Pincus, D. (2001). A framework and methodology for the study of non-linear, self-organizing family dynamics. *Nonlinear Dynamics, Psychology, and Life Sciences, 5,* 139–173.

Pincus, D. (2006). Dynamical systems theory and pain imagery: Bridging the gap between research and practice. *Journal of Mental Imagery, 30*(1–2), 93–112.

Pincus, D., Fox, K. M., Perez, K. A., Turner, J. S., & McGee, A. R. (2008). Nonlinear dynamics of individual and interpersonal conflict in an experimental group. *Small Group Research, 39,* 150–178.

Pincus, D., & Guastello, S. J. (2005). Nonlinear dynamics and interpersonal correlates of verbal turn-taking patterns in a group therapy session. *Small Group Research, 36,* 635–677.

Pincus, D., Wachsmuth-Schlaefer, T., Sheikh, A. A., & Ezaz-Nikpay, S. (2003). Transforming the pain terrain: Theory and practice in the use of mental imagery for the treatment of pain. In A. A. Sheikh (Ed.), *Healing images: The role of imagination in health* (pp. 177–222). New York: Baywood.

Portenoy, R. K. (1994). Opioid therapy for chronic nonmalignant pain: Current status. In H. L. Fields & J. C. Liebeskind (Eds.), *Progress in pain research and management. Pharmacological approaches to the treatment of chronic pain: Vol. 1.* Seattle, WA: International Association for the Study of Pain.

Powers, S. W. (1999). Empirically supported treatments in pediatric psychology: Procedure-related pain. *Journal of Pediatric Psychology, 24,* 131–145.

Prigogine, I., & Stengers, I. (1984). *Order out of chaos: Man's new dialogue with nature.* New York: Bantam Books.

Prochaska, J. O., DiClemente, C.C., & Norcross, J. C. (1992). In search of how people change: Applications to addictive behaviors. *American Psychologist, 47,* 1102–1114.

Rafaeli-Mor, E., & Steinberg, J. (2002). Self-complexity and well-being: A review and research synthesis. *Personality and Social Psychology Review, 6,* 31–58.

Raft, D., Smith, R. H., & Warren, N. (1986). Selection of imagery in the relief of chronic and acute clinical pain. *Journal of Psychosomatic Research, 30,* 481–488.

Reichenbach, H. (1938). *Experience and prediction.* Chicago, IL: University of Chicago Press.

Remen, R. N. (1981). Listening to your symptoms: Turning insight into action. In M.L. Rossman & R. N. Romen (Eds.), *Imagine health: Imagery and insight in self-care* (a booklet and cassettes). Mill Valley, CA: Insight publishing.

Ricards, M. (2003). *Happiness: A guide to developing life's most important skills*. New York: Little, Brown and Company.

Richardson, A. (1969). *Mental imagery*. London: Routledge and Kegan Paul.

Richardson, A. (1983). Imagery: Definition and types. In A.A. Sheikh (Ed.), *Imagery: Current theory, research, and applications* (pp. 3–42). New York: Wiley.

Richardson-Klavehn, A., & Bork, R. A. (1988). Measures of memory. *Annual Review of Psychology, 39,* 475–543.

Rilke, R. M. (1984). *Letters to a young poet* (S. Mitchell, Trans.). New York: Modern Library.

Robinson, M. E., & Riley, J. L. III (1999). The role of emotion in pain. In R. J. & D. C. Turk (Eds.), *Psychosocial factors in pain: Critical perspectives* (pp. 74–88). Guilford: New York.

Rogers, C. (1951). *Client-centered therapy*. Boston: Houghton-Mifflin.

Rogers, C. R. (1975). Empathic: An unappreciated way of being. *Counseling Psychologist, 5,* 2–10.

Ross, L. (1977). The intuitive psychologist and his shortcomings: distortions in the attribution process. In L. Berkowitz (Ed.), *Advances in experimental social psychology* (Vol. 10, pp. 173–220). New York: Academic Press.

Rossi, E. L. (1987). Mind/body communication and the new language of human facilitation. In J. Zeig (Ed.), *The evolution of psychotherapy* (pp. 369–391). New York: Bruner/Mazel.

Rossi, E. L. (1989). Facilitating "creative moments" in hypnotherapy. In S. R. Lankton & J. K. Zeig (Eds.), *Extrapolations: Demonstrations of Ericksonian therapy* (pp. 81–106). New York: Brunner/Mazel.

Rossi, E. L. (1993). *The psychobiology of mind-body healing* (rev. ed.). New York: Norton.

Rossi, E. L. (1994). Ericksonian psychotherapy—then and now: New fundamentals of the naturalistic-utilization approach. In J. K. Zeig (Ed.), *Ericksonian methods: The essence of the story* (pp. 46–76). Philadelphia, PA: Brunner/Mazel.

Rossi, E. L. (1997). Self-organizational dynamics in Ericksonian hypnotherapy: A nonlinear evolution for the psychotherapist of the future. In J. K. Zeig (Ed.), *The evolution of psychotherapy: The third conference* (pp. 151–157). New York: Brunner/Mazel.

Rossi, E. L. (2002). *The psychobiology of gene expressions*. New York: Norton

Rossman, M. L. (2000). *Guided imagery for self-healing*. Novato, CA: H.J. Kramer & New World Library.

Rotter, J. B. (1954). *Social learning and clinical psychology*. Englewood Cliffs, NJ: Prentice-Hall.

Rotter, J. B. (1990). Internal versus external control of reinforcement: A case history of a variable. *American Psychologist, 45,* 489–493.

Salkovskis, P. M. (1996). Somatic problems. In K. Hawton, P. M. Salkovskis, J. Kirk, & D. M. Clark (Eds.), *Cognitive behaviour therapy for psychiatric problems: A practical guide* (pp. 235–276). New York: Oxford University Press.

Samuels, M., & Samuels, N. (1975). *Seeing with the mind's eye*. New York: Random House.

Saudi, F. (2005). A journey through the life and work of Milton Erickson; the world's leading practitioner of medical hypnosis. *European Journal of Clinical Hypnosis, 6*(2), 38–49.

Scarry, E. (1985). *The body in pain: The making and unmaking of the world.* Oxford: Oxford University Press.

Schacter, D. L. (1987). Implicit memory: History and current status. *Journal of Experimental Psychology: Learning, Memory, and Cognition, 13,* 501–518.

Schaverien, J. (2005). Art, dreams and active imagination: A post-Jungian approach to transference and the image. *Journal of Analytical Psychology, 50,* 127–153.

Schechter, N. L., Berde, C. B., & Yaster, M. (Eds.) (2002). *Pain in infants, children, and adolescents* (2nd ed.). Philadelphia, PA: Lippincott Williams & Wilkins.

Scholem, G. (1961). *Jewish mysticism.* New York: Schocken.

Schwartz, J. M., & Begley, S. (2002). *The mind and the brain: Neuroplacticity and the power of mental force.* New York: Regan.

Sheikh, A. A. (1978). Eidetic psychotherapy. In J. L. Singer & K. S. Pope (Eds.), *The power of human imagination: New methods in psychotherapy* (pp. 197–224). New York: Plenum Press.

Sheikh, A. A. (1986). Eidetic psychotherapy techniques. In A. A. Sheikh (Ed.), *Anthology of imagery techniques* (pp. 179–194). Milwaukee, WI: American Imagery Institute.

Sheikh, A. (Ed.). (2002). *Handbook of therapeutic imagery techniques.* Amityville, NY: Baywood.

Sheikh, A. (Ed.). (2003). *Healing images: The role of imagination in health.* New York: Baywood.

Sheikh, A. A., Kunzendorf, R. G., & Sheikh, K. S. (2003). Healing images: Historical Perspective. In A. A. Sheikh (Ed.), *Healing images: The role of imagination in health* (pp. 3-27). Amityville, NY: Baywood.

Sheikh, A. A., Sheikh, K. S. (Eds.). (2007). *Healing with death imagery.* Amityville, New York: Baywood.

Sheikh, A. A., Sheikh, K. S., & Moleski, L. M. (1985). The enhancement of imaging ability. In A. A. Sheikh & K. S. Sheikh (Eds.), *Imagery in education.* Amityville, New York: Baywood.

Shone, R. (1984). *Creative visualization: How to use imagery and imagination for self-improvement.* New York: Thorson's Publishers.

Smith, E. R. (1998). Mental representation and memory. In D. T. Gilbert, S. T. Fiske, & G. Lindzey (Eds.), *The handbook of social psychology* (4th ed., pp. 391–445). New York: McGraw-Hill.

Soelle, D. (1975). *Suffering* (E. R. Kalin, Trans.). Philadelphia, PA: Fortress Press.

Sommer, R. (1978). *The mind's eye: Imagery in everyday life.* New York: Delacorte Press.

Spanos, N. P, Liddy, S. J., Scott, H., Garrard, C., Sine, J., Tirabasso, A., et al. (1993). Hypnotic suggestion and placebo for the treatment of chronic headache in a university volunteer sample. *Cognitive Therapy and Research, 17*(2), 191–205.

Spanos, N. P., & O'Hara, P. A. (1990). Imaginal dispositions and situation-specific expectations in strategy-induced pain reductions. *Imagination, Cognition and Personality, 9,* 147–156.

Sperry, R. W. (1993). The impact and promise of the cognitive revolution. *American Psychologist, 48,* 878–885.

Sprenkle, D. H., & Blow, A. J. (2004). Common factors and our sacred models. *Journal of Marital and Family Therapy, 30,* 113–129.

Stevens, A. (1999). *On Jung.* Princeton, NJ: Princeton University Press.

Stevens, M. J. (1985). Modification of pain through covert positive reinforcement. *Psychological Reports, 56,* 711–717.

Stevens, M. J., Heise, R., & Pfost, K. S. (1989). Consumption of attention versus affect elicited by cognition in modifying acute pain. *Psychological Reports, 64,* 284–286.

Stevens, M. J., Pfost, K. S., & Rapp, B. J. (1987). Modifying acute pain by matching cognitive style with cognitive treatment. *Perceptual and Motor Skills, 65,* 919–924.

Syrjala, K. L., & Abrams, J. R. (1996). Hypnosis and imagery in the treatment of pain. In R. J. Gatchel & D. C. Turk (Eds.) *Psychological approaches to pain management: A practitioner's handbook* (pp. 231–258). New York: Guilford Press.

Syrjala, K. L., & Abrams, J. R. (2002). Hypnosis and imagery in the treatment of pain. In R. J. Gatchel & D. C. Turk (Eds.), *Psychological approaches to pain management: A practitioner's handbook* (2nd ed., pp. 187–209). New York: Guilford Press.

Syrjala, K. L., & Roth-Roemer, S. (1996). Cancer pain. In J. Barber (Ed.), *Hypnosis and suggestion in the treatment of pain: A clinical guide* (pp. 121–157). New York: W.W. Norton.

Tan, S. Y. (1982). Cognitive and cognitive behavioral methods for pain control: A selective review. *Pain, 12,* 201–228.

Ter Kuile, M. M., Spinhoven, P., Linssen, A. C. G., Zitman, F. G., Van Dyck, R., & Rooijmans, H. G. M. (1994). Autogenic training and cognitive self-hypnosis for the treatment of recurrent headaches in three different subject groups. *Pain, 58,* 331–340.

Tolman, E. C. (1940). Spatial angle and vicarious trial and error, *Journal of Comparative Psychology, 30,* 129–135.

Tompkins, P., & Lawley, J. (2000). *Metaphors in mind.* London, England: Developing Company Press.

Tourigny-Dewhurst, D. (1993). Using the self-control triad to treat tension headache in a child. In C. Verduin (Ed.), *Covert conditioning casebook* (pp. 75–81). Belmont, CA: Wadsworth.

Tschacher, W., Scheier, C., & Grawe, K. (1998). Order and pattern formation in psychotherapy. *Nonlinear Dynamics, Psychology, and Life Sciences, 2,* 195–216.

Turk, D. C., & Flor, H. (1999). Chronic pain: A biobehavioral perspective. In R. J. Gatchel & D. C. Turk (Eds.), *Psychosocial factors in pain: Critical perspectives* (pp. 18–34). New York: Guilford.

Turk, D. C., Meichenbaum, D., & Genest, M. (1983). *Pain and behavioral medicine: A cognitive-behavioral perspective.* New York: Guilford Press.

Turk, D. C., & Okifuji, A. (2001). Pain terms and taxonomies of pain. In J. D. Loeser, S. H. Butler, C. R. Chapman, & D. C. Turk (Eds.), *Bonica's management of pain* (3rd ed., pp. 17–25). Philadelphia, PA: Lippincott, Williams, and Wilkins.

Turner, J. A., Lee, J. S., & Schandler, S. L. (2003). An fMRI investigation of hand representation in paraplegic humans. *Neurorehabilitation & Neural Repair, 17,* 37–47.

Turner, J. C. (1989). *Rediscovering the social group: A self-categorization theory.* Oxford, England: Blackwell.

Turner, J. C., & Chapman, C. R. (1982). Psychological interventions for chronic pain: A critical review II, operant conditioning, hypnosis and cognitive behavioral therapy. *Pain, 12,* 23–46.

Turner, J. C., Oakes, P. J., Haslam, S. A., & McGarty, C. (1994). Self and collective: Cognition and social context. *Journal of Personality and Social Psychology, 28,* 135–147.

Tversky, A., & Kahneman, D. (1974). Judgment under uncertainty: Heuristics and biases. *Science, 185,* 1124–1131.

Tynion, J. H. (2002). Gendlin's focusing techniques. In A. A. Sheikh (Ed.), *Handbook of therapeutic imagery techniques* (pp. 193–202). Amityville, NY: Baywood.

Van de Castle, R. L. (1983). Animal figures in fantasy and dreams. In A. Katcher & A. Beck (Eds.), *New perspectives on our lives with companion animals.* Philadelphia, PA: University of Pennsylvania Press.

Van de Castle, R. L. (1994). *Our dreaming mind.* New York: Ballantine Books.

Von Bertalanffy, L. (1968). *General system theory: Foundations, development, applications.* New York: Braziller.

Wall, V. (1991). Developmental considerations in the use of hypnosis with children. In W. C. Wester II & D. J. O'Grady (Eds.), *Clinical hypnosis with children* (pp. 3–18). New York: Bruner/Mazel, Inc.

Walsh, R., & Shapiro, S. L. (2006). The meeting of meditative disciplines and western psychology: A mutually enriching dialogue. *American Psychologist, 61,* 227–239.

Watson, J. B. (1919). *Psychology from the standpoint of a behaviorist.* Philadelphia, PA: JB Lippincott.

Watson, J. B. (1920). Is thinking merely the action of language mechanisms? *British Journal of Psychology, 11,* 87–104.

Weaver, R. (1973). *The old wise woman: A study of active imagination.* New York: G. P. Putnam's Sons.

Wiener, N. (1948). *Cybernetics.* Cambridge, MA: MIT Press.

Weisenberg, M. (1979). Pain and pain control. *Psychological Bulletin, 84,* 1008–1044.

Weisenberg, J. N., & Keefe, F. J. (2002). Personality, individual differences, and psychopathology in chronic pain. In R. J. Gatchel & D. C. Turk (Eds.), *Psychosocial factors in pain: Critical perspectives* (pp. 56–73). New York: Guilford.

West, B. J. (2006). *Where medicine went wrong: Rediscovering the path to complexity.* Hackensack, NJ: World Scientific

West, B. J., & Deering, B. (1995). *The lure of modern science: Fractal thinking.* River Edge, NJ: World Scientific.

Widiger, T. A., Trull, T. J., Hurt, S. W., Clarkin, J., & Frances, A. (1987). A multidimensional scaling of the *DSM-III* personality disorders. *Archives of General Psychiatry, 44,* 557–563.

Wilde, O. (1946). *De profundis.* New York: Penguin Books.

Wilson, C. (2008). *Emergent knowledge: Philosophy.* Retrieved February 4, 2008, from http://www.emergentknowledge.com

Wolpe, J. (1969). *The practice of behavior therapy.* Oxford, England: Pergomon.

Worthington, E. L. Jr. (1978). The effects of imagery content choice of imagery, choice of imagery content, and self-verbalization on the control of pain. *Cognitive Therapy and Research, 2,* 225–240.

Worthington, E. L., & Shumate, M. (1981). Imagery and verbal counseling methods in stress inoculation training for pain control. *Journal of Counseling Psychology, 28,* 1–6.

Wright, L. M. (2005). *Spirituality, suffering and illness.* Philadelphia, PA: F.A. Davis.

Yalom, I. (1980). *Existential psychotherapy.* New York: Basic Books.

Zahourek, R. P. (1988). Imagery. In R. P. Zahourek (Ed.), *Relaxation & imagery: Therapeutic communication and intervention* (pp. 53–83). Philadelphia, PA: W.B. Saunders.

Subject Index

Author Index